HEINEMANN
MODERN DICTIONARY
FOR DENTAL STUDENTS

SECOND EDITION

Compiled by

JENIFER E. H. FAIRPO, B.A., A.L.A.
formerly Librarian
Leeds University School of Dentistry

and

C. GAVIN FAIRPO, B.D.S.
Lecturer in Children's Dentistry
Leeds University School of Dentistry

WILLIAM HEINEMANN MEDICAL BOOKS LTD
LONDON

FIRST PUBLISHED 1962
SECOND EDITION 1973

© by William Heinemann Medical Books Limited

ISBN 0 433 10701 4

PRINTED IN GREAT BRITAIN BY R J ACFORD LTD CHICHESTER

CONTENTS

CONTENTS

PREFACE

This dictionary has been compiled primarily to meet the needs of the dental student, but it is hoped that it may also prove useful to dental nurses, technicians, secretaries, and other workers in the field of dentistry. In view of this the definitions have been kept as simple as possible. Many American terms are included, since the majority of books and periodical articles on dentistry today are published in the United States. A number of obsolete terms have been defined to aid those reading the early literature. Such medical terms have been included as are specifically relevant to dentistry, but it is not, of course, possible to produce an exhaustive list of these in a work of this size. For the benefit of foreign students particular attention has been paid to the pronunciation.

At the end of the dictionary will be found three appendices: anatomical tables of the head and neck, the terminology of which is that approved by the Seventh International Congress of Anatomists, New York 1960, published in *Nomina Anatomica*, 2nd edition (Amsterdam, etc., *Excerpta Medica Foundation*, 1961); an appendix of drugs used in dentistry, which has been prepared by Dr. J. B. Roberts, of Liverpool University, to whom I should like to express my gratitude for the trouble he has taken over it; and a list of dental journals, with their country of origin, frequency, and the official abbreviation according to the International Standard ISO R4, as used in *World Medical Periodicals*, 2nd edition (London, *British Medical Association*, 1957), which it is hoped may prove of value to all concerned with the publication of dental material.

As would be expected in a work of this nature medical and dental dictionaries and many reference books were consulted and I wish to express my indebtedness to all concerned, and especially to the Medico-Dental Publishing Company for permission to reproduce the Classification of tooth cavities from *Operative Dentistry*, 8th edition (1947), by G. V. Black.

I should like to thank most sincerely all those people who have so kindly helped me during the compilation of this work, especially Mr. G. Wreakes, Registrar, Dental Hospital, Leeds, for reading the typescript and for many useful suggestions; Dr. W. J. K. Walls, Reader in Anatomy, University of Leeds, for his careful scrutiny of the anatomical tables; and all the members of staff of the Dental School of Leeds University, who have solved so many of my problems for me. I should also like to acknowledge with gratitude the interest and encouragement which I have received from Mr. B. S. Page, the University Librarian.

vii

My thanks are also due to Mr. Frank Price for his effective line drawings, and to the Dental Manufacturing Company for the loan of the blocks illustrating various dental instruments; to Miss Jean M. Kershaw, formerly Librarian, British Dental Association, for her assistance on various matters and for her hospitality in the Association's Library; to Mr. L. T. Morton, who persuaded me to undertake the work in the first instance, and to Mr. Owen R. Evans, of William Heinemann Medical Books Ltd., for all his patience and help throughout.

Leeds, *January* 1962   J.E.H.F.

PREFACE TO THE SECOND EDITION

In this new edition we have not only added many definitions and corrected errors which had crept into the first edition but we have also tried to revise the terminology used, to bring it into line with the present trend towards more specific and descriptive names. It is hoped, however, that those familiar with the older usage will find these terms adequately cross-referenced. The terminology used for the anatomical tables has been revised in accordance with the recommendations of the Eighth International Congress of Anatomists, Wiesbaden, 1965, published in *Nomina Anatomica*, 3rd edition (Amsterdam, etc., *Excerpta Medica Foundation*, 1966).

In the periodicals section there is an enormous increase in the number of titles. We have now added an indication of those periodicals regularly covered by the *Index to Dental Literature* but we no longer include the international standard abbreviation as there is a growing tendency towards the use of the full title, and, moreover, *World Medical Periodicals*, based on the ISO recommendations, is no longer published.

The appendix of drugs has been revised for this edition by Dr John Eyre of the Institute of Dental Surgery at the Eastman Dental Hospital, London, and we are most grateful to him for the trouble he has taken over the revision.

We should like to thank all our colleagues at the Dental School in Leeds for their unfailing help with our problems, and in particular Professor D. Jackson, Professor H. S. M. Crabb, Mr C. Woodhead, Mr J. F. Gravely and Mr J. N. Kidd, and to acknowledge with gratitude the interest and encouragement of Professor F. E. Hopper, Head of the Dental School. Our thanks are also due to Miss E. M. Read and the staff of the Medical Library, Leeds, and to Miss J. R. Kirk, of the Dental Library, for their hospitality and assistance throughout the work of revision, to Miss E. M. Spencer, Librarian of the British Dental Association, Mr C. H. Fleurent of the *British Medical Journal* and Mr P. Wade, Librarian of the Royal Society of Medicine, for their assistance with the periodical titles; to Amalgamated Dental, London, for their permission to reproduce the blocks of various Ash and other instruments, to Blackwell Scientific Publications for the illustrations of intermaxillary and eyelet wiring from *The dental treatment of maxillo-facial injuries*, by Sir William Kelsey Fry and T. Ward, and to W. B. Saunders Co. for the illustration of Le Fort fracture from *Surgery of facial fractures*, by R. O. Dingman and P. Natvig; to Mr Frank Price for his work on the line drawings, and to Mr Owen R. Evans and Miss L. Schwartz, of William Heinemann Medical Books, who have been a tower of strength and a monument of patience throughout.

J.E.H.F.   C.G.F.

Leeds. *March* 1973

Pronunciation

ā as in pane	ă as in pan
ē as in meet	ĕ as in met
ī as in hide	ĭ as in hid
ō as in coat	ŏ as in cot
ū as in rule	ŭ as in rub

The primary accent is indicated thus ('). In polysyllabic words the secondary accent is, when necessary, indicated (").

In some cases a phonetic equivalent is given.

A vowel followed by a consonant is assumed to be short, and a vowel standing last at the end of a syllable is assumed to be long, unless otherwise marked.

List of commonly used initial abbreviations for Dental Institutions, degrees, etc.

A.D.A. American Dental Association.

ARPA. International Association for Research in Paradentosis.

A.S.O. American Society of Orthodontists.

B.Ch.D. Baccalaureus Chirurgiae Dentalis.
University of Leeds.

B.D.A. British Dental Association.

B.D.S. Bachelor of Dental Surgery.
University of Birmingham, Bristol, Liverpool, London, Manchester, Newcastle upon Tyne, Sheffield, University of Wales–Cardiff, Dundee, Edinburgh, Glasgow, Queen's University, Belfast, National University of Ireland–Dublin and Cork.

B.Dent.Sc. Bachelor in Dental Science.
University of Dublin–Trinity College.

B.N.A. Basle Nomina Anatomica; a list of Latin anatomical terms, adopted as a standard at a conference in Basle in 1895, and since modified.

B.S.I. British Standards Institution.

B.S.S.O. British Society for the Study of Orthodontics.

C.N.S.D. Confédération Nationale des Syndicats Dentaires. This is the

French equivalent of the British Dental Association.

D.Ch.D. Doctor Chirurgiae Dentalis.
University of Wales–Cardiff.

D.D.H. Diploma in Dental Health.
University of Birmingham.

D.D.O. Diploma in Dental Orthopaedics.
Royal College of Physicians and Surgeons, Glasgow.

D.D.P.H. Diploma in Dental Public Health.
Royal College of Surgeons of England.

D.D.S. Doctor of Dental Surgery.
University of Manchester, and of Edinburgh.

D.D.Sc. Doctor of Dental Science.
University of Leeds, Newcastle upon Tyne, Dundee, Glasgow.

D. Orth. Diploma in Orthodontics.
Royal College of Surgeons of England.

D.P.D. Diploma in Public Dentistry.
University of Dundee.

D.S.A. Dental Surgery Assistant.

E.S.O. European Orthodontic Society.

F.D.I. Fédération Dentaire Internationale; International Dental Federation.

F.D.S. Fellow in Dental Surgery.
Royal College of Surgeons of England, Royal College of Physicians and Surgeons of Glasgow, Royal College of Surgeons of Edinburgh.

F.F.D. Fellow in the Faculty of Dentistry.
Royal College of Surgeons in Ireland.

H.D.D. Higher Dental Diploma.
Royal Faculty (*now* College) of Physicians and Surgeons of Glasgow (no longer awarded).

I.A.D.R. International Association for Dental Research.

I.A.D.S. International Association of Dental Students.

L.D.S. Licence in Dental Surgery.
Used to be granted by all those universities which grant dental degrees but is now only granted by University of Bristol and of Sheffield. It is also granted by the Royal College of Surgeons of England, Royal College (*formerly* Faculty) of Physicians and Surgeons of Glasgow, Royal College of Surgeons of Edinburgh, Royal College of Surgeons in Ireland.

L.D.Sc. Licence in Dental Science.
University of Dublin (no longer granted.)

M.Ch.D. Magister Chirurgiae Dentalis.
University of Leeds (no longer awarded).

M.D.S. Master of Dental Surgery.
University of Birmingham, Bristol, Liverpool, London, Manchester, Newcastle upon Tyne, Sheffield, Dundee, Edinburgh (no longer awarded), Glasgow, Queen's

University, Belfast, National University of Ireland–Dublin and Cork.

M.D.Sc. Master of Dental Science.
University of Leeds.

M.Dent.Sc. Master in Dental Science
University of Dublin–Trinity College.

M.Sc. Master of Science.
This degree is awarded by all British Universities.

M.Sc.D. Magister Scientia Dentalis.
University of Wales–Cardiff.

ORCA. Organisme Européen de Coordination des Recherches sur le Fluor et la Prophylaxie de la Carie Dentaire: European Organization for Research on Fluorine and Dental Caries Prevention.

Ph.D. Philosophae doctor.
This degree is granted by all British universities.

PNA Paris Nomina Anatomica. The Latin anatomical terminology approved by the Sixth International Congress of Anatomists, Paris, 1955.

R.C.P.S. Royal College of Physicians and Surgeons of Glasgow (*formerly* Royal Faculty of Physicians and Surgeons of Glasgow).

R.C.S.Ed. Royal College of Surgeons of Edinburgh.

R.C.S.Eng. Royal College of Surgeons of England.

R.C.S.I. Royal College of Surgeons in Ireland.

R.F.P.S. Royal Faculty of Physicians and Surgeons, Glasgow (*now called* Royal College of Physicians and Surgeons of Glasgow).

A

a-, an-. Prefix signifying *without*, *not*.

aa. Abbreviation for *ana—of each*; used in prescription writing.

āāā. Amalgam.

ABC Axiobuccocervical.

ABG Axiobuccogingival.

ABL Axiobuccolingual.

AC Axiocervical.

a.c. Abbreviation for *ante cibum—before meals*; used in prescription writing.

ACTH Adreno-corticotrophic hormone.

AD Axiodistal.

ad. Abbreviation for *adde—add*; used in prescription writing.

ad lib. Abbreviation for *ad libitum—to the desired amount*; used in prescription writing.

ADC Axiodistocervical.

ADG Axiodistogingival.

ADI Axiodistoincisal.

ADO Axiodisto-occlusal.

æq. Abbreviation for *æquales —equal*; used in prescription writing.

aet. Abbreviation for *aetas—age*; used in records and case histories.

AG Axiogingival.

Ag Chemical symbol for silver.

AI Axioincisal.

AL Axiolingual.

Al Chemical symbol for aluminium.

ALa Axiolabial.

ALaG Axiolabiogingival.

ALaL Axiolabiolingual.

ALC Axiolinguocervical.

ALG Axiolinguogingival.

ALO Axiolinguo-occlusal.

alt. dieb. Abbreviation for *alternis diebus*–every other day; used in prescription writing.

alt. hor. Abbreviation for *alternis horis*–every other hour; used in prescription writing.

AMC Axiomesiocervical.

AMD Axiomesiodistal.

AMG Axiomesiogingival.

AMI Axiomesioincisal.

AMO Axiomesio-occlusal.

AO Axio-occlusal.

AP Axiopulpal.

aq. Abbreviation for *aqua—water*.

aq. dest. Abbreviation for *aqua destillata*–distilled water.

Au Chemical symbol for gold.

'A' point. Subspinale (*q.v.*).

ab-. Prefix signifying *away from*.

abacterial (*a-bak-te'-ri-al*). Free from bacteria.

abapical (*ab"-a'-pik-al*). Away from the apex.

abarticulation (*ab-ar-tik-yu-la'-shun*). 1. Dislocation of a joint. 2. Diarthrosis (*q.v.*).

abaxial (*ab-ak'-si-al*). Situated away from the axis.

abducens oris (*ab-du'-senz or'-is*). Levator anguli oris. *See* Table of Muscles.

abducent nerve. Supplies the lateral rectus muscle of the eye. *See* Table of Nerves—abducens.

aberrant (*ab-er'-ant*). Deviating from the normal form or course.

aberration (*ab-er-a'-shun*). 1. Variation from the normal form or course. 2. An abnormal part, in biology.

ablation (*ab-la'-shun*). Removal of a part by excision or amputation.

ablepharous (*a-blef'-ar-us*). Having no eyelids.

ablephary (*a-blef'-ar-ĭ*). Congenital partial or total absence of the eyelids, or of the palpebral fissure.

abnormal (*ab-nor'-mal*). Not normal, deviating in some way from the usual structure, position or state.

abnormality (*ab-nor-mal'-it-ĭ*). Not the normal or usual growth or development.

abocclusion (*ab-ok-lu'-zhun*). Condition where the maxillary and mandibular teeth are not in contact.

aborad (*ab-or'-ad*). Situated or leading away from the mouth.

aboral (*ab-or'-al*). Relating to areas away from or opposite to the mouth.

abradant (*ab-ra'-dant*). An abrasive agent.

abrade (*ab-rād'*). To wear away.

abrasio dentium (*ab-ra'-zĭ-o den'-shĭ-um*). Wearing away of the teeth.

abrasion (*ab-ra'-zhun*). Wearing away; in dentistry, applied to the wearing away of the tooth structure due to an abrasive dentifrice, or to some occupational habit such as biting off sewing thread.

abrasive (*ab-ra'-ziv*). 1. Containing a substance which tends to erode a surface. 2. The actual substance which wears away the surface.

abscess (*ab'-ses*). A collection of pus in a cavity formed by disintegration of tissue as a result of infection.

acute a. One having a short but severe course, producing painful local inflammation, and some fever.

alveolar a. An abscess affecting the alveolar bone, with cellular necrosis and formation of pus.

apical a. An abscess occurring at the apex of a tooth root.

bicameral a. One containing two pockets.

blind a. One having no fistulous opening.

caseous a. An abscess containing cheese-like matter.

chronic a. Any abscess of long duration and slow development; it may be a cold abscess (*q.v.*), or one resulting from the incomplete resolution of a pre-existing acute abscess, or from the presence of pyogenic organisms of low virulence. There is pus formation, but little in-flammation.

circumtonsillar a. Quinsy (*q.v.*).

cold a. A slow-developing tuberculous abscess, generally about a bone or joint, and with little inflammation.

collar-stud a. A superficial abscess connected by a sinus tract to a larger, deep abscess.

congestive a. An abscess forming at a distance from the inflammation, because resistance from the tissues prevents it gathering.

dental a. Any abscess connected with a tooth.

dento-alveolar a. One affecting the tissues round the apex of a non-vital tooth root.

dry a. An abscess which disperses without bursting or coming to a head.

gingival a. An abscess occurring in a periodontal pocket and affecting the gingiva round the cementum of a tooth.

palatal a. An apical abscess of the lateral incisors or the palatal roots of the posterior teeth, pointing towards the palate.

parietal a. A periodontal abscess occurring at any site away from the apex of a tooth root.

parodontal a. An abscess arising in the periodontal membrane.

periapical a. An abscess erupting around the apex of a tooth root.

pericemental a. A parodontal abscess not arising from a diseased pulp or as an extension of a periodontal pocket.

pericoronal a. An abscess arising about the crown of an unerupted tooth.

periodontal a. An abscess formed as a result of periodontal disease.

peritonsillar a. Quinsy (*q.v.*).

root a. An apical granuloma (*q.v.*).

septal a. An abscess forming on the proximal surface of a tooth root.

sterile a. An abscess containing no micro-organisms.

sympathetic a. A secondary abscess arising at some distance from the original focus of infection.

wandering a. An abscess which tracks through the tissues and finally comes to a point some distance from its orginal site.

absorbefacient (*ab-zor-be-fa'-shent*). An agent which promotes absorption.

absorbent (*ab-zor'-bent*). 1. Capable of sucking up or drawing in. 2. Any drug or agent which promotes absorption.

absorbent organ. Vascular tissue lying between the roots of a deciduous tooth and its permanent successor, during resorption of the deciduous roots.

absorption (*ab-zorp'-shun*). 1. The taking up of one substance, or of a fluid, by another substance. 2. Resorption (*q.v.*).

abstraction (*ab-strak'-shun*) *of the jaws:* A form of malocclusion in which the jaws are abnormally distant.

abut (*ă-but'*). To adjoin and touch; to be in contact with.

abutment (*ab-ut'-ment*). A supporting structure.

abutment tooth. A tooth used as support for a false tooth or for one end of a bridge.

acanthion (*ak-an'-thĭ-on*). A craniometric point on the base of the anterior nasal spine.

acanthoameloblastoma (*akan"-tho-am-e"-lo-blast-o'-mă*). A form of ameloblastoma containing squamous or prickle-cell type cells.

acanthoid (*ak-an'-thoyd*). Spinous, spine-like.

acanthoma (*ak-an-tho'-mă*). A form of epidermoid sarcoma containing keratinized epithelium.

accessory (*ak-ses'-or-ĭ*). Auxiliary or supplementary; applied to minor organs which supply major ones.

accessory nerve. Supplies the striated muscles of the pharynx and larynx, and the sternocleidomastoid and trapezius muscles. *See* Table of Nerves—accessorius.

accretion (*ak-re'-shun*). A deposit of foreign matter adhering to a surface.

accretion lines. Retzius' lines (*q.v.*).

acellular (*a-sel'-yu-lar*). Without, free from, cells.

ache (*āk*). A continuous, dull fixed pain.

acheilia (*a-ki'-lĭ-ă*). Congenital absence of a lip or lips.

acheilous (*a-ki'-lus*). Without lips.

achondroplasia (*a-kon-dro-pla'-zi-ă*). A congenital disease affecting the skeletal development and resulting in dwarfism.

acidogenic (*as"-id-o-jen'-ik*). Acid-forming.

acinus (*as'-in-us*) (*pl.* acini). One of the minute sacs, with a narrow lumen, which form the lobules of a compound gland.

aclusion (*a-klu'-zhun*). The condition of having the teeth parted; as opposed to *occlusion*.

acoustic nerve. N. vestibulo-cochlearis. *See* Table of Nerves.

acquired cuticle. Acquired pellicle (*q.v.*).

acquired enamel cuticle. Acquired pellicle (*q.v.*).

acquired pellicle. An acellular layer of organic material deposited on the tooth surface after eruption.

acrocephaly (*ak-ro-sef'-al-ĭ*). Oxycephaly (*q.v.*).

acrodont (*ak'-ro-dont*). Having teeth attached directly to the jaw-bone and not set in sockets; as seen, for example, in lizards.

acromegaly (*ak-ro-meg'-al-ĭ*). Gigantism: associated with hyperfunction of the pituitary body and characterized by enlargement of the bones and soft tissue of the head and the extremities.

acropis (*ak'-ro-pis*). An old term for faulty articulation due to some defect of the tongue.

acrylic (*ak-ril'-ik*). Acrylic resin (*q.v.*).

acrylic mould. A stent used in oral plastic surgery to secure an intraoral skin graft.

acrylic resin. A synthetic form of resin used in the manufacture of dentures, etc.

acrylic splint. A plastic splint or stent used in dental surgery to immobilize fractures of the mandible or the maxilla, or to support bone grafts of the jaw.

acrylic stent. Acrylic splint (*q.v.*).

acrylic veneer crown. A metal crown covered by a thin veneer of acrylic.

actinic carcinoma. Basal-cell type of carcinoma affecting the face and other uncovered body surfaces, caused by prolonged exposure to direct sunlight.

Actinomyces (*ak-tin-o-mi'-sēz*). A genus of the Actinomycetaceae family, vegetable parasites, anaerobic and seen as filamentous rosettes with clubbing of the filaments.

Actinomycetaceae (*ak"-tin-o-mi-se-ta'-se-e*). A family

of micro-organisms of the order Actinomycetales.

Actinomycetales (*ak"tin-o-mi-se-ta'-lēz*). An order of fungi of the class Schizomycetes; mould-like organisms with a tendency to branch.

actinomycosis (*ak-tin-o-mi-ko'-sis*). A chronic infection caused by *Actinomyces bovis*, frequently commensal in the mouth, trauma allowing ingress of the organism; it is characterized by chronic inflammation, formation of granulation tissue, and suppuration discharging through multiple sinuses, the pus containing sulphur granules. It mainly affects the jaw and neck, but may also affect the chest and the abdomen.

activator (*ak'-tiv-a-tor*). 1. Any agent necessary to activate another substance. 2. In orthodontics, an Andresen appliance (*q.v.*).

actual cautery. A white-hot iron used for cauterization.

acusection (*ak-yu-sek'-shun*). Electrosection (*q.v.*).

acute (*ak-yūt'*). 1. Sharp. 2. Of rapid, severe onset and short duration.

acute abscess. An abscess having a short but severe course, producing painful local inflammation, and some fever.

acute periodontitis. An acute inflammation of the periodontium of (usually) a single tooth, arising as a result of acute trauma to the tooth, or, when localized to the periapical area, as a result of irritation from bacterial toxins, drugs or instruments following infection and subsequent root canal therapy.

acutenaculum (*ak-yu-ten-ak'-yu-lum*). A surgical needle-holder.

acutenaculum, Hullihan's. *See* Hullihan's acutenaculum.

ad libitum (*ad lib'-it-um*). Latin for *to the desired amount*; used in prescription writing, and abbreviated *ad lib.*

ad-. Prefix signifying *to, in the direction of.*

-ad. Suffix signifying *towards.*

adamantine (*ad-am-an'-tīn*). Relating to the tooth enamel.

adamantinocarcinoma (*ad-am-an''-tin-o-kar-sin-o'-mă*). A malignant form of ameloblastoma.

adamantinoma (*ad-am-an-tin-o'-mă*). A locally malignant tumour of the jaw, derived from odontogenic epithelium, but not containing any enamel or other dental tissue.

adamantoblast (*ad-am-an'-to-blast*). Ameloblast (*q.v.*).

adamantoblastoma (*ad-am-an''-to-blast-o'-mă*). Adamantinoma (*q.v.*).

adamantoma (*ad-am-an-to'-mă*). Adamantinoma (*q.v.*).

adamas dentis (*ad'-am-as den'-tis*). Tooth enamel.

Adams crib (C. P. Adams, contemporary British orthodontist). A modified form of arrowhead clasp (*q.v.*).

adde (*ad'-dā*). Latin for *add*; used in prescription writing, and abbreviated *ad.*

adduction (*ad-uk'-shun*). A drawing in towards the centre, or to the median line; as opposed to *abduction.*

adenalgia (*ad-en-al'-jĭ-ă*). Pain affecting a gland.

adenectomy (*ad-en-ek'-tom-ĭ*). 1. Surgical removal of a gland. 2. Adenoidectomy (*q.v.*).

adenitis (*ad-en-i'-tis*). Inflammation of a gland.

adeno-. Prefix signifying *gland.*

adenocarcinoma (*ad''-en-o-kar-sin-o'-mă*). A malignant adenoma; a carcinoma derived from glandular tissue and to some extent resembling the organ of its origin.

adenocele (*ad''-en-o-sēl'*). A cystic tumour composed of adenomatous tissue.

adenocyst (*ad''-en-o-sist'*). A glandular cyst.

adenofibroma (*ad''-en-o-fi-bro'-mă*). A tumour composed of fibrous and glandular tissue.

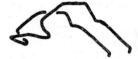

Adams crib

adenoid (*ad'-en-oyd*). 1. Like a gland. 2. *pl.* The adenoid tissue in the nasopharynx.

adenoidectomy (*ad"-en-oyd-ekt'-om-ĭ*). Surgical excision of the adenoids.

adenoiditis (*ad-en-oyd-i'-tis*). Inflammation of the adenoids.

adenolymphoma (*ad"-en-o-limf-o'-mă*). A benign epithelial tumour occurring in the lymph glands.

adenoma (*ad-en-o'-mă*). A benign epithelial tumour of glandlike structure, resembling the organ of its origin.

adenomatome (*ad-en-o'-mat-ōm*). A surgical instrument used for excision of the adenoids.

adhere (*ad-hēr'*). To stick, cling, or become fastened together.

adherent tongue. A tongue which is attached to both the floor and sides of the mouth by folds of mucous membrane.

adhesion (*ad-he'-zhun*). 1. The sticking or fastening together of two adjacent surfaces. 2. In surgery, the abnormal joining of two separate parts by a band of new tissue. 3. The tissue which creates this union. 4. In dentistry, the force which retains a full upper denture in place without the use of vacuum cups.

adhesive (*ad-he'-ziv*). 1. Sticking closely. 2. Characterized by adhesion. 3. A substance used for sticking together.

adhesiveness (*ad-he'-ziv-nes*). The quality of being adhesive.

adipose (*ad'-ip-ōz*). Fat, fatty.

adjustable band. A band which has some form of screw or other mechanism whereby its size can be altered.

adjuvant (*ad'-ju-vant*). An additive which assists the action of a drug.

adnasal (*ad-na'-zal*). Relating to, or situated near, the nose.

adolescent (*ad-ŏ-les'-ent*). 1. Relating to the period from the onset of puberty to the end of somatic development. 2. A person during this period of life.

adoral (*ad-or'-al*). Near to, in the direction of, the mouth.

adrenodontia (*ad-ren-o-don'-shĭ-ă*). Morphological indications of over-activity of adrenal glands, characterized by large pointed canines, and teeth whose occlusal surfaces show a brown discoloration.

adsorption (*ad-zorp'-shun*). The property possessed by certain substances of sucking up fluids.

adult (*ad'-ult*). 1. Fully developed or mature. 2. One who is fully developed or mature.

adventitious (*ad-ven-tish'-us*). 1. Acquired, accidental or foreign; as opposed to natural or hereditary. 2. Found in an abnormal or unusual place.

adventitious cyst. A cyst which forms about a foreign body.

adventitious dentine. Secondary dentine (q.v.).

aequales (ĕ-kwal′-ēz). Latin for *equal*; used in prescription writing, and abbreviated *aeq.*

aerobe (a′-er-ōb). A microorganism requiring air or free oxygen to live and grow.

aerobic (a-er-o′-bik). Requiring air or free oxygen in order to live and grow.

aerodontalgia (a-er-o-dont-al′-ji-ă). Toothache caused by high-altitude flying.

aerodontia, aerodontics (a-er-o-don′-shi-ă). That branch of dentistry which is concerned with the care and treatment of dental conditions caused by a high-altitude flying.

aerodontodynia (a-er-o-dont″-o-din′-i-ă). Aerodontalgia (q.v.).

aetiologic, aetiological (e-tĭ-ol-oj′-ik-al). Relating to aetiology.

aetiology (e-tĭ-ol′-oj-ĭ). The study of the causes of disease.

affection (af-ek′-shun). Any pathologic condition or diseased state.

afferent (af′-er-ent). Carrying to the centre, centripetal; as opposed to *efferent*.

afferent nerve. Any nerve transmitting impulses from the periphery to the centre.

agar (a′-gar). Extract of seaweed of the genus *Gelideum*, used in the preparation of bacteriologic culture media.

agenesis (a-jen′-es-is). Non-development or defective development.

agent (a′-jent). Any substance or power which produces change in the body.

ageusia (a-gu′-si-ă). Loss or absence of a sense of taste.

agger nasi (aj′-er). The anterior portion of the ethmoidal crest, on the maxilla.

agglutination (ag-glu-tin-a′-shun). 1. The grouping together into clumps of particles suspended in fluid. 2. A joining together, as in the physiological process of repair of a wound.

agglutinin (ag-glu′-tin-in). An antibody capable of causing the cells of its specific antigen to become grouped together in clumps.

aglossia (a-glos′-i-ă). Congenital absence of the tongue.

aglossostomia (a-glos-o-sto′-mi-ă). Congenital absence of the tongue and of the mouth opening.

aglutition (a-glu-tĭ′-shun). The condition of being unable to swallow or of experiencing great difficulty in swallowing.

agmatology (ag-mat-ol′-oj-ĭ). The science and study of fractures.

agnathia (ag-na′-thĭ-ă). Complete failure of jaw development.

agomphiasis (a-gom-fĭ′-as-is). 1. Looseness of the teeth. 2. Complete absence of teeth.

agomphious (*a-gom-fi'-us*). Having no teeth.

agomphosis (*a-gom-fo'-sis*). Agomphiasis (*q.v.*).

-agra. Suffix signifying *pain*.

agranular (*a-gran'-yu-lar*). Containing no granules.

Ainsworth's punch (G. G. Ainsworth, 1852-1948. American dentist). Rubber dam punch (*q.v.*).

air chamber. A depression in the palatal portion of an upper denture, once thought to assist in its retention; *also called* a vacuum chamber.

air sinus. Sinus (*q.v.*, 3).

air syringe. A syringe by means of which compressed air may be blown into a cavity or root canal to dry it or to remove loose debris.

airbrasive (*a"-r-bra'-ziv*). An instrument used to cut tooth cavities by means of a mixture of sand and aluminium oxide ejected in a stream of gas under pressure.

airway (*ār'-wa*). 1. The passage by which air is breathed to and from the lungs. 2. The tube used to ensure the free passage of air during recovery after general anaesthesia.

akanthion. *See* acanthion.

ala (*a'-lă*). A wing-like bone process.

ala-tragal line. Camper's line (*q.v.*).

alar (*a'-lar*). Relating to an ala.

alar cartilage. The u-shaped cartilage which forms the tip of the nose.

albation (*al-ba'-shun*.) The bleaching or whitening of teeth or other discoloured matter.

Albers-Schönberg disease (H. E. Albers-Schönberg, 1865-1921. German radiologist). Osteopetrosis (*q.v.*).

Albrecht's bone (K. M. P. Albrecht, 1851-94. German anatomist). An ossicle between the basi-sphenoid and the basi-occipital bones.

alcohol (*al'-kŏ-hol*). Ethyl alcohol, C_2H_5OH, obtained by distillation from fermented sugar, starch, grain or fruits.

Alexander gold (C. L. Alexander, fl. 1923. American dentist). Gold mixed with a vax substance to make it plastic; used for certain types of gold filling.

Alexander's crown (C. L. Alexander, fl. 1923. American dentist). A metal cap crown used as a bridge abutment.

algesia (*al-je'-zĭ-ă*). Sensitivity to pain.

algesic (*al-je'-zik*). Painful.

alginate (*al'-jin-āt*). Any salt of alginic acid; an irreversible colloid used as dental impression material.

algophobia (*al-go-fo'-bĭ-ă*). Morbid fear of pain.

align (*al-īn'*). 1. To arrange in a line. 2. To correct the teeth by bringing them back into the normal arch. 3. To set up teeth in a normal arch for a denture.

aline. *See* align.

alkali (*al'-kal-ĭ*). Any of the class of compounds which form soluble carbonates, and soaps with fats, and which turn litmus blue.

alkaline (*al'-kal-īn*). Relating to or having the characteristics of an alkali.

alkalinity (*al-kal-in'-it-ĭ*). The quality of being alkaline.

all-closing band. A band encircling the whole of a tooth.

Allen's cement (J. Allen, 1810-92. American dentist). A fusible silicous cement used to attach porcelain teeth to a plate.

Allen's root pliers (A. B. Allen, 1862-1943. American dentist). Special pliers designed to remove small pieces of tooth root broken off during extraction.

allergic (*al-er'-jik*). Relating to or characterized by allergy.

allergy (*al'-er-jĭ*). Hypersensitivity to any normally harmless substance, resulting in an exaggerated or abnormal reaction.

allotriodontia (*al-ot-rĭ-o-don'-shĭ-ă*). 1. Transplantation of teeth (*q.v.*). 2. The presence of a tooth in an abnormal place, as in a cyst or tumour.

alloy (*al'-oy*). The substance produced by the fusion of two or more metals.
amalgam a. Shavings or filings of a metal alloy to be mixed with mercury to form an amalgam.

contour a. One suitable for contour fillings.
submarine a. One which can be used in cavities which cannot be kept free from moisture.

alloy, Onion's. *See* Onion's fusible alloy.

alloyage (*al'-oy-āj*). The process of making an alloy.

alternis diebus (*al-ter'-nēs de-a'-bus*). Latin for *every other day;* used in prescription writing and abbreviated *alt.dieb.*

alternis horis (*al-ter'-nēs or'-ēs*). Latin for *every other hour;* used in prescription writing and abbreviated *alt.hor.*

aluminium (*al-yu-min'-ĭ-um*). Chemical symbol: Al. A white, light and ductile metal; formerly used as a denture base.

alundum (*al-un'-dum*). 1. A special form of aluminium used for apparatus in which heat has to be resisted. 2. A trade name for carborundum-type abrasive.

alvealgia (*al-ve-al'-jĭ-ă*). Dry socket (*q.v.*).

alveolabial sulcus. The sulcus between the lips and the alveolar process.

alveolalgia (*al-ve-ol-al'-jĭ-ă*). Dry socket (*q.v.*).

alveolar (*al-ve-o'-lar*). Relating to the alveolus.

alveolar abscess. An abscess affecting the alveolar bone with cellular necrosis and formation of pus.

alveolar angle. The angle between a line running

through a point below the nasal spine and the most prominent point on the lower edge of the maxilla, and the cephalic horizontal line.

alveolar arch. The bow-shape of the alveolar process.

alveolar artery. Supplies blood to the mandibular teeth, floor of the mouth, and buccal mucous membrane (*inferior*), maxillary teeth and antral mucous membrane (*superior*). *Also called* dental artery (British terminology). *See* Table of Arteries —alveolaris.

alveolar canals. Dental canals (*q.v.*).

alveolar crest. One of the highest points on the alveolar process, between the tooth sockets.

alveolar fistula. One leading to a cavity of an alveolar abscess; an alveolar sinus.

alveolar foramen. One of the openings of the alveolar canals on the infratemporal surface of the maxilla, through which the posterior superior alveolar nerves and vessels pass to the molar and premolar teeth. *Also called* posterior superior alveolar foramen.

alveolar index. Gnathic index (*q.v.*).

alveolar line. In cranio-metry, a line from the prosthion to the nasion.

alveolar mucosa. The mucous membrane lining the vestibule of the mouth.

alveolar nerve. Supplies the teeth and alveolar processes. *Also called* dental nerve (British terminology). *See* Table of Nerves—alveolaris.

alveolar osteomyelitis. Pyorrhoea alveolaris (*q.v.*).

alveolar pericementitis. Pyorrhoea alveolaris (*q.v.*).

alveolar periostitis. Pyorrhoea alveolaris (*q.v.*).

alveolar point. The mid-point, between the central incisors, on the maxillary alveolar arch.

alveolar process. A bony ridge on the border of the maxilla or the mandible containing the tooth sockets.

alveolar ridge. The crest remaining in an edentulous mouth after the resorption of the alveolar process.

alveolar septum. Inter-alveolar septum (*q.v.*).

alveolar wiring. Immobilization of a jaw fracture by wires passed through the alveolar bone; used in edentulous patients or those with no suitable teeth to support a splint.

alveolectomy (*al-ve-o-lect'-om-i*). Surgical correction of bone deformity and removal of bone in the alveolar process.

alveolingual (*al-ve-o-lin'-gwal*). Relating to the alveolar process and the tongue.

alveolingual groove. A groove between the lower jaw and the tongue.

alveolingual sulcus. The sulcus between the tongue

and the alveolar process and the teeth.

alveolitis (*al-ve-o-li'-tis*). Inflammation of an alveolus, as of a tooth socket, or of the alveolar process.

alveolobasilar line. In craniometry, a line from the prosthion to the basion.

alveoloclasia (*al"-ve-o-lo-kla'-zĭ-ă*). The break-down of the alveolar process by disintegration or absorption, causing loosening of the teeth.

alveolocondylean (*al-ve-o"-lo-kon-di-le'-an*). Relating to the alveolus and the condyle.

alveolodental (*al"-ve-o-lo-den'-tal*). Relating to the alveolar process and the teeth.

alveolodental canal. An old term for dental canal (*q.v.*).

alveolo-labial (*al"-ve-o-lo-la'-bĭ-al.*) Relating to the alveolar process and the lips.

alveololabialis (*al-ve-o"-lo-la-bĭ-a'-lis*). Buccinator muscle. *See* Table of Muscles.

alveolo-lingual (*al"-ve-o-lo-lin'-gwal*). Alveolingual (*q.v.*).

alveolomaxillary (*al-ve-o"-lo-mak-sil'-ar-ĭ*). The buccinator muscle. *See* Table of Muscles.

alveolomerotomy (*al-ve"-o-lo-mer-ot'-om-ĭ*). Surgical removal of part of the alveolar process; alveolectomy.

alveolonasal (*al-ve"-o-lo-na'-zal*). Craniometric term relating to the alveolar point and the nasion.

alveolonasal line. Alveolar line (*q.v.*).

alveolopalatal (*al"-ve-o-lo-pal-a'-tal*). Relating to the alveolar process and the palate.

alveoloplasty (*al-ve-o'-lo-plast"-ĭ*). Surgical alteration and improvement of the alveolar process for denture construction.

alveolosubnasal (*al-ve-o"-lo-sub-na'-zal*). In craniometry, relating to the alveolar point and the acanthion.

alveolotomy (*al"-ve-ol-ot'-om-ĭ*). Surgical incision of an alveolus or of the alveolar process.

alveolus (*al-ve-o'-lus*). (*pl.* alveoli). *In dentistry:* The bony socket in which the tooth is held.

alveolysis (*al-ve-o-li'-sis*). Resorption of the alveolar bone.

amalgam (*am-al'-gam*). 1. Any alloy of mercury with another metal or metals. 2. Any plastic alloy.
binary a. An amalgam containing mercury and one other metal.
dental a. Any amalgam used for filling teeth; it usually contains silver, tin, and mercury.

amalgam alloy. Shavings or filings of a metal alloy to be mixed with mercury to form an amalgam.

amalgam carrier. A syringe-like instrument used to transfer small quantities of amalgam to a cavity.

amalgam die. A model cast in amalgam from an impression, and from which inlays or crowns may be fabricated.

amalgam manipulator. An instrument used to contour an amalgam.

amalgam matrix. A matrix used to provide a temporary tooth wall to support and assist in the contouring of plastic fillings.

amelification (*am-el-if-ik-a'-shun*). Amelogenesis (*q.v.*).

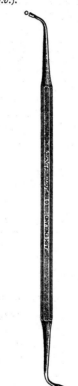

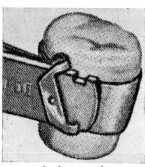

Amalgam matrix

amalgam plugger. An instrument used to condense amalgam in a cavity.

amalgamation (*am-al-gam-a'-shun*). The formation of an amalgam.

amasesis (*am-az-e'-sis*). Inability to chew.

Amalgam plugger

ameloblast (*am-e'-lo-blast*). One of the germ cells developed in the epithelium, from which the enamel organ is formed.

ameloblastic process. A projection of cytoplasm from an enamel cell, about which calcification occurs.

ameloblastoma (*am-e"-lo-blast-o'-mă*). Adamantinoma (*q.v.*).

ameloblastosarcoma (*am-e"-lo-blast"-o-sar-ko'-mă*). A malignant tumour arising from the epithelial odontogenic tissues.

amelocemental (*am-e"-lo-se-ment'-al*). Cemento-enamel (*q.v.*).

amelo-dentinal junction (*am-e"-lo-dent-e'-nal*). The line marking the join between the enamel and the dentine.

amelogenesis (*am-e"-lo-jen'-is-is*). The formation of enamel.

amelogenesis imperfecta. An hereditary defect in enamel formation characterized by a brown colouring of the teeth.

amelogenic (*am-e-lo-jen'-ik*). Enamel-forming.

amnalgesia (*am-nal-je'-zi-ă*). A method of abolishing pain and the memory of pain either by drugs or hypnosis.

amnion (*am'-ni-on*). The innermost of the foetal membranes forming the fluid-filled sac enclosing the foetus and also a sheath for the umbilical cord.

amniotic (*am-ni-ot'-ik*). Relating to the amnion.

amorphous (*a-mor'-fus*). Shapeless; without form.

amphiarthrosis (*am-fi-arth-ro'-sis*). A joint in which the bone surfaces are connected by synovial membrane or by fibro-cartilagenous disks, and in which there is little movement.

amphidiarthrosis (*am"-fi-di-arth-ro'-sis*). A joint which is both ginglymoid and arthrodial, such as the temporo-mandibular joint.

ampoule (*am'-pul*). A small glass container which can be hermetically sealed, used to hold sterile drug preparations.

ampule (*am'-pyul*). Ampoule (*q.v.*).

ampullary nerve. Supplies the ampullae of the semi-circular ducts. *See* Table of Nerves—ampullaris.

amputation (*am-pyu-ta'-shun*). The surgical removal of a limb or part of a limb, or of any other projecting part.
pulp a. Pulpotomy (*q.v.*)
root a. Surgical excision of the apical portion of a tooth root.
subperiosteal a. Amputation in which the stump of bone is covered by a periosteal flap.

amygdala (*a-mig'-dal-ă*). 1. An almond. 2. A tonsil.

amygdaloglossus (*am-ig-dal-o-glos'-us*). The muscle which raises the base of the tongue. *See* Table of Muscles.

amyloid (*am'-il-oyd*). 1. Starch-like. 2. A white, insoluble protein found in the tissues as an abnormal deposit.

amylosis (*am-il-o'-sis*). The digestion of starch or its conversion to glucose.

amylolytic (*am-il-o-lit'-ik*). Relating to or causing the digestion of starch.

amyxorrhoea (*a-miks-or-e'-ă*). Deficiency of mucous secretion.

anabolism (*an-ab'-ol-izm*). The process of assimilation of nutriment and its conversion to living tissue.

anachoresis (*an-ak-or-e'-sis*). The attraction of micro-organisms towards a local tissue lesion, associated with increased immunity to infections other than that of the lesion.

anaemia (*an-e'-mi-ă*). A deficiency in the blood, either qualitative or quantative.

anaemic (*an-e'-mik*). Relating to or affected with anaemia.

anaerobe (*an'-er-ōb*). A micro-organism which can live and grow without air or free oxygen.

anaerobic (*an-er-o'-bik*). Capable of living and growing without air or free oxygen.

anaesthesia (*an-es-the'-zi-ă*). Loss of sensation or feeling.
block a. Anaesthetic block (*q.v.*, 1).

facial a. Loss of sensation in an area of the face as a result of trauma or of a pathological process affecting either the central nervous system or the sensory nerves supplying the area.

general a. Anaesthesia of the whole body.

infiltration a. Local anaesthesia produced by the infiltration of an anaesthetic agent into the surrounding tissue.

inhalation a. General anaesthesia induced by the inhaling of gaseous or volatile liquid anaesthetic agents.

intra-oral a. Local anaesthesia produced by an injection into the oral tissues from within the mouth.

intraosseous a. Anaesthesia of a tooth produced by introducing the anaesthetic agent directly into the alveolar bone in the region of the tooth apex.

intravenous a. General anaesthesia induced by the introduction of an anaesthetic agent into the blood stream by injection into a vein.

local a. Anaesthesia of a circumscribed area of the body.

regional a. Anaesthetic block (*q.v.*, 1).

surface a. Local anaesthesia produced by the application of an agent externally before injection or some other operation liable to cause pain.

topical a. Surface anaesthesia (*q.v.*).

anaesthesiology (*an-es-the-zī-ol′-oj-ĭ*). The study of anaesthesia and anaesthetics.

anaesthetic (*an-es-thet′-ik*). 1. Relating to, or marked by, anaesthesia. 2. Any drug which produces anaesthesia.

anaesthetic block. 1. The injection of an anaesthetic agent into or around a major nerve. 2. The interruption of the nerve supply to an area because of trauma or a pathological lesion.

analgesia (*an-al-je′-zĭ-ă*). Insensibility to pain.
surface a. Surface anaesthesia (*q.v.*).

analgesic (*an-al-je′-sik*). 1. Not sensitive to pain. 2. Pain-relieving. 3. Any agent which relieves pain.

analysis (*an-al′-is-is*). 1. The separation and identification of the various constituents in a compound body or substance. 2. The application of accepted statistical tests to numeric data.

anamnesis (*an-am-ne′-sis*). 1. Memory. 2. A case history.

anaphylaxis (*an-af-il-aks′-is*). An antigen—antibody reaction produced by the parenteral injection of an antigen, causing hypersensitivity.

anaplasia *of tooth enamel* (*an-ă-pla′-zĭ-ă*). Defective development of the tooth enamel extending from the incisal edge or cuspal tip to the cemento-enamel junction.

anaraxia (*an-ar-aks′-ĭ-ă*). Malocclusion (*q.v.*).

anastomosis (*an-as-to-mo′-sis*). 1. A communication between two vessels. 2. A communication between two normally separate hollow parts or organs, either caused by disease or created by surgery.

anastomotic (*an-as-tom-ot′-ik*). Relating to an anastomosis.

anatomic, anatomical (*an-at-om′-ik*). Relating to anatomy.

anatomical articulator. An articulator in which an attempt is made to reproduce the relationships of the upper and lower jaws in all positions and movements.

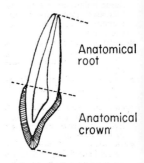

Anatomical crown and root

anatomical crown. That part of a tooth which is covered with enamel.

anatomical root. That portion of a tooth which is covered by cementum.

anatomy (*an-at'-om-ĭ*). The study of the body structure of any organism.

anchor band. A band placed on one tooth to serve as anchorage for the movement of another, in orthodontics.

anchor splint. A splint used in fracture of the jaw, which has metal loops fitting over the teeth.

anchorage (*an'-kor-āj*). 1. The means of retention of a filling. 2. The means of retention of a bridge or artificial crown. 3. The teeth used for supports with an orthodontic regulating appliance.

anchylosis. *See* ankylosis.

Andresen appliance (V. Andresen, 20th century Danish orthodontist). A solid functional orthodontic appliance used mainly for the treatment of Class II, div. I, malocclusion, and occasionally for the treatment of Class III malocclusion. *Also called* the Norwegian appliance, activator, or monobloc.

anemia. *See* anaemia.

anesthesia. *See* anaesthesia.

aneurysm (*an'-yur-izm*). A circumscribed dilatation of an artery wall, forming a pulsating, blood-containing swelling.

angeitis (*an-jĕ-i'-tis*). Angiitis (*q.v.*).

angiitis (*an-jĭ-i'-tis*). Inflammation affecting either a blood or a lymph vessel.

angina, Ludwig's. *See* Ludwig's angina.

angina, Plaut's. Acute ulcerative tonsillitis (*q.v.*).

angina, Vincent's. Acute ulcerative tonsillitis (*q.v.*).

angiofibroma (*an"-jĭ-o-fĭ-bro'-mă*). A fibroma containing blood vessels or lymph vessels.

angiology (*an-jĭ-ol'-oj-ĭ*). The study of blood vessels and lymphatics.

angioma (*an-jĭ-o'-mă*). A tumour composed of blood or lymphatic vessels.

angle (*an'-gl*). 1. The inclination of one line or plane to another, expressed in degrees or radians. 2. The point of meeting of two lines or the line of intersection of two planes.

alveolar a. In craniometry, the angle between a line running through a point below the nasal spine and the most prominent point on the lower edge of the maxilla, and the cephalic horizontal line.

buccal a. In dentistry, any angle formed by the junction of a buccal tooth surface, or a cavity wall, in a posterior tooth, with any other tooth surface or cavity wall.

cavity a. The angle formed by the walls of a tooth cavity, named according to the walls which form it.

cavosurface a. The angle formed between a cavity

wall and the surface of a tooth.

craniofacial a. In craniometry, the angle between the basicranial and basifacial axes at the spheno-ethmoid suture.

cusp. a The angle of incline of the sides of a cusp made with the perpendicular line bisecting the cusp, measured mesiodistally or buccolingually.

distal a. In dentistry, any angle formed by the junction of a distal tooth surface, or cavity wall, with any other tooth surface or cavity wall.

facial a. In craniometry, the the angle between a line joining the nasion and the prosthion and one passing through the orbital opening and the auricular point; it indicates the degree of protrusion of the chin.

genial a. The angle formed between the ramus and the body of the mandible.

gonial a. Gonion (*q.v.*).

incisal a. In dentistry, any angle formed by the junction of an incisal edge, or cavity wall, in an anterior tooth, with any other tooth surface or cavity wall.

labial a. In dentistry, any angle formed by the junction of a labial tooth surface, or cavity wall, in an anterior tooth, with any other tooth surface or cavity wall.

line a. An angle formed at the junction of two tooth surfaces or of two cavity walls.

lingual a. In dentistry, any angle formed by the junction of a lingual tooth surface or cavity wall with any other tooth surface or cavity wall.

mandibular a. The angle of the jaw; the angle between the base of the body of the mandible and the ramus, on either side.

maxillary a. The angle formed at the point of contact of the central incisors by the intersection of lines from the ophryon and the most prominent point of the mandible.

mesial a. In dentistry, any angle formed by the junction of a mesial tooth surface, or a cavity wall, with any other tooth surface or cavity wall.

occipital a. The angle formed at the junction of lines connecting the lambda and the point of the external occipital protuberance with the point on the sagittal curvature of the occipital bone.

occlusal a. In dentistry, any angle formed by the junction of an occlusal surface or cavity wall with any other tooth surface or cavity wall.

orifacial a. In craniometry, the angle formed by the facial line with the upper occlusal plane.

parietal a. The angle formed at the junction of lines

connecting the bregma and the lambda to the highest point on the sagittal curvature above the horizontal plane passing through them.

point a. An angle formed at the junction of three tooth surfaces or cavity walls.

tooth a. The angle formed by the surfaces of the tooth, named according to the surfaces which form it.

uranal a. The angle formed at the junction of lines connecting the highest point on the sagittal curvature of the palate with the premaxillary point and with the posterior nasal spine.

For eponymous angles *see* under the name of the person by which the angle is known.

angle *of the mouth.* The angle at the junction of the upper and lower lips on either side of the mouth.

Angle band (E. H. Angle, 1835-1930. American orthodontist). An orthodontic clamp band, having the clamp on the lingual side.

Angle's chin retractor (E. H. Angle, 1835-1930. American orthodontist). A metal chin-cup connected by elastic bands to a head cap.

Angle's classification of malocclusion (E. H. Angle, 1855-1930. American orthodontist). See under *malocclusion.*

Angle's fracture bands (E. H. Angle, 1835-1930. American orthodontist). Anchor bands which have provision for the attachment of wires or elastic bands for intermaxillary fixation in jaw fracture.

Angle's splint (E. H. Angle, 1855-1930. American orthodontist). Angle's fracture bands (*q.v.*).

angular artery. Supplies the inferior portion of M. orbicularis palpebrum and the lacrimal sac. *See* Table of Arteries—angularis.

angulis oris (*an'-gu-lis or'-is*). The angle of the mouth (*q.v.*).

anisodont (*an-i'-so-dont*). Having unequal and irregular teeth.

anisognathous (*an-i-sog'-nath-us*). Having the upper jaw of much greater width than the lower.

ankylocheilia (*an''-ki-lo-ki'-li-ă*). Adhesion of the lips.

ankyloglossia (*an-ki-lo-glos'-i-ă*). Tongue-tie.

ankylosis (*an-ki-lo'-sis*). 1. The type of tooth attachment where the tooth is directly connected to the bone, with no intervening soft tissue. 2. Abnormal stiffness or immobility of a joint.

bony a. Complete joint fixation through bone fusion.

fibrous a. Stiffness due to fibrous adhesions or fibrosis of the joints.

ankylotomy (*an-ki-lot'-om-i*). An operation for releasing tongue-tie.

anlage (*an'-lāj; an'-lah-gĕ*). The primary collection of cells from which any distinct organ or part of the embryo is developed.

anneal (*an-ēl'*). The process of softening a metal by heat and cooling, rendering it more malleable and ductile, and less brittle.

annular (*an'-yu-lar*). In the shape of a ring.

anodontia (*an-o-don'-shĭ-ă*). Absence of teeth.

anodontism (*an-o-dont'-izm*). Absence of all dental organs.

anodyne (*an'-o-dīn*). 1. Pain-relieving. 2. Any drug used to ease pain.

anomalous (*an-om'-al-us*) Relating to an anomaly; irregular.

anomaly (*an-om'-al-ĭ*). Deviation or irregularity compared with the normal.
developmental a. An anomaly due to defective development.

anomodont (*an-om'-o-dont*). An extinct reptile, of the order Anomodontia, having long canines, a horny beak in place of incisors, and irregular molars.

anonymous vein. Brachiocephalic vein. *See* Table of Veins—brachiocephalica.

anorexia (*an-or-eks'-ĭ-ă*). Lack of appetite.

anosmia (*an-os'-mĭ-ă*). Absence of sense of smell.

anostosis (*an-os-to'-sis*). Defective bone development.

anoxia (*an-oks'-ĭ-ă*). Lack of oxygen either in the tissues or the blood.

ansa (*an'-să*). Anatomical term denoting a loop.

ansa, Haller's. *See* Haller's ansa.

ansa cervicalis. Supplies omohyoid, sternohyoid and sternothyroid muscles. *See* Table of Nerves.

ansa hypoglossi. Ansa cervicalis (*q.v.*).

antagonist (*an-tag'-on-ist*). 1. Any muscle which acts against or in opposition to another muscle. 2. Any drug which counteracts or interferes with the action of another drug administered at the same time. 3. The tooth of one jaw which occludes with one in the other jaw.

ante cibum (*an'-tĕ si'-bum*). Latin for *before meals*; used in prescription writing, and abbreviated *a.c.*

antelabium (*an-te-la'-bi-um*). The procheilon (*q.v.*).

antenatal (*an''-tĕ-na'-tal*). Before birth; relating to anything occurring before birth.

anterior (*an-te'-rĭ-or*). In front; as opposed to *posterior.*

anterior facial vein. Facial vein. *See* Table of Veins—facialis.

anterior open-bite. Open-bite (*q.v.*) in which the anterior teeth do not come into contact.

anterior teeth. The incisors and canines.

anterocclusion (*an-ter-ok-lu'-zhun*). A form of malocclusion in which the mandibular teeth are forward of their normal position in the arch.

anthracosis linguae. Black tongue (q.v.).

anti-. Prefix signifying *opposed to*.

antibiosis (*an″-ti-bi′-os-is*). An antagonistic association between two micro-organisms, to the detriment of one of them.

antibiotic (*an-ti-bi-ot′-ik*). 1. Relating to antibiosis. 2. Destructive of life; applied to certain agents, such as penicillin, used against infections caused by micro-organisms.

antibody (*an′-ti-bod-i*). Any one of a class of substances produced in the body as a reaction to a specific antigen, and with which it reacts in some observable way to produce a specific effect such as inactivation, agglutination, flocculation, etc.

anticalculous (*an″-ti-kal′-kyu-lus*). Inhibiting the formation or deposition of calculus.

anticariogenic (*an″-ti-ka-ri-o-jen′-ik*). Relating to anything which prevents or delays the onset of caries.

anticarious (*an″-ti-ka′-ri-us*). Inhibiting dental caries.

antidote (*an′-ti-dōt*). An agent used to counteract or prevent the action of a poison.

antigen (*an′-ti-jen*). Any substance which, when introduced into the body, excites the formation of specific antibodies.

antiodontalgic (*an-ti-o-dont-al′-jik*). Counteracting toothache, or any agent which relieves toothache.

antiphlogistic (*an″-ti-floj-ist′-ik*). 1. Counteracting inflammation and fever. 2. An agent used to allay inflammation and fever.

antipyretic (*an″-ti-pi-ret′-ik*). 1. Fever-reducing. 2. Any substance or form of treatment which reduces fever.

antisepsis (*an-ti-sep′-sis*). The prevention of sepsis by the destruction, or inhibition of growth, of pathogenic micro-organisms.

antiseptic (*an-ti-sep′-tik*). 1. Relating to antisepsis. 2. Any substance which produces antisepsis.

antisialagogue (*an″-ti-si-al′-ă-gog*). 1. Saliva-inhibiting. 2. Any agent which inhibits excessive flow of saliva.

antisialic (*an″-ti-si-al′-ik*). 1. Checking the flow of saliva. 2. An agent which checks salivary secretion.

antitoxin (*an-ti-toks′-in*). A substance produced in the body, or which may be injected into it, which is antagonistic to a specific toxin and will neutralize it.

antitrismus (*an-ti-triz′-mus*). Muscular spasm preventing the closing of the mouth.

antodontalgic (*ant″-o-dont-al′-jik*). Antiodontalgic (q.v.).

antracele (*an′-tră-sēl*). Antrocele (q.v.).

antral (*an′-tral*). Relating to an antrum.

antral fistula. A fistula leading from an antral abscess or from a bone cavity.

antritis (*an-tri'-tis*). Inflammation of the maxillary sinus (or antrum).

antrocele (*an'-tro-sēl*). An accumulation of fluid in the maxillary sinus (or antrum).

antrolith (*an'-tro-lith*). A concretion or calculus in the maxillary sinus (or antrum).

antronasal (*an-tro-na'-zal*). Relating to the maxillary sinus (or antrum) and the nose.

antro-oral (*an-tro-or'-al*). Relating to the maxillary sinus (or antrum) and the mouth.

antroscope (*an'-tro-skōp*). An instrument for inspecting the maxillary sinus (or antrum).

antrotome (*an'-tro-tōm*). An instrument used to cut open an antrum.

antrotomy (*an-trot'-om-ĭ*). Surgical opening of the maxillary sinus (or antrum) for drainage.

antrum (*an'-trum*). An air cavity, generally in bone; also called a *sinus* (def. 3). *maxillary a.* Maxillary sinus (*q.v.*).

antrum of Highmore (N. Highmore, 1613-85. English anatomist). The maxillary sinus (*q.v.*).

anvil (*an'-vil*). An iron block, steel-faced, on which, in a dental laboratory, metals may be hammered or forged.

apectomy (*a-pek'-tom-ĭ*). Apicectomy (*q.v.*).

aperture (*ap'-er-tyur*). An opening.

orbital a. One of the openings in the facial bones which contain the eyeballs.

piriform a. The pear-shaped nasal opening in the skull.

apex (*a'-peks*) (*pl.* apices). *In dentistry*, the extreme point of a tooth root.

apexograph (*a-peks'-o-graf*). An instrument used to locate the apex of a tooth root.

aphonia (*a-fo'-nĭ-ă*). Hoarseness, loss of voice.

aphtha (*af'-thă*) (*pl.* aphthae). 1. Any small ulcer. 2. An irregular whitish ulcer occurring in the mouth.

aphthae, Bednar's. *See* Bednar's aphthae.

aphthae, Riga's. *See* Riga's aphthae.

aphthosis (*af-tho'-sis*). Any condition characterized by the formation of aphthae.

aphthous (*af'-thus*). Relating to or characterized by aphthae.

aphthous stomatitis. A form of stomatitis, often recurring, characterised by painful aphthae affecting the oral mucous membranes.

aphthous ulcer. Aphthae (*q.v.*) which break down into a shallow and painful ulcer.

apical (*a'-pik-al*). Relating to or affecting the apex of a tooth root.

apical abscess. An abscess occurring at the apex of a tooth root.

apical foramen. The small opening at the apex of the tooth root by which the nerve and blood supply of the pulp enter.

apical granuloma. A dental granuloma (q.v.) associated with the apical area of a tooth.

apical space. The area between the bony wall of the tooth socket and the apex of the tooth root; the site of an apical abscess.

apicectomy (a-pi-sek'-tom-i). Surgical removal of the apex of a tooth root.

apico-. Prefix signifying apex.

apicoectomy (a-pi-ko-ek'-tom-i). Apicectomy (q.v.).

apicolocator (a"-pik-o-lo-ka'-tor). An instrument used to locate the apex of a tooth root.

aplasia (a-pla'-zi-ă). Failure of, or defect in the development of, an organ or tissue; agenesis.

aplastic (a-plast'-ik). Relating to or affected by aplasia.

apo-. Prefix signifying from.

aponeurosis (ap-o-nyur-o'-sis). A flat tendon investing or serving as attachment to muscles.
epicranial a. The scalpal aponeurosis; galea aponeurotica (q.v.).
palatine a. The fibrous extension of the tensor palati muscles forming the anterior part of the soft palate and to which other palatal muscles are attached.

apophysis (ap-of'-is-is). An outgrowth or projection, used especially of a bone process.

apostema (ap-os-te'-mă). An abscess (q.v.).

apoxemena (ap-ok-sem'-en-ă). The material removed from periodontal pockets in the treatment of pericemento-clasia.

apoxesis (ap-oks-e'-sis). Curettage (q.v., 2).

appliance (ap-li'-ans). Any device in the mouth used to move or to immobilize the teeth in order to correct or prevent malocclusion, or to supply missing teeth or serve as an obturator.
fixed a. An orthodontic regulating appliance which is attached to the supporting teeth so that it cannot be removed by the wearer.
removable a. Any orthodontic or prosthetic appliance which can be easily removed by the wearer.
For eponymous appliances *see* under the personal name by which the appliance is known.

applicator (ap'-lik-a-tor). Any instrument used for making local applications of a medicament.

apposition (ap-o-zish'-un). The contact between two opposed surfaces, and their fitting together.

approximate (ap-roks'-im-āt). 1. To bring into close contact. 2. Situated close together, used of adjoining tooth surfaces.

approximate (ap-roks'-im-āt). Only roughly calculated, not precise and accurate.

aptyalism (a-ti'-al-izm). Lack or deficiency of saliva.

apyetous (*a-pi-ě'-tus*). Not pus-producing.

apyogenous (*a-pi-oj'-en-us*). Not produced by or because of pus.

apyous (*a-pi'-us*). Apyetous (*q.v.*).

apyrexia (*a-pi-reks'-i-ă*). Absence or temporary reduction of fever.

aqua (*ak'-wă*). Latin for *water*; abbreviated *aq.*

aqua destillata (*ak'-wă des-til-a'-tă*). Latin for *distilled water*; abbreviated *aq. dest.*

aqueduct of Fallopius. Facial canal (*q.v.*).

aqueous (*a'-kwe-us*). Relating to or mixed with water.

arch (*artch*). 1. A curved or bow-shaped structure. 2. A form of orthodontic appliance.

alveolar a. The bow shape of the alveolar process.

dental a. The bow-shaped arrangement of the teeth in the mandible and the maxilla.

expansion a. An orthodontic appliance used to assist in the lateral movement of teeth.

glossopalatine a. Palatoglossal arch (*q.v.*).

lingual a. An orthodontic wire appliance conforming to the lingual aspect of the dental arch.

mandibular a. 1. The first branchial arch, from which the jaws and parts of the face develop. 2. The dental arch of the mandible.

palatal a. The roof of the mouth.

palatoglossal a. The anterior pillar of the fauces.

palatopharyngeal a. The posterior pillar of the fauces.

ribbon a. An orthodontic appliance of flattened wire conforming to the dental arch, used for anchorage in the movement of teeth; a type of expansion arch.

superciliary a. The slight bulge over the medial part of the supra-orbital margin of the frontal bone.

zygomatic a. The arch formed by the zygoma and the zygomatic process of the maxilla and the temporal bone.

arch, Johnson twin wire. *See* Johnson twin wire arch.

arch bar. An orthodontic appliance consisting of a wire extending round the dental arch, to which intervening teeth may be attached.

arch bridge. Fixed bridge (*q.v.*).

archwire (*artch'-wīr*). In an orthodontic appliance, any wire which follows closely the lingual or labial outline of the dental arch.

arctation (*ark-ta'-shun*). Narrowing or contracture of a canal or other opening.

areola (*ar-e-o'-lă*). A small space or interstice in tissue.

areolar (*ar-e-o'-lar*). Relating to areolae.

ariboflavinosis (*a-ri-bo-fla-vin-o'-sis*). Deficiency of

riboflavin, one of the vita-
min-B complex, producing
cheilosis, scaly seborrhoeic
desquamation, glossitis, etc.

Arkansas stone. A specially
hard stone used to sharpen
the cutting edges of dental
instruments.

Arkövy's mixture (J. Arkövy,
fl. 1923. Hungarian dentist).
A preparation containing
8 gm. phenol, 4 gm. cam-
phor, and 4 cc. eucalyptus
oil, used in the treatment of
putrescent root canals.

armamentarium (*ar-mă-
ment-a'-ri-um*). The instruments, books and appliances,
and other equipment possessed by a medical or dental
practitioner for use in his
profession.

Arnold's nerve (F. Arnold,
1803-90. German anato-
mist). N. auricularis. *See*
Table of Nerves.

arrowhead clasp. A form of
orthodontic attachment consisting of a wire clasp round
a molar tooth, fitting under
the mesial and distal bulge,
to which removeable appliances may be fastened. The
Adams crib is a modified
form of arrowhead clasp.

artefact (*ar'-tĕ-fakt*). An
artificial product. Used in
histology to mean a de-
fect or distortion produced
by some artificial means, resulting in a misleading
appearance.

arteria auditiva. A. labyrinthi. *See* Table of Arteries.

arterial (*ar-te'-rĭ-al*). Relating to an artery.

arteriole (*ar-te'-rĭ-ōl*). A
minute branch of an artery.

arteriorrhexis (*ar-te"-rĭ-
or-eks'-is*). Rupture of an
artery.

arteriosclerosis (*ar-te"-rĭ-
o-skler-o'-sis*). A condition
characterized by loss of
elasticity and thickening of
the artery walls.

arteriostenosis (*ar-te"-rĭ-o-
sten-o'-sis*). The narrowing
of the calibre of an artery.

arteriostosis (*ar-te"-rĭ-os-
to'-sis*). Arterial ossification.

artery (*ar'-ter-ĭ*). One of the
blood vessels which carries
oxygenated blood from the
heart.
  pulmonary a. The artery
which conveys deoxygenated
blood from the heart to the
lungs.

**artery of the pterygoid
canal.** Supplies palatine
muscles and upper portion
of pharynx. *See* Table of
Arteries—canalis pterygoidea.

arthral (*ar'-thral*). Relating
to a joint.

arthralgia (*ar-thral'-jĭ-ă*).
Pain affecting a joint.

arthritis (*ar-thri'-tis*). Inflammation of a joint.
  dental a. Inflammation
affecting the periodontal
membrane.

arthrochondritis (*ar"-thro-
kon-dri'-tis*). Inflammation
of joint cartilage.

arthrodia (*ar-thro'-dĭ-ă*). A
joint of which the articulation is a gliding movement
of the surfaces.

arthrodial (*ar-thro'-dĭ-al*). Resembling an arthrodia.

arthrodynia (*ar-thro-din'-ĭ-ă*). Pain affecting a joint; arthralgia.

arthrolith (*ar'-thro-lith*). A calcareous deposit in a joint.

arthrology (*ar-throl'-oj-ĭ*). The study of joints.

arthropathy (*ar-throp'-ath-ĭ*). Any joint disease.

arthroplasty (*ar'-thro-plast-ĭ*). 1. Plastic surgery of a joint. 2. The construction of an artificial joint.

arthrosis (*ar-thro'-sis.*). 1. Any joint. 2. A joint disease.

arthrosteitis (*ar-thros-te-i'-tis*). Inflammation affecting the bony structures of a joint.

arthrosynovitis (*ar''-thro-si-no-vi'-tis*). Inflammation affecting the synovial membrane of a joint.

articular (*ar-tik'-yu-lar*). Relating to a joint.

articular disc. A fibrous plate between articulating bone surfaces in a joint.

articulating paper. Carbon paper which, when bitten on, records the contact points of the teeth.

articulation (*ar-tik-yu-la'-shun*). 1. A joint (*q.v.*). 2. The jointed movement of the upper and lower teeth in contact. 3. The arrangement of artificial teeth to fit the mouth and function like the natural dentition. 4. The production of sounds in speech.

articulator (*ar-tik'-yu-la-tor*). *In dentistry:* An instrument

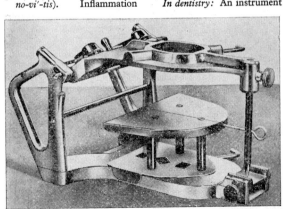

Anatomical articulator

to which models are attached in order to simulate the relationship between the upper and lower jaws in centric relation and, to a varying extent, in opening and closing movements, in protrusion and in lateral excursion.

anatomical a. An articulator in which an attempt is made to reproduce the relationships of the upper and lower jaws in all positions and movements.

articulator, Gysi's. *See* Gysi's articulator.

articulomachelian bar (*ar-tik'-yu-lo-mak-e'-lĭ-an*). Embryonic cartilage from which the mandible develops.

artifact. *See* artefact.

artificial (*ar-tĭ-fish'-al*). Made by art; as opposed to *natural*.

artificial denture. Any appliance designed to replace natural teeth.

artificial palate. An obturator used to close a cleft palate.

artificial velum. An appliance used in prosthetic treatment of a cleft of the soft palate.

aryepiglotticus muscle. Inconstant fascicle of oblique arytenoid muscle. *See* Table of Muscles—aryepiglotticus.

arytenoid muscle. Closes inlet of larynx and approximates arytenoid cartilages. *See* Table of Muscles—arytenoideus.

asbestos (*as-bes'-tos*). A fibrous calcium or magnesium silicate, non-combustible. In dentistry it is used, mixed with plaster, as an investment material in soldering.

asepsis (*a-sep'-sis*). Absence of infection or of putrefaction.

aseptic (*a-sep'-tik*). Relating to asepsis; free from infection.

Ash's dowel crown. A crown made of porcelain baked onto a platinum tube, and held in position by a fluted dowel.

asialia (*a-si-al'-ĭ-ă*). Aptyalism (*q.v.*).

asphyxia (*as-fiks'-ĭ-ă*). Suffocation; deprivation of oxygen causing anoxia and the accumulation of carbon dioxide in the blood, with resultant coma.

aspirate (*as'-pir-āt*). 1. To suck up or to breathe in. 2. To remove fluid or gas from a body cavity by suction.

aspirating needle. A long hollow needle used to withdraw fluid from a cavity.

aspiration (*as-pir-a'-shun*). 1. The act of breathing in. 2. The removal of gas or liquid from a cavity by means of suction.

asporous (*a-spor'-us*). Having no spores.

Assezat's triangle (J. Assezat, 1832-76. French anthropologist). A craniometric triangle bounded by lines joining the basion, the alveolar point, and the nasion; the facial triangle.

assimilable (*as-im'-il-abl*). Capable of assimilation.

assimilate (*as-im'-il-āt*). To absorb and change into body tissue.

assimilation (*as-im-il-a'-shun*). The processes whereby food is absorbed and changed into body tissue.

asthenic (*as-then'-ik*). Lacking strength and vigour; weak.

astomatous (*a-sto'-mat-us*). Without a mouth.

astomia (*a-sto'-mi-ă*). Congenital absence of a mouth opening.

astringent (*as-trinj'-ent*). 1. Capable of causing contraction, or of drawing together. 2. An agent producing organic contraction, or arresting discharge.

asymmetrical (*a-sim-et'-rik-al*). Relating to asymmetry; not symmetrical.

asymmetry (*a-sim'-et-ri*). Dissimilarity or irregularity of normally similar or corresponding parts; lack of symmetry.

asymptomatic (*a-simp-tom-at'-ik*). Without any symptoms.

ataxia (*a-taks'-ĭ-ă*). Lack of muscular co-ordination.

atelo-. Prefix signifying *faulty development*, or *incomplete development*.

atelocheilia (*at"-el-o-ki'-li-ă*). Defective development of the lip.

ateloglossia (*at"-el-o-glos'-i-ă*). Congenital defect of the tongue.

atelognathia (*at"-el-og-na'-thi-ă*). Congenital defect of the jaw.

ateloprosopia (*at"-et-o-pro-so'-pi-ă*). Faulty or incomplete development of the facial processes.

atelostomia (*at"-el-o-sto'-mi-ă*). Deficient or faulty development of the mouth.

atlantoaxial (*at-lan"-to-ak'-si-ăl*). Relating to the atlas and the axis.

atlantoepistrophic (*at-lan"-to-ep-is-trof'-ik*). Atlantoaxial (*q.v.*).

atlas (*at'-las*). The first cervical vertebra.

atomizer (*at'-om-i-zer*). An instrument for ejecting a liquid as a fine spray.

atonic (*a-ton'-ik*). Lacking in normal tone, slack or relaxed; used particularly of muscles.

atoxic (*a-toks'-ik*). Non-poisonous.

atrophic (*at'-rof-ik*). Affected by, or relating to, atrophy.

atrophy (*at'-rof-i*). A reduction in size of tissue or of an organ due to a decrease in the size or number of its constituent cells; it may be physiological or pathological.

attachment (*at-atch'-ment*). 1. The means by which one thing is fastened to another. 2. Any clasp, hook, or cap used to fasten a partial denture or an appliance to a natural tooth.

epithelial a. The epithelium at the base of the gingival crevice or periodontal pocket, lying in close proximity to the tooth surface and "attaching" the gingiva to the tooth. It is thought to originate from the cells of the reduced enamel epithelium.

precision a. A prefabricated form of attachment for the retention of a bridge or partial denture; it consists of a male and a female portion, one being incorporated in the prosthesis and the other in the retainer cemented to the supporting tooth or root.

attachment, Roach's. *See* Roach's attachment.

attraction (*at-rak'-shun*) *of the jaws.* A form of malocclusion in which the jaws are abnormally close together.

attrition (*at-rish'-un*). Rubbing or wearing away; in dentistry, applied to the mechanical wearing down of the tooth surface in mastication.

atypical (*a-tip'-ik-al*). Not typical, irregular, not corresponding to the accepted norm.

audio-analgesia (*aw''-di-o-an-al-je'-zi-ă*). A method of producing insensibility to pain by means of music and background sounds to which the patient listens through earphones.

auditory (*aw'-dit-or-i*). Relating to hearing or to the organs of hearing.

auditory artery. A. labyrinthi. *See* Table of Arteries.

auditory canal, internal. The internal auditory meatus (*q.v.*).

auditory meatus, *external:* The external auditory canal from the concha to the tympanic membrane in the ear. *internal:* The canal from the tympanic membrane through the petrous bone, giving passage to the facial and auditory nerves and the internal auditory artery.

auditory nerve. N. vestibulocochlearis. *See* Table of Nerves.

auditory tube. External auditory meatus (*q.v.*).

augnathus (*aw-gna'-thus*). A foetus having a double lower jaw; a rare anomaly.

aural (*aw'-ral*). Relating to the ear and hearing.

auric (*aw'-rik*). Relating to or containing gold.

auricle (*awr'-ikl*). 1. One of the two upper chambers of the heart. 2. The pinna, or external ear.

auricular (*aw-rik'-yu-lar*). Relating to the auricle.

auricular artery. Supplies digastric and other muscles, parotid gland, external auditory meatus, mastoid cells, etc.; three branches—posterior, anterior, deep. *See* Table of Arteries—auricularis.

auricular muscle. Draws auricle or pinna forward or back, or raises it. *See* Table of Muscles—auricularis.

auricular nerve. Supplies auricle or pinna and external auditory meatus. *See* Table of Nerves—auricularis.

auriculare (*aw-rik'-yu-lah-rē*). The central point of the external auditory meatus.

auriculo-infraorbital plane. Frankfort plane (*q.v.*).

auriculo-nasal plane. Camper's plane (*q.v.*).

auriculo-orbital plane. Frankfort plane (*q.v.*).

auriculotemporal nerve. Supplies skin over temple and scalp. *See* Table of Nerves — auriculotemporalis.

aurinasal (*aw"-ri-na'-zal*). Relating to the ear and the nose.

auto-. Prefix signifying *self*.

autoclave (*aw'-to-klāv*). A high-pressure steam type of sterilizer.

autogenous (*aw-toj'-en-us*). Produced within the body itself; self-generated.

automallet (*aw-to-mal'-et*). Automatic mallet (*q.v.*).

automatic mallet. An instrument used to condense gold or amalgam in restorations; the blow is produced either by hand operation, with a dental engine, or with compressed air.

autonomic (*aw-to-no'-mik*). 1. Independent in function. 2. Spontaneous.

autonomic nerve. Any nerve of the autonomic nervous system.

autopolymer (*aw"-to-pol'-im-er*). A plastic substance which polymerizes without the use of external heat, by the addition of a catalyst and an activator.

autotrophic (*aw-to-tro'-fik*). Relating to micro-organisms which can obtain nourishment from carbon dioxide in an inorganic environment; as opposed to *heterotrophic*.

avulsion (*ă-vul'-shun*). Complete detachment of a tooth from its socket.

axial (*aks'-i-al*). Relating to, or in relation to, an axis.

axial wall. That wall lying nearest the pulp in cavities on an axial surface.

axio-. Prefix signifying *axis*, especially the long axis of a tooth.

axiobuccal (*aks"-i-o-buk'-al*). Buccoaxial (*q.v.*).

axiobuccocervical (*aks"-i-o-buk"-o-ser-vi'-kal*). Gingivobuccoaxial (*q.v.*).

axiobuccogingival (*aks"-i-o-buk"-o-jin'-jiv-al*). Gingivobuccoaxial (*q.v.*).

axiobuccolingual plane. A plane through the buccal and lingual surfaces of a tooth parallel to its axis.

axioclusal (*aks"-i-ok-lu'-zal*). Axio-occlusal (*q.v.*).

axiocervical (*aks"-i-o-ser-vi'-kal*). Axiogingival (*q.v.*).

axiodistal (*aks"-i-o-dis'-tal*). Relating to the axial and distal walls of a buccal or lingual cavity in a molar or premolar.
a. angle. The angle formed at the junction of these walls; a *line* angle.

axiodistocclusal (*aks''-ĭ-o-dis-tok-lu'-zal*). Axiodisto-occlusal (*q.v.*).

axiodistocervical (*aks''-ĭ-o-dis''-to-ser-vi'-kal*). Axiodistogingival (*q.v.*).

axiodistogingival (*aks''-ĭ-o-dis''-to-jin'-jiv-al*). Relating to the axial, distal and gingival walls of a buccal or lingual cavity in a molar or premolar.
a. angle. The angle formed at the junction of these walls; a *point* angle.

axiodistoincisal (*aks''-ĭ-o-dis''-to-in-si'-zal*). Relating to the axial, distal and incisal walls of a labial or lingual cavity in an incisor or canine.
a. angle. The angle formed at the junction of these walls; a *point* angle.

axiodisto-occlusal (*aks''-ĭ-o-dis''-to-ok-lu'-zal*). Relating to the axial, distal, and occlusal walls of a buccal or lingual cavity in a molar or premolar.
a. angle. The angle formed at the junction of these walls; a *point* angle.

axiogingival (*aks''-ĭ-o-jin'-jiv-al*). Relating to the axial and gingival walls of a mesial, distal or proximo-occlusal cavity in an incisor or canine, or of a buccal or lingual cavity in a molar or premolar.
a. angle. The angle formed at the junction of these walls; a *line* angle.

axioincisal (*aks''-ĭ-o-in-si'-zal*). Relating to the axial and incisal walls of a mesial or distal cavity in an incisor or canine.
a. angle. The angle formed at the junction of these walls; both a *line* angle and a *point* angle.

axiolabial (*aks''-ĭ-o-la'-bĭ-al*). Relating to the axial and labial walls of a mesial, distal or proximo-incisal cavity in an incisor or canine.
a. angle. The angle formed at the junction of these walls; a *line* angle.

axiolabiocervical (*aks''-ĭ-o-la''-bĭ-o-ser-vi'-kal*). Axiolabiogingival (*q.v.*).

axiolabiogingival (*aks''-ĭ-o-la''-bĭ-o-jin'-jiv-al*). Relating to the axial, labial, and gingival walls of a mesial, distal or proximo-incisal cavity in an incisor or canine.
a. angle. The angle formed at the junction of these walls; a *point* angle.

axiolabiolingual (*aks''-ĭ-o-la''-bĭ-o-lin'-gwal*). Incisal (*q.v.*).

axiolabiolingual plane. A plane through the labial and lingual surfaces of a tooth parallel to its axis.

axiolingual (*aks''-ĭ-o-lin'-gwal*). Relating to the axial and lingual walls of a mesial, distal or proximo-incisal cavity in an incisor or canine.
a. angle. The angle formed at the junction of these walls; a *line* angle.

axiolinguoocclusal (*ask″-ĭ-o-lin-gwok-lu′-zal*). Axiolinguo-occlusal (*q.v.*).

axiolinguocervical (*aks″-ĭ-o-lin″-gwo-ser-vi′-kal*). Axiolinguogingival (*q.v.*).

axiolinguogingival (*aks″-ĭ-o-lin″-gwo-jin′-jiv-al*). Relating to the axial, lingual and gingival walls of a mesial, distal, or proximoincisal cavity in an incisor or canine.

a. angle. The angle formed at the junction of these walls; a *point* angle.

axiolinguo-occlusal (*aks″-ĭ-o-lin″-gwo-ok-lu′-zal*). Relating to the axial, lingual and occlusal walls of a tooth cavity.

axiomesial (*aks″-ĭ-o-me′-zĭ-al*). Relating to the axial and mesial walls of a buccal or lingual cavity in a molar or premolar.

a. angle. The angle formed at the junction of these walls; a *line* angle.

axiomesiocclusal (*aks″-ĭ-o-me-zi-ok-lu′-zal*). Axio-mesio-occlusal (*q.v.*).

axiomesiocervical (*aks″-ĭ-o-me″-zĭ-o-ser-vi′-kal*). Axiomesiogingival (*q.v.*).

axiomesiodistal plane. A plane through the mesial and distal surfaces of a tooth parallel to the axis.

axiomesiogingival (*aks″-ĭ-o-me″-zĭ-o-jin′-jiv-al*). Relating to the axial, mesial and gingival walls of a buccal or lingual cavity in a molar or premolar.

a. angle. The angle formed at the junction of these walls; a *point* angle.

axiomesioincisal (*aks″-ĭ-o-me″-zĭ-o-in-si′-zal*). Relating to the axial, mesial and incisal walls in a labial or lingual cavity in an incisor or canine.

a. angle. The angle formed at the junction of these walls; a *point* angle.

axiomesio-occlusal (*aks″-ĭ-me″-zĭ-o-ok-lu′-zal*). Relating to the axial, mesial and occlusal walls of a buccal or lingual cavity in a molar or premolar.

a. angle. The angle formed at the junction of these walls; a *point* angle.

axio-occlusal (*aks″-ĭ-o-ok-lu-zal.*) Relating to the axial and occlusal walls of a buccal or lingual cavity in a molar or premolar.

a. angle. The angle formed at the junction of these walls; a *line* angle.

axiopulpal (*aks″-ĭ-o-pul′-pal*). Relating to the axial and pulpal walls in the step portion of a proximo-occlusal cavity in a molar or premolar.

a. angle. The angle formed at the junction of these walls; a *line* angle.

axis (*aks′-is*). 1. The line about which a body revolves. 2. In anatomy, the second cervical vertebra.

axle tooth. Azzle tooth (*q.v.*).

azzle tooth (*az′-el*). An old term for a molar tooth.

B

B Buccal.

BA Buccoaxial.

BAC Buccoaxiocervical.

BAG Buccoaxiogingival.

BC Buccocervical.

BD Buccodistal.

b.d. Abbreviation for *bis die*—twice a day; used in prescription writing.

BG Buccogingival.

b.i.d. Abbreviation for *bis in die*—twice a day; used in prescription writing.

bib. Abbreviation for *bibe*—drink; used in prescription writing.

BL Buccolingual.

BM Buccomesial.

BO Bucco-occlusal.

BP Buccopulpal.

B.P. British Pharmacopoeia; used in descriptions of drugs, to indicate the source of the formula in a prescription.

B.P.C. British Pharmaceutical Codex.

B.T.U.; B.Th.U. British thermal unit; a measurement of heat. May also be written *Btu*.

'B' point. Supramentale (*q.v.*).

Babbitt metal (I. Babbitt, 1799-1862. American inventor). An alloy sometimes used in dentistry; it contains copper, tin and antimony.

bacciform (*bak'-si-form*). Shaped like a berry.

Bacillaceae (*bas-il-a'-se-e*). A family of rod-shaped micro-organisms of the order Eubacteriales.

bacillary (*bas-il'-ar-ĭ*). Relating to or affected by a bacillus.

bacillicide (*bas-il'-is-īd*). Any agent used to destroy bacilli.

bacilliform (*bas-il'-i-form*). In the shape of a bacillus.

bacillus (*bas-il'-us*). A term used, loosely, to denote any rod-shaped micro-organism of the class Schizomycetes.

bacillus, Vignal's. Leptotrichia buccalis (*q.v.*).

Bacillus (*bas-il'-us*). A genus of the Bacillaceae family, Gram-positive and aerobic, seen as rod-shaped organisms.

backing (*bak'-ing*). *In dentistry:* The metal plate to which a porcelain tooth-facing is attached.

bacteraemia (*bak-ter-e'-mĭ-ă*). A condition characterized by the transient presence of bacteria in the bloodstream.

bacteria (*bak-te'-rĭ-ă*). Microscopic unicellular vegetable organisms; the fission fungi, or Schizomycetes.

Bacteriaceae (*bak-ter-i-a'-se-e*). A family of bacteria of the order Eubacteriales.

bacterial (*bak-te'-ri-al*). Relating to or characterized by bacteria.

bacterial endocarditis, sub-acute. A type of endocarditis caused by *Streptococcus viridans*, and having a prolonged course.

bacterial plaque. Dental plaque (*q.v.*, 1).

bactericide (*bak-ter'-is-īd*). Any agent used for the destruction of bacteria.

bacteriology (*bak-te-rĭ-ol-oj-ĭ*). The study of bacteria.

bacteriolysis (*bak-te-rĭ-ol'-is-is*). The destruction or disintegration of bacteria.

bacteriolytic (*bak-te-rĭ-o-lit'-ik*). Relating to bacteriolysis.

bacteriophage (*bak-te'-rĭ-o-fāj*). A micro-organism which attacks bacteria, sometimes resulting in their destruction.

bacteriostasis (*bak-te"-rĭ-o-sta'-sis*). The process of prevention or hindrance of growth of bacteria.

bacteriostat (*bak-te'-rĭ-o-stat*). Any agent which inhibits the growth and multiplication of bacteria, such as any of the sulphonamide group of drugs.

bacteriostatic (*bak-te"-rĭ-o-stat'-ik*). Relating to bacteriostasis.

bacteritic (*bak-ter-it'-ik*). Characterized or caused by bacteria.

Bacterium (*bak-te'-rĭ-um*). A genus of Bacteriaceae, Gram-negative, and seen as rod-shaped or ellipsoid organisms.

bacteroid (*bak-ter'-oyd*). Resembling bacteria.

Baelz's disease (E. von Baelz, 1845-1913. German physician). A disease characterized by the presence of painless papules on the labial mucous membrane.

bake (*bāk*). To harden by means of heat, as of dental porcelain.

balance (*bal'-ans*). 1. An apparatus used for weighing. 2. Equilibrium.

balanced occlusion. 1. The ideal interdigitation of the teeth, in which there is no cuspal interference in lateral excursions of the mandible. 2. In prosthetic dentistry, the simultaneous contact of all occlusal areas to prevent the tipping or rotating of the denture base.

balancing contacts. The contacts of the upper and lower teeth on the balancing side of a denture.

balancing side. The side away from which the mandible has moved, during mastication.

bald tongue. A clean, smooth tongue having no prominent papillae on its surface, seen in conditions such as vitamin B deficiency.

bald tongue, Sandwith's. *See* Sandwith's bald tongue.

band (*band*). 1. Any structure or appliance which binds. 2. In dentistry, a thin metal strip formed to encircle the crown or root of a natural tooth.
  adjustable b. A band which has some form of screw or mechanism whereby its size can be altered.
  all-closing b. A band encircling the whole of a tooth.
  anchor b. A band placed on one tooth to serve as

anchorage for the movement of another, in orthodontics.

clamp b. A band which is held in place by means of a screw and a nut.

contoured b. A band shaped to the tooth.

lip furrow b. Vestibular lamina (q.v.).

matrix b. Matrix (q.v., 3).

pier b. Any band constructed to fit an abutment tooth.

seamless b. A band stamped out from a metal tube, having no joins.

bandage (*band'-āj*). A strip of gauze, muslin, or other soft material, either in the form of a roll, or triangular, or tailed, bound round a part to hold dressings in place, to support or immobilize a part, or to apply pressure. For eponymous bandages *see* under the personal name by which the bandage is known.

band-driver (*band-dri'-ver*). An instrument used in orthodontics to seat a band over a tooth crown.

bands, Angle's fracture. See Angle's fracture bands.

bar (*bahr*). 1. A band or strip. 2. In dentistry, a metal rod or wire used either in prosthetics or orthodontics as part of an appliance. 3. That portion of the gums in the upper jaw of a horse which bears no teeth.

arch b. An orthodontic appliance consisting of a wire extending round the dental arch, to which the intervening teeth may be attached.

articulomachelian b. Embryonic cartilage from which the mandible develops.

labial b. A metal connector conforming to the labial mandibular arch and joining two parts of a lower partial denture.

lingual b. A metal bar fitted to the lingual arch of the lower jaw, and connecting two parts of a partial denture.

palatal b. A metal bar extending across the hard palate, connecting and strengthening two parts of an upper partial denture.

bar, Passavant's. See Passavant's bar.

bar clasp. A type of clasp in which the arms are a direct extension of the connector bars of the denture.

barb (*bahrb*). A fine backward-projecting point on a dental instrument, preventing its withdrawal.

barodontalgia (*bar-o-dont-al'-ji-ă*). Pain in the teeth experienced as a result of high-altitude flying; aerodontalgia.

barrel (*bar'-el*). 1. The band of a metal tooth crown. 2. The reservoir of a hypodermic or other syringe.

bartholinitis (*bahr″-thol-in-i'-tis*). Inflammation affecting Bartholin's duct.

Bartholin's duct (C. Bartholin, 1655-1738. Danish

anatomist). The larger of the sublingual ducts.

Barton's bandage (J. R. Barton, 1794-1871. American surgeon). A figure-of-eight bandage used in fracture of the mandible.

basal (*ba'-sal*). Relating to a base.

basal bone. The bone tissue of the mandible and maxillae, with the exception of their alveolar processes.

basal layer, Weil's. *See* Weil's basal layer.

basal ridge. Cingulum (*q.v.*).

basal seat. The tissue area on which the denture base rests.

basal vein. Formed by the union of the anterior cerebral, and deep middle cerebral veins. *See* Table of Veins—basalis.

basal-cell carcinoma. Locally malignant carcinoma developing from the basal-cell layer of the epithelium and retaining its characteristics.

base (*bās*). *In dentistry:* That part of a denture which rests on the alveolar ridges, and which may extend over the palate, and to which the artificial teeth are attached.

base plane. An imaginary plane used to estimate the retention in the construction of artificial dentures.

base plate. Base (*q.v.*).

basialveolar line (*ba''-si-al-ve-o'-lar*). In craniometry, the line joining the basion and the alveolar point.

basicranial (*ba''-si-kra'-ni-al*) Relating to the base of the skull.

basifacial (*ba''-si-fa'-shi-al*). Relating to the lower part of the face.

basilar (*bas'-il-ar*). Relating to the base.

basilar artery. Supplies cerebellum and cerebrum. *See* Table of Arteries—basilaris.

basilar pit. A pit in the crown of a maxillary incisor above the cervix.

basilar plexus. A venous plexus into which drain the inferior petrosal sinuses. *See* Table of Veins—plexus basilaris.

basilomental (*bas-il''-o-men'-tal*). Relating to the base of the skull and the chin.

basilosubnasal (*bas''-il-o-sub-na'-zal*). Basinasal (*q.v.*)

basinasal (*ba''-si-na'-zal*). Relating to the basion and the nasion.

basinasal line. In craniometry, a line from the basion to the nasion.

basioccipital (*ba''-si-ok-sip'-it-al*). Relating to the basilar part of the occipital bone.

basitemporal (*ba''-si-tem'-por-al*). Relating to the lower part of the temporal bone.

basion (*ba'-si-on*). The central point of the anterior edge of the foramen magnum.

basket crown. A form of three-quarter crown, with an acrylic facing, used as a semi-permanent restoration for a fractured incisor in a school-child.

batrachoplasty (*bat-rak-o-plast'-ĭ*). Plastic surgery in the cure of ranula.

Bazin's disease (A. P. E. Bazin, 1807-78. French physician). Leukoplakia (buccalis) (*q.v.*).

beak (*bēk*). The projecting jaws of pliers or forceps.

Bean crown. Split-dowel crown (*q.v.*).

Béchard's triangle (P. A. Béchard, 1785-1825. French anatomist). The area comprised within the posterior border of the hyoglossus muscle, the greater cornu of the hyoid bone and the posterior belly of the dygastric muscle.

Bechterew. *See* Bekhterev.

Bednar's aphthae (A. Bednar, 1816-88. Austrian physician). Two ulcers appearing symmetrically one on either side of the midline of the hard palate in cachetic infants.

Beers' crown (J. B. Beers, fl. 1873). Morrison crown (*q.v.*).

Bekhterev's reflex (V. M. Bekhterev, 1857-1927. Russian neurologist). Irritation of the mucosa on one side of the nasal cavity producing facial contraction on the same side.

bell-crown. A crown of a tooth in which the diameter, mesiodistally, is much greater at the occlusal surface than at the cervix.

Bell's palsy (Sir C. Bell, 1774-1842. Scottish physiologist). Peripheral facial paralysis.

belly (*bel'-ĭ*) *of a muscle*. The bulging, fleshy part of a muscle.

benign (*ben-īn'*). Not malignant or recurrent; not endangering life or health.

Bennett angle (Sir N. G. Bennett, 1870-1947. British dentist). The angle, during lateral movement of the mandible, between the sagittal plane and the path of the condyle.

Bennett movement (Sir N. G. Bennett, 1870-1947. British dentist). The movement of the mandible to left or right during mastication.

Berry-Franceschetti syndrome (Sir G. A. Berry, 1853-1940. English ophthalmologist; A. Franceschetti, b. 1896). Mandibulo-facial dysostosis (*q.v.*).

bevel (*bev'-el*). 1. An outward inclination cut or ground on any surface. 2. The outward inclination of the enamel edges of a prepared tooth cavity. 3. The act of making such an inclination.

bi-. Prefix signifying *two*, or *twice*.

bibe (*bī'-bĕ*). Latin for *drink*; used in prescription writing, and abbreviated *bib*.

bibeveled (*bi-bev'-eld*). Be ing beveled on two sides.

bicameral abscess. An abscess containing two pockets.

Bichat's fossa (M. F. X. Bichat, 1771-1802. French anatomist). Pterygomaxillary fossa (q.v.).

Bickel's ring (G. Bickel, fl. 19th century. German physician). The area of lymphoid tissue comprised by the pharyngeal and lingual tonsils and the lymphoid tissue of the soft palate.

biconcave (bi-kon'-kāv). Having two concave surfaces.

biconvex (bi-kon'-veks). Having two convex surfaces.

bicuspid (bi-kus'-pid). 1. Having two cusps. 2. A premolar tooth.

bicuspidal, bicuspidate (bi-kus'-pid-al; bi-kus'-pid-āt). Having two cusps.

bidental, bidentate (bi-den'-tal; bi-den'-tāt). Having, or affecting, two teeth.

bifid (bi'-fid). Split into two branches, or parts.

bifid tongue. A tongue which is split into two down the midline from its tip.

biforate (bi-for'-āt). Having two openings or foramina.

bifurcate (bi-fur'-kāt). Forked, as the roots of molar or other teeth.

bifurcation (bi-fur-ka'-shun). Division into two branches, as of tooth roots.

bihora (bi-or'-ă). Latin for *two hours*; used in prescription writing.

bilateral (bi-lat'-er-al). Occurring on, or relating to, two sides.

biligulate (bi-lig'-yu-lāt). Resembling two tongues;

having two tongue-like processes.

bilophodont (bi-lof'-o-dont). Having teeth with two transverse ridges forming the crown.

bimaxillary (bi-maks-il'-ar-i). Relating to both jaws.

binangle (bi-nan'-gl). *Of an instrument:* Having two angles in the shank.

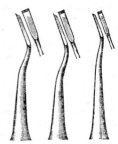

Binangle instruments

binary (bi'-nar-i). 1. *In chemistry:* Composed of two elements. 2. *In anatomy:* Divided into two branches or parts. 3. *In mathematics:* To the base 2; i.e. a number system based on 0 and 1. This is used especially with digital computers.

binary amalgam. An amalgam containing mercury and one other metal.

Bing bridge (B. J. Bing, fl. 1865. American dentist). A bridge for a single tooth, attached to the adjoining teeth.

bio-. Prefix signifying *life*.

biochemistry (*bi''-o-kem'-ist-ri*). The chemistry of living organisms.

biological chemistry. Biochemistry (*q.v.*)

biometrics, biometry (*bi-o-met'-riks*). The application of statistical methods to biological sciences.

bio-occlusion (*bi''-o-ok-lu'-zhun*). Normal occlusion.

bioplasis (*bi-o-pla'-sis*). Anabolism (*q.v.*).

biopsy (*bi-op'-si*). Microscopic examination of tissue from a living body, generally for purposes of diagnosis.

bis in die (*bis in de'-a*). Latin for *twice a day*; used in prescription writing, and abbreviated *b.i.d. Also* written as *bis die*, abbreviated *b.d.*

biscuit (*bis'-kit*). Porcelain after it has been baked once, but before it has been glazed.

bisect (*bi-sekt'*). To divide into two parts by cutting.

bistoury (*bis'-tu-ri*). A long, narrow surgical knife, which may be either straight or curved.

bite (*bit*). 1. To grasp or to cut anything with the teeth. 2. An impression, in some plastic material, of the teeth or the gums in occlusion, to show their relationship; used for making artificial dentures. 3. A skin wound made by the teeth, especially those of insects.
check b. An impression taken in hard wax or in modelling compound to record the various occlusal positions of the teeth in the mouth, and used to check these positions in artificial dentures in an articulator.
close-b. A form of malocclusion in which there is abnormally deep overlap of the incisors when the jaws are closed.
counter-b. The bite which opposes that taken of the teeth in one jaw.
cross b. A form of malocclusion caused by an abnormality of the lateral relationship of the jaws to each other, thus preventing normal occlusion.
edge-to-edge b. A form of malocclusion in which the anterior teeth occlude along the incisal edges and do not overlap.
end to end b. Edge-to-edge bite (*q.v.*).
jumping the b. The forcible movement forward of a retruded mandible to obtain normal occlusion.
locked b. Interlocking of the teeth in occlusion so that lateral movement of the mandible is restricted or prevented.
mush b. Squash bite (*q.v.*).
open b. See open-bite.
over b. See overbite.
rest b. See restbite.
squash b. A bite taken to register the relationship of the cusps of the upper and lower teeth, but not to give any clear reproduction of the teeth.

underhung b. A form of malocclusion in which the mandibular anterior teeth occlude with the labial surfaces of their maxillary antagonists.

bite block. Occlusal rim (*q.v.*).

bite gauge. An instrument designed to aid in the establishment of a correct bite in dentistry.

bite lock. A device which can be attached to the bite rims of a denture to retain them in the same position out of the mouth as they occupied in it.

bite plane. 1. Occlusal plane (*q.v.*). 2. Bite plate (*q.v.*, 2).

bite plate. 1. A temporary base plate of rigid material, carrying a rim of wax or plastic (occlusal rim) on which the bite is recorded. 2. An orthodontic appliance designed to correct an abnormal bite by interposing a ledge of metal, vulcanite or acrylic behind the maxillary incisors, on which the mandibular incisors strike. Where the ledge is sloped and not flat this appliance is known as a *bite plane.*

bite rim. Occlusal rim (*q.v.*).

bitewing (*bit'-wing*). A form of individual *x*-ray film, held in place in the mouth by a central wing on which the teeth can close. It shows the crowns of both the upper and lower teeth on one film.

bizygomatic (*bi"-zi-go-mat'-ik*). Relating to the most

prominent point on either zygomatic arch.

black tongue. Black patches of pigmentation on the tongue, composed of hypertrophied filiform papillae and micro-organisms.

Black's amalgam (G. V. Black, 1836-1915. American dentist). A quaternary amalgam (*q.v.*).

Black's classification of cavities (G. V. Black, 1836-1915. American dentist).

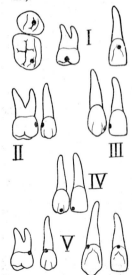

Black classification

Class 1. Cavities beginning in structural defects in the teeth; pits and fissures. These are located in the occlusal surfaces of the bicuspids and molars, in the occlusal two-thirds of the buccal surfaces of the molars, in the lingual surfaces of the upper incisors, and occasionally in the lingual surfaces of the upper molars.

Class 2. Cavities in the proximal surfaces of bicuspids and molars.

Class 3. Cavities in the proximal surfaces of the incisors and cuspids which do not involve the removal and restoration of the incisal angle.

Class 4. Cavities in the proximal surfaces of the incisors and cuspids which do require the removal and restoration of the incisal angle.

Class 5. Cavities in the gingival third—not pit cavities—of the labial, buccal or lingual surfaces of the teeth.

Black's crown (G. V. Black, 1836-1915. American dentist). A porcelain-faced crown for an anterior tooth, attached by a threaded post screwing into a gold-lined root canal.

blade (*blād*). The cutting portion of a knife or a pair of scissors.

bland (*bland*). 1. Mild. 2. Soothing.

Blandin's gland (P. F. Blandin, 1798-1849. French surgeon). A mixed salivary gland near the tip of the tongue, on its under surface. *Also called* Nuhn's gland.

Blandin's operation (P. F. Blandin, 1798-1849. French surgeon). An operation for the correction of double harelip by excision of a triangular wedge from the vomer, with reduction of the projecting maxillary process.

blank (*blank*). In orthodontics, a short, slightly curved strip of metal used in banding.

Blasius' duct (G. Blasius, *or* Blaes, 1626 (?)-82. Dutch anatomist). Stensen's duct (*q.v.*).

blastoma (*blast-o'-mă*). A true tumour, exhibiting independent localized growth.

bleach (*blētch*). 1. To whiten by means of chemicals; discoloured teeth may be so treated. 2. Any agent used for this purpose.

bleb (*bleb*). A bulla or other skin blister filled with blood or serous fluid.

bleeding (*ble'-ding*). Haemorrhage (*q.v.*).

blennoid (*blen'-oyd*). Mucuslike.

blennostasis (*blen-os'-tas-is*). Suppression of excessive mucous discharge.

blepharal (*blef'-ar-al*). Relating to the eyelid.

blepharon (*blef'-ar-on*). The eyelid.

blind abscess. An abscess having no fistulous opening.

blind fistula. A fistula which has an opening at one end only; a *sinus* (*q.v.*, 4).

blister (*blis'-ter*). A vesicle caused by a localized accumulation of fluid beneath the skin.

block (*blok*). 1. A stoppage or obstruction. 2. A solid mass of material.

anaesthetic b. 1. The injection of an anaesthetic agent into or around a major nerve. 2. The interruption of the nerve supply to an area because of trauma or a pathological lesion.

block anaesthesia. Anaesthetic block (*q.v.*, 1).

blood (*blŭd*). The red fluid in the vessels of the circulatory system, which conveys oxygen and nutritive material to the tissues and removes carbon dioxide and waste matter.

blood poisoning. Septicaemia (*q.v.*).

blood pressure. The pressure exerted by the blood on the artery walls, dependent on the force of the heart action, the elasticity of the vessel walls, capillary resistance, and the volume and viscosity of the blood.

blood vessel. Any of the tubes which carries blood through the body.

blue line. Lead line (*q.v.*)

blunderbuss canal (*blun'-der-bus*). Term used to describe an incompletely formed root having the apical third of the root canal wider in diameter than the upper part.

Bochdalek's ganglion (V. A. Bochdalek, 1801-83. Austrian anatomist). The ganglion situated in the maxilla, and formed by the junction of the middle and superior dental nerves.

Bock's pharyngeal nerve (A. C. Bock, 1782-1833. German anatomist and surgeon). The pterygopalatine or pharyngeal branch of Meckel's ganglion.

Bodecker's index. The ratio between the number of tooth surfaces affected by caries, and the total number of surfaces which might be so affected.

Bohn's epithelial pearls, Bohn's nodules. Epstein's pearls (*q.v.*).

boil (*boyl*). A localized skin abscess, usually at the site of a hair follicle.

Boley gauge. A finely calibrated instrument used for intra-oral measurements.

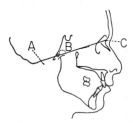

Bolton plane

A Bolton point.
B Bolton plane.
C Nasion.

Bolton plane, Bolton-Broadbent plane (C. B. Bolton, sponsor; B. H. Broadbent, contemporary American orthodontist). The imaginary plane marking the division between the face and the skull, lying about a line from the Bolton point (q.v.) to the nasion.

Bolton point (C. B. Bolton, who, with Mrs. C. C. Bolton, his mother, sponsored the research work of B. H. Broadbent which resulted in the designation of this point). The deepest point on the postcondylar notch of the occipital bone, seen on a lateral radiograph and marking the height of the curvature.

bolus (bo'-lus). 1. A rounded mass of food ready to be swallowed. 2. A large, rounded pill.

bone (bōn). 1. The material of the skeleton of most vertebrates, consisting of connective tissue containing ossein and impregnated with calcium salts. 2. Any separate part of the skeleton; see under the names of the individual bones for those of the skull.

basal b. The bone tissue of the mandible and maxillae, with the exception of their alveolar processes.

bone, Albrecht's. See Albrecht's bone.

bone, Eysson's. See Eysson's bone.

bone, Goethe's. See Goethe's bone.

bone fibres. Sharpey's fibres (q.v.).

bone marrow. See marrow.

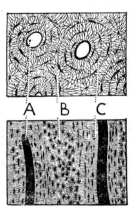

Bone

A Haversian canal.
B Bone cell between interstitial lamellae.
C Bone cell.

Bonwill crown (W. G. A. Bonwill, 1833-99. American dentist). A porcelain crown attached to the tooth root by a threaded post, and held in position by amalgam.

Bonwill triangle (W. G. A. Bonwill, 1833-99. American dentist). The adaptation and measurement of the mandible and mandibular arch as an equilateral triangle, with angles at the centre of each condyle and at the mesial contact area of the mandibular central incisors.

bony (*bo'-ni*). Relating to or resembling bone.

bony ankylosis. Complete joint fixation through bone fusion.

bony palate. Hard palate (*q.v.*).

border (*bor'-der*). An edge or boundary round an organ or tissue mass.
vermilion b. The red margin of the lips.

border moulding. The shaping of impression material, either by hand or by tissue action, to the outline adjacent to the edges of the impression.

border seal. The fit of a denture border with the adjacent tissues so that nothing can pass between.

boss (*bos*). A rounded, knob-like prominence on the surface of a bone or a tumour.

Bowen's disease of the mouth (J. T. Bowen, 1857-1941. American dermatologist). A skin disease affecting the oral mucosa and characterized by reddish papules covered by a thick keratinized layer.

boxed cast. An impression cast in a box or cup which has been built up round it of strips of soft metal or of wax, thus providing a cast which needs little trimming and which can be well vibrated.

boxing (*boks'-ing*) *of an impression.* The process of building up walls round an impression to produce a cast of the desired size and form, and to preserve the principal landmarks of the impression.

brachiocephalic trunk. The blood supply for the right upper limb, and the right side of the head and neck. *Also called* the innominate artery. *See* Table of Arteries—truncus brachiocephalicus.

brachiocephalic vein. The vein found in the median portion of the root of the neck, deep to the sternocleidomastoid muscle, and draining into the superior vena cava. *See* Table of Veins—brachiocephalica.

brachiofaciolingual (*brak''-i-o-fa''-shi-o-lin'-gwal*). Relating to or affecting the arm, the face and the tongue.

brachy-. Prefix signifying *short*.

brachycephalic (*brak-i-sef-al'-ik*). Having an abnormally short head.

brachycheilia (*brak''-i-ki'-li-ă*). Shortness of the lip or lips; *also called* microcheilia.

brachyfacial (*brak-i-fa'-shi-al*). Having an abnormally short and broad face.

brachyglossal (*brak-i-glos'-al*). Having an abnormally short tongue.

brachygnathia (*brak-ig-na'-thi-ă*). Abnormal shortness of the mandible.

brachygnathous (*brak-ig-na'-thus*). Having an abnormally small jaw.

brachyodont (*brak'-ĭ-o-dont*). Having teeth with short crowns and long roots.

brachyprosopic (*brak"-ĭ-pro-sop'-ik*). Having an abnormally short face.

brachypyrosopic (*brak-ĭ-pi-ro-sop'-ik*). Brachyfacial (*q.v.*).

brachyrhinia (*brak"-ĭ-ri'-nĭ-ă*). Abnormal shortness of the nose.

brachyrhynchus (*brak"-ĭ-rin'-kus*). Abnormal shortness of both the nose and the maxilla.

brachystaphyline (*brak"-ĭ-staf"-il-in*). Having an abnormally short alveolar arch or palate.

brachyuranic (*brak"-ĭ-yuran'-ik*). Having an abnormally short and wide palate, with a palatomaxillary index above 115.

bracket (*brak'-et*). A type of downward-facing hook or clip on an orthodontic tooth band, used to attach ribbon arch-wire to banded teeth.

Brackett's probes (C. A. Brackett, 1850-1927. American dentist). Delicate, flexible probes, made of silver wire, used to explore fistulae of alveolar abscesses.

brady-. Prefix signifying *slow*.

bradyglossia (*brad"-ĭ-glos'-ĭ-ă*). Abnormal slowness of speech, due to difficulty in tongue movement.

bradylalia (*brad"-ĭ-lal'-ĭ-ă*). Slowness of speech, due to a central lesion.

brain (*brān*). That part of the central nervous system within the cranium of vertebrates.

branch (*bransh*). An offshoot from the main trunk or stem, as of blood vessels or nerves.

brass (*brahs*). An alloy of copper and zinc.

breathing (*bre'-īthing*). Respiration (*q.v.*).

bregma (*breg'-mă*). The junction of the coronal and sagittal sutures; the site of the anterior fontanel.

bridge (*bridj*). *In dentistry*: An appliance, attached to remaining natural teeth, designed to restore aesthetics and function where teeth have been removed or failed to erupt.
   arch b. Fixed bridge (*q.v.*).
   cantilever b. A bridge of which one end only is attached to an abutment and the other is seated on the alveolar ridge.
   dentine b. A layer of dentine which reseals an exposed pulp or forms over the excised surface after pulpotomy.
   extension b. A dental bridge having a free pontic attached at one end beyond the point of anchorage.
   fixed b. A dental bridge which is fixed in place permanently to its abutments.
   removable b. A dental bridge which can be removed

by the wearer for cleaning or other purposes.

span b. Fixed bridge (*q.v.*).

bridge of the nose. The bridge formed at the junction of the two nasal bones; the upper part of the nose.

broach (*brōtch*). A fine tapered instrument, either smooth or barbed, used to remove tooth pulp in the treatment of infected root canals, and as a reamer to enlarge root canals.

watchmaker's b. A tapered broach, sharp-angled and having four or five sides, used to enlarge root canals.

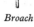

Broach

broach, Donaldson's. *See* Donaldson's broach.

bromopnoea (*bro"-mop-ne'-ă*). Foetid breath.

bronchospasm (*bron-ko'-spazm*). Spasmodic contraction of the bronchial tubes.

Brophy's operation (T. W. Brophy, 1848-1928. American surgeon). An operation for the closure of cleft palate by means of wire tension sutures held in place by lead plates, drawing the edges of the cleft together.

Brown crown (E. P. Brown, 1844-1916. American dentist). A porcelain crown with a convex base, into which is baked a platinum post for attachment to the tooth root.

brown pellicle. Acquired pellicle (*q.v.*).

bruise (*brūz*). A superficial injury caused by a blow, and producing discoloration of the skin and subcutaneous tissue.

bruxism (*bruks'-izm*). Grinding or gnashing of the teeth during sleep.

bruxomania (*bruks-o-ma'-ni-ă*). A nervous disorder characterized by grinding of the teeth.

brycomania (*bri-ko-ma'-ni-ă*). Insane tooth-grinding.

brygmus (*brig'-mus*). Grinding of the teeth.

bucca (*buk'-ă*). The cheek, especially the inner side in the mouth.

buccal (*buk'-al*). Relating to the cheek.

buccal angle. Any angle formed by the junction of a buccal tooth surface or a cavity wall, in a posterior tooth with any other tooth surface or cavity wall.

buccal artery. Supplies buccinator muscle, buccal mucous membrane and skin of cheek. *Also called* buccinator artery. *See* Table of Arteries—buccalis.

buccal embrasure. The space between molars or premolars, opening towards the cheek.

buccal glands. The mixed salivary glands of the buccal mucosa.

buccal hiatus. A transverse facial cleft.

buccal involution. The inward folding of the ectoderm in the embryo which forms the stomodeum.

buccal nerve. The sensory fibres of the buccinator nerve, supplying the skin and mucous membrane of the cheek. *See* Table of Nerves—buccalis.

buccal raphe. The line marking the union of those parts of the cheek derived from the maxillary process with those derived from the mandibular process.

buccal wall. That wall of a tooth cavity which faces the buccal surface of the tooth.

buccellation (buk-sel-a'-shun). The arrest of bleeding by means of a lint pad.

buccilingual (buk"-sĭ-lin'-gwal). Relating to the cheek and the tongue.

buccinator (buk'-sin-a-tor). 1. The cheek muscle. *See*

Table of Muscles. 2. The artery supplying the buccal mucosa, the skin of the cheek, and the buccinator muscle. *See* Table of Arteries —buccalis. 3. The nerve supplying the buccinator muscle. *See* Table of Nerves. *Sensory* fibres are called *buccalis.*

bucco-. Prefix signifying *cheek.*

buccoaxial (buk"-o-aks'-ĭ-al). Relating to the buccal and axial walls in the mesial or distal portion of a proximoocclusal cavity in a molar or premolar.

b. angle. The angle formed at the junction of these walls; a *line* angle.

buccoaxiocervical (buk"-o-aks"-ĭ-o-ser-vi'-kal). Gingivobuccoaxial (q.v.).

buccoaxiogingival (buk"-o-aks"-ĭ-o-jin'-jiv-al). Gingivobuccoaxial (q.v.).

buccobranchial (buk-o-bran'-ki-al). Buccopharyngeal (q.v.).

buccocclusal (buk-ok-lu'-zal). Bucco-occlusal (q.v.).

buccocervical (buk"-o-ser-vi'-kal). 1. Buccogingival (q.v.). 2. Relating to the cheek and the neck.

buccocervical ridge. A ridge on the buccal surface of a deciduous molar near to the cervix of the tooth.

buccodistal (buk"-o-dis'-tal). 1. Relating to the buccal and distal surfaces of a tooth. 2. Relating to the buccal and distal walls in the step portion of a proximo-occlusal cavity in a molar or pre-molar.

b. angle. The angle formed at the junction of these walls; *a line angle.*

buccofacial (*buk″-o-fa′-shĭ-al*). Relating to the cheek and the face.

buccofacial obturator. An appliance used to close an opening through the cheek into the mouth.

buccogingival (*buk″-o-jin′-jiv-al*). 1. Relating to the cheek and the gums. 2. Relating to the buccal and gingival walls in the mesial or distal portion of a proximo-occlusal cavity in a molar or premolar.

b. angle. The angle formed at the junction of these walls; *a line angle.*

buccogingival ridge. Bucco-cervical ridge (*q.v.*).

buccoglossopharyngitis sicca (*buk″-o-glos″-o-far-in-ji′-tis*). Inflammation and dryness of the buccal and pharyngeal mucous membranes and of the tongue. Part of a syndrome complex known as *Sjögren's syndrome.*

buccolabial (*buk″-o-la′-bĭ-al*). Relating to the cheek and the lip.

buccolingual (*buk″-o-lin′-gwal*). Relating to the buccal and lingual surfaces of a tooth.

buccolingual plane. Any plane passing through both the buccal and lingual surfaces of a tooth.

buccomaxillary (*buk″-o-maks-il′-ar-ĭ*). 1. Relating to

the cheek and the maxilla. 2. Relating to the buccal cavity and the maxillary sinus.

buccomesial (*buk″-o-me′-zĭ-al*). Relating to the buccal and mesial surfaces of a molar or premolar, or to the buccal and mesial walls in the step portion of a proximo-occlusal cavity.

b. angle. The angle formed at the junction of these walls; *a line angle.*

bucconasal (*buk″-o-na′-zal*). Relating to the cheek and the nose.

bucconasopharyngeal (*buk″-o-na″-zo-far-in′-jĕ-al*). Relating to the cheek, the nose, and the pharynx.

bucco-occlusal (*buk″-o-ok-lu′-zal*). Relating to the buccal and occlusal surfaces of a molar or premolar tooth, or to the corresponding walls of a cavity.

buccopharyngeal (*buk″-o-far-in′-jĕ-al*). Relating to the cheek and the pharynx.

buccopharyngeal membrane. That area of the primitive embryo which later develops into the mouth and the pharynx.

buccopharyngeal muscle. Part of constrictor pharyngis superior. *See* Table of Muscles—buccopharyngeus.

buccoplacement (*buk″-o-pla′-sment*). Displacement of a tooth buccally.

buccopulpal (*buk″-o-pul′-pal*). Relating to the buccal and pulpal walls in an occlusal cavity, or in the step portion

of a proximo-occlusal cavity in a molar or premolar.
b. angle. The angle formed at the junction of these walls; a *line* angle.

buccoversion (*buk-o-ver'-shun*). The position of a tooth which is inclined outwards towards the cheek.

buccula (*buk'-yu-lă*). The fleshy fold which forms a ' double chin '.

bud (*bud*). 1. A knob-like structure, the early stage in the growth of any plant, leaf or branch. 2. Any small anatomic structure resembling a bud.

bulboid (*bul'-boyd*). Shaped like a bulb.

bulbous (*bul'-bus*). Resembling a bulb in either shape or nature; arising from or producing a bulb.

bulla (*bul'-ă*) (*pl.* bullae). A large vesicle.

bullous (*bul'-us*). Relating to or characterized by bullae.

bunodont (*bu'-no-dont*). Having rounded cusps or cones on the molar teeth.

bunolophodont (*bu''-no-lo'-fo-dont*). A paleontological term for teeth having rounded crests.

bunoselenodont (*bu''-no-sel-e'-no-dont*). A paleontological term for teeth having longitudinal rounded crests.

bur (*bur*). A rotary cutting instrument used in a dental handpiece for the preparation of cavities and the trimming of restorations.

burn (*burn*). The injury resulting from the application of excessive heat, electric current, friction, or caustics to the skin or mucous membrane.

Bur

burnish (*bur'-nish*). To smooth or polish by friction either to obtain a high gloss or to secure the adaptation of two corresponding substances at a join.

burnisher (*bur'-nish-er*). An instrument used to finish and to polish fillings, crowns, or dentures.

bursa, Fleischmann's, See Fleischmann's bursa.

Burton's line (H. Burton, 1799-1849. British physician). Lead line (*q.v.*).

Buttner crown. A porcelain-faced shell crown attached to the root by a post and a metal band.

C

c. Abbreviation for *cum*—with: used in prescription writing.

C. Abbreviation for *canine*, in the permanent dentition.

C Cervical.

C Chemical symbol for carbon.

CA 1. Cervicoaxial. 2. Chronological age.

Ca Chemical symbol for calcium.

cap. Abbreviation for *capsula*— a capsule; used in prescription writing.

cc. Abbreviation for *cubic centimetres*.

CLA Cervicolinguoaxial.

cm. Abbreviation for *centimetre*.

Cr Chemical symbol for chromium.

Cu Chemical symbol for copper.

cable (*ka'-bl*). The flexible arm of a dental engine, which transmits power to the instrument to be used.

cachectic (*kak-ek'-tik*). Relating to cachexia.

cachet (*kash'-a*). A hollow capsule of rice paper enclosing a dose of some unpleasant medicine.

cachexia (*kak-eks'-ĭ-ă*). Generalized state of ill health due to some constitutional disorder.

cachou (*kash-u'*). A tablet or pill for deodorizing or scenting the breath.

caco-. Prefix signifying *bad, diseased*.

cacodontia (*kak-o-don'-shĭ-ă*). Any condition characterized by diseased teeth.

cacogeusia (*kak-o-gu'-sĭ-ă*). A bad taste.

cacoglossia (*kak-o-glos'-ĭ-ă*). The condition of having a diseased or gangrenous tongue.

cacostomia (*kak-o-sto'-mĭ-ă*). Any diseased condition of the mouth.

caecal (*se'-kal*). 1. Relating to a blind tube or passage. 2. Relating to the caecum.

caecal foramen *of the tongue*. A depression above the root and dorsum of the tongue, the site of the former opening of the thyroglossal duct.

caecum (se'-kum). 1. Any blind pouch, tube, or passage. 2. The blind dilated pouch which is the beginning of the large intestine.

calcareous (*kal-ka'-rĕ-us*). Relating to or containing calcium or calcium salts; chalky.

calcareous degeneration. Degeneration accompanied by deposit of calcareous material in the degenerate tissue.

calcific (*kal-sif'-ik*). Lime-forming.

calcification (*kal-sif-ik-a'-shun*). The deposition in organic tissue of calcium salts, causing hardening.

calcification lines. Retzius' lines (*q.v.*).

calcified (*kal'-sif-īd*). Hardened by the deposition of calcium salts.

calcination (*kal-sin-a'-shun*). The reduction of a substance to powder, or the removal of volatile constituents from a compound by heat.

calcine (*kal-sīn'*). To reduce to powder, roast, or dry, by heat.

calcinosis (*kal-sin-o'-sis*). A condition characterized by either localized or general depositions of calcium salts in nodules in the soft tissues.

calcium (*kal'-si-um*). A bivalent metal, symbol Ca, the basic component of lime, and occurring in almost all organic tissue.

calcular (*kal'-kyu-lar*). Relating to calculus.

calculous (*kal'-kyu-lus*). Relating to or resembling a calculus.

calculus (*kal'-kyu-lus*) (*pl.* calculi). An abnormal concretion occurring in the body, generally in the urinary system, bile duct, gall bladder, or salivary glands; it usually contains calcium salts.

dental c. A deposit of calcium salts in an organic matrix attached to the teeth.

salivary. c. 1. An abnormal concretion occuring in a salivary gland or duct. 2. Supragingival calculus (*q.v.*).

serumal, seruminal c. Subgingival calculus (*q.v.*).

subgingival c. Dental calculus attached to the tooth within the gingival pocket.

supragingival c. Dental calculus attached to the tooth above the gingival margin.

Caldwell-Luc operation (G. W. Caldwell, 1866-1946. American surgeon; H. Luc, 1855-1925. French laryngologist). An operation for the relief of severe infection of the maxillary sinus by creating an opening into the supradental fossa.

calibration (*kal-ib-ra'-shun*). 1. The measurement of the diameter of a canal or tube. 2. The marking of graduations on a measuring instrument, from a given standard.

calipers (*kal'-ip-ers*). An instrument, similar to a pair of compasses, having curved legs, and used to measure diameters of cylindrical bodies.

Callahan's method (J. R. Callahan, 1853-1918. American dentist). A method of root canal cleansing in which the application of sulphuric acid is used to aid in opening the canal and in the destruction of putrescent pulp.

calvaria, calvarium (*kal-va'-ri-ă*; *kal-va'-ri-um*). The bony skull cap or cranium.

camera (*kam'-er-ă*). A box or chamber, especially the equipment used to take photographs.

camera pulp. The pulp chamber of a tooth.

Camper's angle (P. Camper, 1722-89. Dutch anatomist). Maxillary angle (*q.v.*).

Camper's line (P. Camper, 1722-89. Dutch anatomist). A line extending from the external auditory meatus to a point below the nasal spine.

Camper's plane (P. Camper, 1722-89. Dutch anatomist). A horizontal plane passing through the tragale and sub-nasale on either side of the face, and usually parallel with occlusal plane.

campylognathia (*kam-pil-o-na'-thi-ă*). Malformation of the jaw or lip in a rabbit-like appearance.

canal (*kan-al'*). Any channel or duct which affords a passage, usually through bone.

alveolar c's. Dental canals (*q.v.*).

alveolodental c. An old term for a dental canal (*q.v.*).

auditory c., internal. The internal auditory meatus (*q.v.*).

blunderbuss c. Term used to describe an incompletely formed root having the apical third of the root canal wider in diameter than the upper part.

carotid c. A passage in the petrous portion of the temporal bone, through which passes the internal carotid artery.

circulatory c. Nutrient canal (*q.v.*).

condylar c.; *condyloid c.*

   anterior: A passage for the hypoglossal nerve through the occipital bone; *also called* the hypoglossal canal.

   posterior: An occasional canal in the floor of the condylar fossa, through which passes a vein from the transverse sinus.

dental c's. Any of the canals in the maxilla or in the mandible which afford passage to the vessels or

nerves supplying the teeth. The *superior* dental canals are those in the maxilla, and the *inferior* dental canals are those in the mandible.

dentinal c. Dentinal tubule (*q.v.*).

ethmoid c's. Canals between the ethmoid and frontal bones, through which pass the posterior ethmoid and the nasociliary nerves and the ethmoid vessels.

facial c. A canal extending from the petrous portion of the temporal bone to the stylo-mastoid foramen, through which passes the facial nerve.

hypoglossal c. The anterior condylar canal (*q.v.*).

incisive c. A canal in the maxilla leading from the incisive fossa to the floor of the nasal cavity.

infraorbital c. One of the passages from the infra-orbital grooves to the infra-orbital foramen in the maxilla, through which pass the infraorbital arteries and nerves.

interdental c. Nutrient canal (*q.v.*).

mandibular c. The inferior dental canal (*q.v.*).

maxillary c. The superior dental canal (*q.v.*).

nasolacrimal c. The canal in which runs the naso-lacrimal duct.

nasopalatine c. One of the passages from the nasal cavity to the palate, normally occluded in man.

nutrient c. One of the tubular

canals or grooves occurring in the alveolar bone structure of the maxilla and of the mandible, through which pass anastomosing blood vessels.

palatine c. greater, or anterior: The canal running from the pterygopalatine fossa to the greater palatine foramen, in the side wall of the nasal cavity, between the maxilla and the palatine bone, through which pass the greater palatine artery and nerve. *lesser, or posterior:* One of the branches of the greater palatine canal conveying branches of the greater palatine vessels to the tissues of the soft palate. *pterygopalatine c.* The posterior palatine canal (*q.v.*). *pulp c.* Root canal (*q.v.*). *root c.* The canal, containing dental pulp, running through the root of the tooth to the pulp chamber. *zygomatico-orbital c.* A passage through the orbital process of the zygoma, through which pass the facial and temporal branches of the zygomatic nerve.

canal, Hirschfeld. Nutrient canal (*q.v.*).

canaliculus (*kan-al-ik'-yu-lus*). A minute canal.

canaliculus dentalis. One of the minute canals carrying the processes of the cemento-blasts to developing cementum.

canalis pterygoidei, nerve. See Table of Nerves.

cancellous (*kan'-sel-us*). Having a lattice-like, spongy structure; applied to bone tissue.

cancer (*kan'-ser*). Any malignant form of tumour; a lay term.

cancrum (*kan'-krum*). A gangrenous ulcer.

cancrum nasi. Gangrene of the nasal mucous membrane.

cancrum oris. Noma; gangrene of the mouth.

Candida (*kan'-did-ă*). A genus of yeast-like, pathogenic bacterial fungi; also called *Monilia*.
C. albicans. A species which produces moniliasis.

canine eminence. The ridge on the anterior surface of the maxilla, occurring over the canine tooth socket.

canine fossa. A depression on the external surface of the maxilla, immediately distal to the canine tooth socket.

canine muscle. M. levator anguli oris. *See* Table of Muscles.

Canine tooth

canine tooth (*kan'-in*). A single-cusped tooth, resembling a dog's, found between the lateral incisor and the first molar or premolar. There is one in each quadrant in both the deciduous and the permanent dentitions in man.

caniniform (*kan-in'-ĭ-form*). In the shape of or resembling a canine tooth.

canker (*kan'-ker*). Ulceration, especially of the mouth and lips; aphthous stomatitis.

cantilever bridge (*kan'-tĭ-le-ver*). A bridge of which one end is attached to an abutment but the other is only seated on the alveolar ridge.

cap (*kap*). *In dentistry:* Any substance or structure covering an exposed pulp.
enamel c. The enamel covering the top of a developing tooth papilla.

cap crown. Shell crown (*q.v.*).

cap splint. A cast metal dental splint fitting accurately over the crowns and occlusal surfaces of the teeth and cemented in place; used to assist in immobilizing jaw fractures.

capillary (*kap-il'-ar-ĭ*). 1. very fine, thread-like blood vessels, connecting the veins and arteries. 2. Used to describe any very fine tube.

capitulum (*kap-it'-yu-lum*). A small head; a bony articulating eminence.

capitulum mandibulae. The articulating head of the lower jaw; the mandibular condyle.

capsula (*kap'-syul-ă*). Latin for *capsule*; used in prescription writing, and abbreviated *cap*.

capsular (*kap'-syu-lar*). Relating to a capsule.

capsule (*kap'-syul*). 1. The fibrous or membranous sheath or covering of an organ or part. 2. A soluble casing for enclosure of a drug.
enamel c. Primary enamel cuticle (*q.v.*).
nasal c. The cartilagenous structure around the embryonic nasal cavity.

Carabelli's tubercle (G. C. Carabelli, 1787-1842. Austrian dentist). A small tubercle sometimes found on the lingual surface of a maxillary molar; usually hereditary.

carbohydrate (*kar"-bo-hi'-drāt*). An organic substance containing carbon, hydrogen and oxygen; included in this class of compounds are sugars, starches, dextrins, and celluloses.

carbuncle (*kar'-bun-kl*). A staphylococcal infection of the sweat glands or hair follicles, causing inflammation of the surrounding subcutaneous tissues and discharging pus through several openings, finally sloughing away.

carcinogen (*kar-sin-o'-jen*). 1. Any substance or agent producing a carcinoma. 2. Used more loosely for any agent producing a malignant tumour of any kind.

carcinogenesis (*kar″-sin-o-jen′-is-is*). The production of cancer.

carcinoma (*kar-sin-o′-mă*). A malignant epithelial tumour, giving rise to metastases.

actinic c. Basal-cell type of carcinoma affecting the face and other uncovered body surfaces, caused by prolonged exposure to direct sunlight.

basal-cell c. Locally malignant carcinoma developing from the basal-cell layer of the epithelium and retaining its characteristics.

epidermoid c. A form of carcinoma derived from the stratified squamous epithelium; it can be differentiated into various types.

squamous-cell c. Carcinoma developing from the squamous epithelium; a type of epidermoid carcinoma.

carcinomatoid (*kar-sin-o′-mat-oyd*). Resembling a carcinoma.

carcinomatous (*kar-sin-o′-mat-us*). Relating to or affected by carcinoma.

carcinosarcoma (*kar″-sin-o-sar-ko′-mă*). A mixed tumour containing characteristics of both carcinoma and sarcoma.

cardinal tongue. A tongue which has a bright red appearance, being denuded of epithelium.

cardio-. Prefix signifying heart.

caries (*ka′-rez*). Inflammatory decay of bone tissue.

dental c. Localized decay and disintegration of tooth enamel, dentine and/or cementum.

cariogenic (*ka-ri-o-jen′-ik*). Caries-producing.

carious (*ka′-ri-us*). Relating to, or characterized by, caries.

Carmichael crown (J. P. Carmichael, 1856-1946. American dentist). A three-quarter crown (*q.v.*).

carnassial (*kar-nas′-i-al*). Relating to flesh eating; applied to those teeth designed to tear flesh.

carnivore (*kar′-niv-or*). Any animal which eats meat.

carnivorous (*kar-niv′-or-us*). Meat-eating.

caroticotympanic artery. Branch of internal carotid supplying the tympanic cavity. *See* Table of Arteries—caroticotympanica.

caroticotympanic nerve. *See* Table of Nerves—caroticotympanicus.

carotid artery. Common carotid, from the brachiocephalic trunk and the aortic arch, divides into the external and internal carotid arteries, supplying the brain and meninges, face, neck, side of head, and tongue. *See* Table of Arteries—carotis communis, carotis externa, carotis interna.

carotid canal. A passage in the petrous portion of the temporal bone, through which passes the internal carotid artery.

carotid nerve. Supplies filaments to the glands and smooth muscles of the head. *See* Table of Nerves—caroticus.

carotid sheath. The envelope containing the common carotid artery, the internal jugular vein, and the vagus nerve.

carpule (*kar'-pūl*). A patent type of glass cartridge containing one dose of a drug solution, which can be loaded directly into a special hypodermic syringe for injection.

cartilage (*kar'-til-āj*). A form of elastic, non-vascular connective tissue attached to articular bone surfaces and also forming some parts of the skeleton.
alar c. The u-shaped cartilage which forms the tip of the nose.
lateral nasal c. One of the two wing-like expansions of the septal cartilage, attached to the nasal bones and to the maxillae.
septal c. The cartilage lying within the nasal septum, dividing the right and left nasal cavities.

cartilage, Meckel's. *See* Meckel's cartilage.

cartilagenous (*kar-til-aj'-in-us*). Consisting of or relating to cartilage.

caruncle, caruncula (*kar-unkl'*). A small fleshy elevation.
sublingual c. Caruncula sublingualis (*q.v.*).

caruncula (*kar-un'-kyu-lă*). Caruncle (*q.v.*).

caruncula salivaris; caruncula sublingualis. A small elevation on either side of the lingual fraemun, at the apex of which is the opening of the sublingual gland.

carver (*kar'-ver*). Any instrument used for carving and modelling, especially in the making of inlays, crowns and dentures.

caseous (*ka'-sē-us*). Cheese-like.

caseous abscess. An abscess containing cheese-like matter.

cassette (*kas-et'*). In radiography, a holder for an *x*-ray plate or film.

cast (*kast*). A postive likeness of an object produced by the introduction of a plastic substance into a mould or impression of that object; e.g. a cast of the mouth made during the construction of dentures.
boxed c. An impression cast in a box or cup which has been built up round it of strips of soft metal or of wax, thus providing a cast which needs little trimming and which can be well vibrated.

casting (*kast'-ing*). 1. The forcing of molten metal into a mould. 2. The solid metal shape this produces. 3. The process of making a cast.

catabasis (*kat-ab'-as-is*). The abatement of a disease.

catabolism (*kat-ab'-ol-izm*). The process of break-down of complex compounds by the body; destructive metabolism, as opposed to *anabolism*.

cataleptic (*kat-al-ep'-tik*). Relating to catalepsy.

catalepsy (*kat'-al-ep-si*). An unconscious state, often associated with hypnosis, which is characterized by rigidity and loss of voluntary motion, the limbs of the patient remaining in any position in which they may be placed.

cataphasia (*kat-af-a'-zi-ă*). A speech disorder in which the sufferer constantly repeats the same word or phrase.

cataplexy (*kat'-ap-lek-si*). A state of muscular rigidity which may be caused by shock, by loss of muscle tone, or as a result of hypnosis.

catarrh (*kat-ahr'*). Inflammation of the mucous membranes, especially those of the nose and throat, with a discharge of mucus.

catarrhal (*kat-ahr'-al*). Relating to or affected by catarrh.

catenoid (*kat'-en-oyd*). Chainlike; having a chain-like arrangement.

catgut (*kat'-gut*). Suture thread prepared from the lining of a sheep's intestine, cleansed, treated and rendered aseptic.

catheter (*kath'-et-er*). A surgical tube used to evacuate fluid from body cavities,

or to distend a canal or vessel.

catodont (*kat'-o-dont*). One who has mandibular teeth only.

cauda (*kaw'-dă*). A tail or tail-like appendage.

caudal (*kaw'-dal*). 1. Relating to a cauda. 2. Relating to the tail end of a body, as opposed to *rostral*.

caustic (*kaw'-stik*). 1. Burning; destructive of tissue substance. 2. Any agent used to burn or to destroy tissue.

cauterization (*kaw-ter-i-za'-shun*). 1. The application of a cautery or caustic. 2. The result of such an application.

cautery (*kaw'-ter-i*). 1. The destruction of tissue by burning with a caustic substance or a hot iron. 2. The substance or iron used for cauterization.
actual c. A white-hot iron used for cauterization.
chemical c. A chemical caustic used for cauterization.
cold c. The use of extreme cold, such as carbon dioxide snow, for cauterization.
electrocautery. See electrocautery.
galvanocautery. Electrocautery (*q.v.*).

caval (*ka'-val*). Relating to a cavity.

cavernous (*kav'-er-nus*). Containing hollow spaces.

cavernous sinus. A venous sinus at the side of the pituitary fossa, into which the ophthalmic and cerebral veins drain. *See* Table of Veins—sinus cavernosus.

cavilla (*kav-il'-ă*). The sphenoid bone.

cavitas pulpae. The pulp cavity (*q.v.*).

cavity (*kav'-it-ĭ*). A hollow or space; in a tooth, the space either caused by caries or cut out to remove caries. *pulp c.* The cavity at the core of a tooth, comprising the pulp chamber and the root canal.

cavity angle. Any angle formed by the adjacent walls of a tooth cavity, named according to the walls which form it.

cavity classification. *See* Black's cavity classification.

cavity liner. Material used in dentistry to protect and insulate the tooth tissues after the excavation of caries before the placing of a restoration in a prepared cavity.

cavity preparation. Those operative procedures in conservative dentistry which are necessary to remove carious matter from a tooth and to shape the resultant cavity for filling.

cavity primer. Cavity liner (*q.v.*).

cavity walls. The walls which form the outline of a tooth cavity; they are named after the tooth surface towards which they face: *i.e.* mesial, distal, buccal, lingual, pulpal, axial, gingival, occlusal, incisal, labial.

cavosurface angle. The angle formed between a cavity wall and the surface of a tooth.

cavum dentis. The pulp cavity (*q.v.*).

cebocephaly (*se-bo-sef'-al-ĭ*). A congenital malformation of the head, marked by the absence of a nose, and with the orbital cavities close together, giving a general monkey-like appearance.

cell (*sel*). One of the minute masses of protoplasm, containing a nucleus, which form the basis of all animal and plant structure. *embryonal c.* One of the developmental cells. *enamel c.* Ameloblast (*q.v.*). *epithelial attachment c's.* Reduced enamel epithelium (*q.v.*). *epithelial c.* One of the cells which make up the epithelium. *giant c.* A large, multinuclear cell, such as an osteoclast. *prickle c.* One having delicate fibrous processes connecting it to neighbouring cells.

cellular (*sel'-yu-lar*). Composed of cells.

cellulitis (*sel-yu-li'-tis*). Diffuse inflammation, often purulent, of the intercellular tissue and especially of subcutaneous tissue.

cement (*sem-ent'*). 1. A substance which will unite two opposed surfaces. 2. A plastic material which sets hard, used in dentistry to secure an inlay in a cavity, or as a filling material. 3. Cementum (q.v.).

cementation (se-men-ta'-shun). The process of attaching restorations or fillings with cement.

cementicle (sem-ent'-ikl). A small calcareous body developing in the periodontal membrane.

cementitis (se-men-ti'-tis). Inflammation of the cementum.

cementoblast (sem-ent'-o-blast). A germ cell from which cementum is eventually formed.

cementoblastoma (se-men"-to-blast-o'-mă). A benign tumour of odontogenic origin, composed of cemento-blasts and cementum.

cementoclasia (se-ment-o-kla'-zi-ă). Resorption of the cementum.

cementocyte (sem-ent'-o-sīt). One of the cells incorporated in cementum.

cementodentinal (sem-en"-to-den-te'-nal). Relating to both the cementum and the dentine of a tooth.

cemento-enamel. (sem-ent'-to-en-am'-el). Relating to both the cementum and the enamel of a tooth.

cemento-enamel junction. The line where the cementum of the root joins the enamel of the crown; the cervix of the tooth.

cemento-exostosis (se-ment''-o-eks-os-to'-sis). Cementosis (q.v.).

cementoma (se-ment-o'-mă). A tumour composed of cementum.

cementopathia (sem-en-to-path'-i-ă). Periodontosis (q.v.).

cementoperiostitis (sem-en"-to-per-i-os-ti'-tis). Pyorrhoea alveolaris (q.v.).

cementosis (se''-men-to'-sis). Localized deposition of cementum.

cementum (se-men'-tum). Bony tissue, a layer of which surrounds the dentine of the root of a tooth in man.

cementum exostosis (eks-os-to'-sis). Cementosis (q.v.).

cementum hyperplasia (hi''-per-pla'-zi-ă). Localized deposition of cementum; cementosis.

cementum inostosis (in-os-to'-sis). A pathological thickening of cementum developing inwards into the dentine.

centi-. Prefix signifying one-hundredth.

centigrade (sen'-ti-grād). 1. Denoting a thermometric scale on which freezing point is 0° and boiling point is 100°. 2. A term used by G. V. Black in his instrument formula ; 1 centigrade =3.6°.

central artery of the retina. Branch of the ophthalmic artery supplying the retina. Also called Zinn's artery. See Table of Arteries—centralis retinae.

centric occlusion. The relationship of the upper and lower dental arches when the teeth are brought into contact from centric relation (*q.v.*).

centric relation. The relation of the jaws which obtains when the condyles are in the most retruded unstrained position in the glenoid fossa from which lateral excursions of the jaw can be made. In an edentulous mouth it is applied to the position of the alveolar processes with the jaws at rest.

centrifugal (*sen-tri-fyu'-gal*). Moving away from the centre.

centripetal (*sen-trip'-et-al*). Moving towards the centre.

cephalalgia (*sef-al-al'-ji-ă*). Headache.

cephalic (*sef-al'-ik*). Relating to, or in the direction of, the head.

cephalic index. The ratio of

$$\frac{\text{cranial breadth} \times 100}{\text{cranial length}}$$

which gives an indication of the shape and size of a head.

cephalic triangle. Formed by lines from the chin to forehead and occiput, and a line joining occiput to forehead.

cephalo-. Prefix signifying *head*.

cephalometry (*sef-al-om'-et-ri*). The science of measurement of the head, used in orthodontics and in facial plastic surgery.

cephalostat (*sef'-al-o-stat*). An apparatus designed to ensure the location of the head in a constant plane so that a series of *x*-ray photographs, taken over a long period, may be accurately superimposed for purposes of comparison.

cera (*se'-ră*). Wax.

ceramics (*ser-am'-iks*). The art of making porcelain objects, and of processing porcelain.
    dental c. The art of making porcelain teeth, crowns, and inlays.

ceramodontics (*ser-am-o-don'-tiks*). Dental ceramics (*q.v.*).

ceratopharyngeal muscle. Part of constrictor pharyngis medius. *See* Table of Muscles—ceratopharyngeus.

cerebellar (*ser-eb-el'-ar*). Relating to the cerebellum.

cerebellar artery. Supplies the cerebellum, the medulla and vermiform process; three branches: anterior inferior, posterior inferior, and superior. *See* Table of Arteries—cerebelli.

cerebellum (*ser-eb-el'-um*). That part of the brain which controls and co-ordinates movement; situated behind the cerebrum.

cerebral (*ser'-eb-ral*). Relating to the cerebrum.

cerebral artery. Supplies blood to the brain; three branches: anterior, middle, and posterior. *See* Table of Arteries—cerebri.

cerebral vein. One of the veins draining the cerebrum. *See* Table of Veins—cerebri.

cerebralgia (*ser-eb-ral'-ji-ă*). Headache.

cerebrum (*ser'-eb-rum*). The main part of the brain, occupying the upper part of the cranium.

cereous (*ser'-ě-us*). Composed of wax.

cervical (*ser-vi'-kal*). Relating to the cervix, or neck; especially to the neck of a tooth.

cervical artery. Supplies neck muscles, spinal cord and vertebrae; three branches: ascending, deep, and superficial (variable). *See* Table of Arteries—cervicalis.

cervical line. The line formed at the cemento-enamel junction.

cervical nerves. *See* Table of Nerves—cervicales.

cervical third *of a tooth.* That portion of the crown or root adjacent to the cervical line.

cervicoaxial (*ser-vi"-ko-aks'-i-al*). Axiogingival (*q.v.*).

cervicobuccal (*ser-vi'-ko-buk'-al*). 1. Relating to the buccal surface of the cervix of a posterior tooth. 2. Buccogingival (*q.v.*).

cervicobuccoaxial (*ser-vi"-ko-buk"-o-aks'-i-al*). Gingivobuccoaxial (*q.v.*).

cervicofacial (*ser-vi"-ko-fa'-shi-al*). Relating to the neck and the face.

cervicolabial (*ser-vi"-ko-la'-bi-al*). 1. Relating to the labial surface of the cervix of an anterior tooth. 2. Labiogingival (*q.v.*).

cervicolingual (*ser-vi"-ko-lin'-gwal*). 1. Relating to the lingual surface of a tooth cervix. 2. Linguogingival (*q.v.*).

cervix (*ser'-viks*). *In dentistry:* The neck of a tooth; the narrowed part where the tooth enters the gum, at the cemento-enamel junction.

chalinoplasty (*kal'-in-o-plast-i*). Plastic surgery operation at the angles of the mouth.

chamber (*chăm'-ber*). 1. Any enclosed space. 2. In anatomy, a small or clearly defined cavity.
air c. A depression in the palatal portion of an upper denture, and once thought to assist in its retention; a vacuum chamber.
pulp c. The cavity at the core of a tooth crown, surrounded by dentine and containing dental pulp.
relief c. A recess in the surface of a denture base to reduce pressure on a specific area in the mouth.
suction c. Air chamber (*q.v.*).
vacuum c. Air chamber (*q.v.*).

chamecephalic (*kam-ě-sef-al'-ik*). Having a flattened skull.

chameprosopic (*kam-ě-pros'-op-ik*). Having a broad, low face.

chamfer (*cham'-fer*). To bevel.

chancre (*shan'-ker*). The primary syphilitic lesion, starting as a small papule and rapidly developing into an erosive ulcer.

chart (*chart*). 1. A visible record of data relating to a patient's illness, progress or treatment. 2. To record such data on a visible record. *dental c.* A diagrammatic representation of the tooth surfaces of the upper and lower jaws, on which may be recorded details of cavities, fillings, extractions, or other relevant information.

check bite. An impression taken in hard wax or in modelling compound to record the various occlusal positions of the teeth in the mouth, and used to check these positions in artificial dentures in an articulator.

cheek (*chēk*). The side of the face, below the eye. *cleft c.* A developmental anomaly caused by the failure of some of the facial processes to unite.

cheekbone (*chēk'-bōn*). The zygoma (*q.v.*).

cheilalgia (*ki-lal'-ji-ă*). Neuralgic pain affecting the lip or lips.

cheilectomy (*ki-lek'-tom-ĭ*). The surgical removal of part of a lip.

cheilectropion (*ki-lek-tro'-pi-on*). Eversion of the lip.

cheilion (*ki'-li-on*). The angle of the mouth.

cheilitis (*ki-li'-tis*). Inflammation of the lip. *impetiginous c.* Impetigo affecting the lip. *migrating c.* Cheilosis (*q.v.*).

cheilitis actinica. Cheilitis caused by exposure to sunlight.

cheilitis exfoliativa. Recurrent crust formation which affects the vermilion border of the lip, and peels off.

cheilitis glandularis. Inflammation of the labial glands, causing swelling and hardening of the lips.

cheilitis venenata. Contact dermatitis caused by cosmetic or chemical irritants.

cheilocarcinoma (*ki"-lo-kar-sin-o'-mă*). Cancer of the lip.

cheilognathopalatoschisis (*ki"-lo-na"-tho-pal-at-os'-kis-is*). Congenital malformation marked by fissure of the upper lip, the maxillary alveolar process and the palate; hare-lip and cleft palate.

cheilognathoprosoposchisis (*ki"-lo-na"-tho-pros-op-os'-kis-is*). A fissure involving the upper lip and the maxilla, associated with an oblique facial cleft.

cheilognathoschisis (*ki"-lo-na-thos'-kis-is*). Congenital fissure of the upper lip and the maxillary alveolar process.

cheilognathouranoschisis (*ki"-lo-na"-tho-yur-an-os'-kis-is*). Hare-lip and cleft palate.

cheilognathus (*ki-lo-na'-thus*). Hare-lip.

cheiloncus (*ki-lon'-kus*). A tumour of the lip.

cheilopalatognathus (*ki"-lo-pal"-at-o-na'-thus*). Congenital fissure of the maxillary alveolar process combined with cleft palate.

cheilophagia (*ki-lo-fa'-ji-ă*). Biting the lips.

cheiloplasty (*ki'-lo-plast-i*). The repair of a lip defect by plastic surgery.

cheilorrhaphy (*ki-lor'-af-i*). Suture of the lips.

cheiloschisis (*ki-los'-kis-is*). Hare-lip.

cheilosis (*ki-lo'-sis*). A condition caused by riboflavin deficiency and marked by lesions on the lips and at the angles of the mouth; perlèche.

cheilostomatoplasty (*ki"-lo-sto-mat'-o-plast-i*). The repair of lip and mouth damage by plastic surgery.

cheilotomy (*ki-lot'-om-i*). Excision of part of a lip.

cheloid (*ke'-loyd*). *See* keloid.

chemical (*kem'-ik-al*). Relating to chemistry.

chemical cautery. A chemical caustic used for cauterization.

chemico-parasitic theory of caries. A theory of the cause of dental decay advanced in 1889; it postulated that caries was the result of decalcification of the tooth enamel due to the action of acids produced by bacteria.

chemistry (*kem'-ist-ri*). The science and study of the composition of matter, and the analysis and transformation of substances.

biological c. Biochemistry (q.v.).

histological c. Histochemistry (q.v.).

pharmaceutical c. The chemistry of drugs.

chemoprophylaxis (*kem"-o-prof-il-aks'-is*). The use of chemical drugs in the prevention of disease.

chemotherapy (*kem-o-ther'-ap-i*). The treatment of disease by chemicals which affect the pathogenic organism without harming the patient.

cheoplastic (*ke-o-plast'-ik*). Relating to cheoplasty.

cheoplasty (*ke'-o-plast-i*). The moulding of artificial teeth by means of low-fusing alloys; now obsolete.

cherubism (*cher'-u-bizm*). The round, chubby features and upturned eyes characteristic of facial fibrous dysplasia.

chiasm (*ki'-azm*). Chiasma (q.v.).

chiasma (*ki-az'-mă*) (*pl.* chiasmata). 1. Any crossing over; a decussation. 2. The crossing of the fibres of the optic nerve; the optic chiasm.

chiasmal, chiasmatic, chiasmic (*ki-az'-mal; ki-az-mat'-ik; ki-az'-mik*). Relating to a chiasma.

Chievitz's organ (J. H. Chievitz, 1850-1901. Danish anatomist). The mandibular branch of the parotid duct.

child (*chīld*). Human young, up to the age of puberty.

chilitis (*ki-li'-tis*). *See* cheilitis.

chill (*chil*). A cold sensation with shivering, often characteristic of the onset of fever.

chin (*chin*). The central prominence of the lower jaw.

chin reflex. Jaw jerk reflex (*q.v.*).

chin retractor, Angle's. *See* Angle's chin retractor.

chirurgical (*ki-rur'-jik-al*). Relating to surgery.

chisel (*chiz'-el*). An instrument used in surgery for chipping away bone, and in dentistry for cutting tooth enamel; it is bevelled on one side of the blade only.

chloroma (*klor-o'-mă*). A condition characterized by multiple myeloid tumours, of a greenish colour, affecting particularly the face and skull, and associated with a blood picture of leukaemia.

chlorosarcoma (*klor"-o-sar-ko'-mă*). Chloroma (*q.v.*).

choana (*ko-a'-nă*). 1. Any funnel-shaped opening. 2. One of the posterior nasal orifices; a nostril.

chondral (*kon'-dral*). Relating to cartilage.

chondrocranium (*kon"-dro-kra'-ni-um*). The cartilagenous cranium of the embryo.

chondrofibrosarcoma (*kon"-dro-fi"-bro-sar-ko'-mă*). Chondrosarcoma (*q.v.*).

chondroglossal muscle. Draws back and depresses

tongue. *See* Table of Muscles—chondroglossus.

chondroliposarcoma (*kon"-dro-lip"-o-sar-ko'-mă*). Chondrosarcoma (*q.v.*).

chondroma (*kon-dro'-mă*). A tumour composed of cartilagenous tissue.

chondromalacia (*kon"-dro-mal-a'-shi-ă*). A condition characterised by abnormal softness of cartilage.

chondropharyngeal muscle. Part of constrictor pharyngis medius. *See* Table of Muscles — chondropharyngeus.

chondrosarcoma (*kon-dro-sar-ko'-mă*). A malignant, cartilagenous sarcoma.

chondrosis (*kon-dro'-sis*). Cartilage formation.

chorda tympani nerve. *See* Table of Nerves.

choroid artery. Supplies the choroid plexus of the lateral ventricle. *See* Table of Arteries—choroidea.

chrome (*krōm*). Chromium (*q.v.*).

chromium (*kro'-mi-um*). A hard, brittle, silvery metal used mainly as protective plating. Chemical symbol Cr.

chronic (*kron'-ik*). Long continued; as opposed to *acute*.

chronic abscess. Any abscess of long duration and slow development; it may be a cold abscess (*q.v.*)., or one resulting from incomplete resolution of a pre-existing acute abscess, or from the presence of pyogenic organisms of low virulence. There is pus formation, but little inflammation.

chronic periodontitis. A form of periodontitis in which the progress of the condition is slow and usually generalised.

cicatricial (*sik-at-rish'-ĭ-al*). Relating to a cicatrix or scar.

cicatrix (*sik'-at-riks*). A scar.

cicatrization (*sik"-at-riz-a'-shun*). The process of wound-healing which leaves a scar.

ciliary artery. Supplies blood to the eyeball; three branches: anterior, long posterior, short posterior (*also called* uveal). *See* Table of Arteries—ciliaris.

ciliary muscle. Muscle of accommodation of vision. *See* Table of Muscles—ciliaris.

ciliary nerve. Supplies the eyeball and ciliary muscles. *See* Table of Nerves—ciliaris.

ciliated (*sil'-ĭ-a-ted*). Having hair-like processes, or a fringe of hair.

ciliiform (*sil'-ĭ-form*). Hairlike.

ciliiform teeth. Very fine, closely set teeth, as found in certain fish.

cingulum (*sin'-gyu-lum*). Basal ridge in the cervical third on the lingual surface of the anterior maxillary teeth.

circa (*sir'-kă*). Latin for *about*; abbreviated *c*.

circle of Willis (T. Willis, 1621-75. English anatomist

and physician). The circular arterial system at the base of the brain, formed by the anterior and posterior cerebral, the anterior and posterior communicating, and the internal carotid arteries.

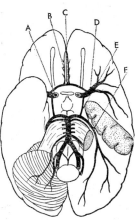

Circle of Willis

A Internal carotid.
B Anterior cerebral.
C Anterior communicating.
D Middle cerebral.
E Posterior communicating.
F Posterior cerebral.

circular (*sir'-kyu-lar*). In the shape of or resembling a circle.

circulatory (*sir-kyu-la'-tor-ĭ*). Relating to circulation;

applied especially to the circulation of the blood.

circulatory canal. Nutrient canal (q.v.).

circulus arteriosus (*sir'-kyu-lus ar-ter-i-o'-sus*). The circle of Willis (q.v.).

circulus arteriosus halleri. A circle of arteries round the entrance of the optic nerve in the sclera; Zinn's circle.

circumcoronitis (*sir-kum-kor-on-i'-tis*). Pericoronitis (q.v.).

circumferential clasp. A clasp which surrounds more than half of the abutment tooth.

circumferential wiring. A method of immobilization of a jaw fracture in an edentulous mandible where the vulcanite or other splint is held in place by wires passed over the bone and through the soft tissues.

circumoral (*sir-kum-or'-al*). Around the mouth.

circumtonsillar (*sir-kum-ton'-sil-ar*). About a tonsil.

circumtonsillar abscess. Quinsy (q.v.).

circumvallate (*sir-kum-val'-āt*). Surrounded by a wall, as the circumvallate, or vallate, papillae of the tongue.

circumvallate papilla. Vallate papilla (q.v.).

clamp (*klamp*). 1. A screw or spring type of device for holding anything in position. 2. A surgical device used to apply compression.

clamp band. A band which is held in place by means of a screw and a nut.

Clapton's line. A greenish line on the gums, seen in copper poisoning.

Clarke's tongue (Sir Charles M. Clarke, 1782-1857. British physician). The fissured tongue of syphilitic glossitis sclerosa.

clasp (*klasp*). Any hook or band attached to a natural tooth and used to anchor a partial denture or any orthodontic appliance.
arrowhead c. A form of orthodontic attachment consisting of a wire clasp round a molar tooth, fitting under the mesial and distal bulge, to which removable appliances may be fastened. An Adams crib is a modified form of this clasp.
bar c. A type of clasp in which the arms are a direct extension of the connector bars of the denture.
circumferential c. A clasp which surrounds more than half of the abutment tooth.
continuous c. Continuous bar retainer (q.v.).

class (*klas*). The primary division in biological classification, subdivided into orders.

cleat (*klēt*). Occlusal rest (q.v.).

cleft (*kleft*). A fissure.

cleft, Stillman's. *See* Stillman's cleft.

cleft cheek. A developmental anomaly caused by the

failure of some of the facial processes to unite.

cleft palate. Congenital fissure of the palate, due to defective development in embryo; it may be associated with harelip. There is a wide range of deformity, from a bifid uvula to complete bilateral cleft of both palate and lip.

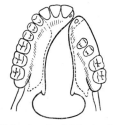

Cleft palate (and cleft alveolus)

cleidocranial (*kli-do-kra´-ni-al*). Relating to the clavicle and the cranium.

cleidocranial dysostosis. A rare form of dysostosis characterized by defective formation of the cranial bones and partial or complete absence of the clavicles; eruption of the teeth is often affected, and there may be partial anodontia.

cleoid (*kle´-oyd*). A claw-like instrument used in cavity excavation.

cliche metal. A fusible alloy of tin, lead, antimony and bismuth, used in dentistry.

clinical (*klin´-ik-al*). 1. Relating to a clinic. 2. Relating to the observation and treatment of disease in the patient, as opposed to theoretical and experimental investigation.

clinical crown. That part of the tooth crown which projects above the gum surface.

clinical root. That portion of a tooth which is embedded in the gums, from the gingival sulcus.

clinocephalic (*kli´´-no-sef-al´-ik*.) Saddle-headed; having a congenital defect of the skull, in which there is a concavity in the vertex.

clonic (*klon´-ik*). Relating to or characteristic of a clonus.

clonus (*klo´-nus*). Convulsive spasm, with alternating contraction and relaxation of muscles.

close-bite, closed bite (*klōs´-bīt*). A malocclusion in which there is abnormally deep overlap of the incisors when the jaws are closed.

Clostridium (*klos-trid´-i-um*). A genus of the Bacillaceae family, anaerobic, Gram-positive, spore-bearing, seen as spindle- or rod-shaped organisms.

clutch (*klutch*).
dental c. A metal casting of the dental arch with space for the tooth crowns, which can be fitted over the teeth, leaving the occlusal surfaces free, and following the indentations of the teeth on both the lingual and

buccal surfaces; it is used as attachment for a face-bow or other measuring instrument.

coagulation (*ko-ag-yu-la'-shun*). The process of clotting.

coalesce (*ko-al-es'*). To fuse or unite separate parts.

coalescence (*ko-al-es'-ens*). The fusion or union of parts previously separate.

coated tongue. A whitish covering of the tongue surface containing food particles, epithelial debris and bacteria.

cobblestone tongue. Hypertrophy of the lingual papillae and a whitish coating, associated with leukoplakia and glossitis.

coccal (*kok'-al*). Relating to or resembling a coccus.

coccus (*kok'-us*). A spherical micro-organism of the family Coccaceae.

cochlea (*kok'-le-ă*). A spiral tube forming part of the inner ear.

cochlear (*kok'-le-ar*). Relating to the cochlea.

cochlear nerve. Supplies the spiral organ of the cochlea. *See* Table of Nerves—cochlearis.

coffer dam. Rubber dam (*q.v.*).

Coffin split plate (C. R. Coffin, 1826-91. American dentist). An orthodontic appliance used formerly for expanding the dental arch by means of a divided plate, constructed to exert controlled lateral pressure on the lingual edges of the arch.

cohesion (*ko-he'-zhun*). The force which unites the molecules of a substance.

cohesive (*ko-he'-ziv*). Relating to cohesion; sticking together.

cohesiveness (*ko-he'-ziv-nes*). The quality of being cohesive.

cold abscess. A slow-developing tuberculous abscess, generally about a bone or joint, and with little inflammation.

cold cautery. The use of extreme cold, such as carbon dioxide snow, for cauterization.

cold sore. Herpes labialis (*q.v.*).

collagen (*kol'-aj-en*). An albuminoid, one of the main constituents of bone, cartilage, and connective tissue.

collagenous (*kol-aj'-en-us*). Relating to collagen.

collar (*kol'-ar*). A band which encircles, generally round the neck, or a tooth cervix.

collar crown. An artificial crown attached to the tooth root by a metal band.

collar-stud abscess. A superficial abscess connected by a sinus tract to a larger, deep abscess.

collet (*kol'-et*). A collar (*q.v.*).

colloid (*kol'-oyd*). 1. A state of matter in which individual particles of one substance, either as large single molecules or collections of smaller molecules (the disperse phase), are uniformly distributed in a dispersion medium of another substance. 2. Glue-like. 3. The colourless, gelatinous secretion of the thyroid gland.

colloidal (*kol-oyd'-al*). Relating to or having the properties of a colloid.

coma (*ko'-mǎ*). A state of complete unconsciousness from which a patient cannot be roused even by determined external stimulation.

comatose (*ko'-mat-ōz*). The condition of being in a coma.

commensal (*kom-en'-sal*). An organism which lives on or within another organism to its own advantage and without detriment to the host.

comminuted (*kom-in-yu'-ted*). Broken into small pieces.

commissure (*kom-is'-shur*). The point of union between similar parts or bodies. *labial c.* The corners of the mouth where the upper and lower lips join.

communicating artery. Forms part of the circle of Willis. *See* Table of Arteries —communicans.

complex muscle. M. semispinalis capitis. *See* Table of Muscles.

complex pocket. A periodontal pocket involving more than one tooth surface but having an outlet on only one surface.

composite odontome. One made up of various elements of the tooth germ.

compound. *See* impression compound.

compound pocket. A periodontal pocket involving more than one tooth surface.

compression moulding. The process of shaping under pressure in a mould.

compressor naris muscle. Compresses nostril. *See* Table of Muscles.

concave (*kon-kāv'*). Having an inward curve or a hollowed surface.

concha (*kon'-shǎ*) (*pl.* conchae). Any anatomic structure resembling a shell, as the centre of the external ear, or the turbinate bone.

concrement (*kon'-krě-ment*). Concretion (*q.v.*).

concrescence (*kon-kres'-ens*). The joining of the roots of two adjacent teeth by a deposit of cementum.

concretion (*kon-kre'-shun*). Any hardened or solidified mass in the tissues; a calculus.

concussion (*kon-kush'-un*). 1. A violent blow or shock; generally used of a blow on the head. 2. The condition resulting from such a blow.

condensation (*kon den-sa'-shun*). 1. The act of making more compact or denser. 2. In dentistry, the act of packing a filling into a tooth cavity, used particularly of a gold foil filling.

condenser (*kon-den'-ser*). *In dentistry:* An instrument with a blunt, serrated edge, used for packing and compressing gold-foil or amalgam fillings.

conditioned reflex. A reflex which is not normal and instinctive but which is developed as a result of repeated association.

condylar (*kon'-di-lar*). Relating to a condyle.

condylar canal. A passage for the hypoglossal nerve through the occipital bone.

condylar foramen. Condylar canal (*q.v.*).

condylar fossa, condyloid fossa. One of the two small depressions on the occipital bone, situated behind one of the condyles.

condylar plane. The plane passing through the most posterior points on the condylar head and on the ascending ramus in the region of the angle of the mandible, and perpendicular to the sagittal plane.

condyle (*kon'-dīl*). A rounded articulating prominence, especially one of the rounded articulating prominences of the mandible.

condylectomy (*kon-di-lek'-tom-i*). Surgical removal of a condyle.

condylion (*kon-di'-li-on*). A point on the lateral tip of the mandibular condyle.

condyloid (*kon'-dil-oyd*). Relating to or resembling a condyle.

condyloid process. One of the two mandibular condyles.

condylotomy (*kon-di-lot'-om-i*). Surgical division of or incision into a condyle.

cone, silver. Silver point (*q.v.*).

cone-socket instrument. One in which the shank and blade or nib are separate from the handle, and screw into it.

congenital (*kon-jen'-it-al*). Present at birth.

congenital epulis. A granular cell tumour which develops *in utero*.

congestive abscess. An abscess forming at a distance from the inflammation because resistance from the tissues prevents it gathering.

conical (*kon'-ik-al*). Cone-shaped.

conjunctiva (*kon-junk-ti'-vă*). The mucous membrane covering the front of the eyeball and lining the eyelid.

conjunctival (*kon-junk-ti'-val*). Relating to the conjunctiva.

conjunctival arteries. Supply the conjunctiva. *See* Table of Arteries—conjunctivalis.

conjunctivitis (*kon-junk-tiv-i'-tis*). Inflammation of the conjunctiva.

connector (*kon-ek'-tor*). Any part of a partial denture whose function is to link two of the major components of the denture.

conoides (*kon-oyd'-ez*). Canine teeth, so named from their cone-like shape.

conversation (*kon-ser-va'-shun*). Restoration and

preservation of health, or of injured parts, such as teeth.

conservative dentistry. That branch of dentistry which is concerned with the preservation of the teeth and the restoration of injured or diseased teeth; this includes removal of caries, filling of cavities, crown- and bridgework.

constitution (*kon-stit-yu'-shun*). *In medicine:* The functional habit of the body, taking into account inherited qualities and the effects of environment on the physical and mental development.

constitutional (*kon-stit-yu'-shun-al*). Relating to or affecting the constitution as a whole.

constriction (*kon-strik'-shun*). A contraction or drawing together in one part; tightness.

constrictor pharyngis muscle. Constricts pharynx. *See* Table of Muscles.

contact points. The areas of contact on the proximal surfaces of adjacent teeth.

contagious disease. A disease which is communicated by direct contact with an affected person, with any object with which such a person has been in contact, or with his secretions.

contaminate (*kon-tam'-in-āt*). To soil or make impure by the addition of foreign material or organisms.

contamination (*kon-tam-in-a'-shun*). The condition of being soiled or impure as a result of the addition of foreign material or organisms.

continuous bar retainer. A metal bar along the lingual surfaces of the teeth, used in prosthetic dentistry to stabilize them and to act as an indirect retainer.

continuous clasp. Continuous bar retainer (*q.v.*).

continuous gum denture. An obsolete form of denture constructed by fusing a porcelain base and teeth on to a platinum matrix.

contour (*kon'-tor*). 1. The external shape of any object. 2. To carve or otherwise create the external form, as of artificial teeth or fillings.

contour alloy. One suitable for contour fillings.

contour lines of Owen. *See* Owen's contour lines.

contoured band. A band shaped to the tooth.

contra-angle (*kon'-tră-an'-gl*). A double angle or a series of angles in the shank of an instrument bringing its point or edge into line with the axis of the handle.

contraction (*kon-trak'-shun*). 1. A decrease in size, either of length, area, or volume. 2. The shortening and tensing of a muscle.

contusion (*kon-tyu'-zhun*). A bruise (*q.v.*).

convex (*kon-veks'*). Having an outward curve or a domed surface.

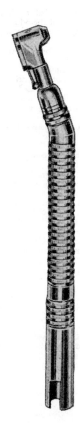

Contra-angle handpiece

cope (*kōp*). A metal plate used to cover the root of a tooth before attaching an artificial crown; a diaphragm.

coping (*ko'-ping*). 1. A thin metal cap. 2. A cope.

copper (*kop'-er*). A reddish metallic element, chemical symbol, Cu, soft and malleable, with poisonous salts; it is much used in alloys.

copper line. A greenish line or a red line on the edge of the gums, seen in copper poisoning.

copula (*kop'-yu-lă*). 1. Any connecting structure. 2. An elevation on the tongue, in the embryo, formed by the joining of the second branchial arches, and representing the future root of the tongue.

cord (*kord*). Any long, circular and flexible structure.

enamel c. A temporary structure in the developing tooth linking the enamel knot to the outer dental lamina.

cordate (*kor'-dāt*). Heart-shaped.

corium (*kor'-ĭ-um*). The layer of connective tissue between the epidermis and the subcutaneous tissue; the dermis or true skin.

cornu (*kor'-nu*) (*pl.* cornua). A horn or horn-shaped process.

cornual (*kor'-nu-al*). Relating to a cornu.

coronal (*kor-o'-nal*). 1. Relating to a crown. 2. In the direction of the coronal suture.

corone (*kor-o'-nĕ*). The coronoid process of the mandible (*q.v.*).

coronion (*kor-o'-nĭ-on*). In craniometry, the point or tip of the coronoid process of the mandible.

coronofacial (*kor''-on-o-fa'-shi-al*). Relating to the crown of the head and the face.

coronoid (*kor'-on-oyd*). 1. Crown-shaped. 2. Curved, like a beak.

coronoid process. A thin and flattened projection of bone from the anterior upper border of the ascending ramus of the mandible into which the temporal muscle is inserted.

Corrigan's line (Sir D. J. Corrigan, 1802-80. Irish physician). A purple line on the gums, seen in copper poisoning.

corrugator supercilii muscle. Draws eyebrow down and wrinkles forehead. *See* Table of Muscles.

cortex (*kor'-teks*). 1. The external layer of an organ, within the capsule. 2. The outer layer of gray matter of the brain.

cortical (*kor'-tik-al*). 1. Relating to a cortex. 2. Relating to the bark of a tree; applied to the outer bone tissue.

cortical plate. The superficial outer layer of bone in the alveolar process.

Corynebacterium (*kŏ-rī''-ne-bak-te'-rĭ-um*). A genus of the Mycobacteriaceae family; Gram-positive, aerobic, slender rod-shaped organisms.

coryza (*kor-i'-ză*). The common cold; a catarrhal inflammation of the nasal mucous membrane.

Costen's syndrome (J. B. Costen, b. 1895. American otolaryngologist). Referred pain associated with temporomandibular joint destruction through faulty occlusion, occurring in the head, the eye, the tongue, and nasal sinuses; there may also be painful muscle spasm during mastication.

cotton wool roll. A small and tightly packed roll of cotton wool used in the mouth to absorb saliva and assist in keeping the operative field dry.

Cotunnius' nerve (D. Cotugno (Cotunnius), 1736-1822. Italian anatomist). The nasopalatine nerve (*q.v.*).

counter-bite. The bite which opposes that taken of the teeth in one jaw.

counterdie (*kown'-ter-di*). The reverse image of a die.

counter-irritant (*kown-ter-ir'-it-ant*). 1. Producing or causing counter-irritation. 2. Any agent used to produce counter-irritation.

counter-irritation (*kown-ter-ir-it-a'-shun*). The deliberate production of superficial irritation in order to mask or relieve an existing irritation or pain.

countersink (*kown'-ter-sink*). 1. A bevelled depression in a surface to accommodate the head of a screw or rivet. 2. The instrument used to make this depression.

cranial (*kra'-ni-al*). Relating to the cranium.

cranial index. Cephalic index (*q.v.*).

cranial nerve. Any one of twelve pairs of peripheral nerves arising directly from the brain stem. *See* Table of Nerves—craniales.

cranial nerves. *See* Table of Nerves—craniales.

cranio-. Prefix signifying *cranium.*

craniobuccal (*kra''-ni-o-buk'-al*). Relating to the cranium and the oral cavity.

craniocleidodysostosis (*kra''-ni-o-kli''-do-dis-os-to'-sis*). Cleidocranial dysostosis (*q.v.*).

craniofacial (*kra''-ni-o-fa'-shi-al*). Relating to the cranium and the face.

craniofacial angle. The angle between the basicranial and basifacial axes at the spheno-ethmoid suture.

craniofacial dysjunction. Le Fort fracture of the maxilla, Class III (*q.v.*).

craniofacial notch. A notch in the bony partition between the nasal and orbital cavities.

craniomalacia (*kra''-ni-o-mal-a'-shi-ă*). A condition characterized by softness of the bones of the skull; seen usually in infants.

craniomandibular (*kra-ni-o-man-dib'-yu-lar*). Relating to the skull and mandible.

craniometric point. Any one of the landmarks on the skull used in craniometry.

craniometry (*kra-ni-om'-et-ri*). The science of measuring the skull for the comparative study of racial types in man, and variations with other primates.

craniostosis (*kra-ni-os-to'-sis*). Ossification of the cranial sutures, occurring prematurely.

cranium (*kra'-ni-um*). The skull.

cranter (*kran'-ter*). A third molar; an obsolete term.

crazing (*kra'-zing*). A pattern of minute cracks which may appear on the surface of plastic or porcelain teeth.

crepitation (*krep-it-a'-shun*). Crepitus (*q.v.*).

crepitus (*krep'-it-us*). A crackling noise; occurring in joints, in the lungs when affected by certain diseases, and in other parts.

crest (*krest*). A prominent raised edge or border.

alveolar c. One of the highest points on the alveolar process, between the tooth sockets.

dental c. Kölliker's dental crest (*q.v.*).

gingival c. Gingival margin (*q.v.*).

nasal c. of the maxilla. A ridge on the medial border

of the maxillary palatal process, articulating with the vomer.

nasal c. of the palatine bone. A ridge on the medial border of the palatal bone, articulating with the vomer.

palatine c. A thin transverse ridge of bone across the back of the hard palate.

crest, dental, Kölliker's. See Kölliker's dental crest.

crevice (krev′-is). A narrow split or fissure in a tooth.

gingival c. The space lying between the inner aspect of the free gingiva and the tooth enamel or cementum, depending on the level of the epithelial attachment.

crevicular (krev-ik′-yu-lar). Relating to a crevice, particularly applied to the gingival crevice.

crib (krib). A removable form of anchorage used with orthodontic appliances.

crib, Adams. See Adams crib.

crib, Jackson. See Jackson crib.

cribriform (krib′-ri-form). Perforated like a sieve.

cricoarytenoid muscle. Opens or narrows rima glottidis. See Table of Muscles—cricoarytenoideus.

cricopharyngeal muscle. Part of constrictor pharyngis inferior. See Table of Muscles—cricopharyngeus.

cricothyroid artery. Supplies the cricothyroid muscle. See Table of Arteries—cricothyroidea.

cricothyroideus muscle. Tenses the vocal folds. See Table of Muscles.

crocodile tongue. Scrotal tongue (q.v.).

cross-bite (kros′-bīt). A malocclusion in which the buccolingual relationships of opposing teeth are the reverse of normal.

cross-cut bur. Dentate bur (q.v.).

cross-pin teeth. Artificial teeth which are attached by pins running at right-angles to the long axis of the tooth.

crown (krown). 1. That part of a tooth, covered by enamel, which is exposed above the gum. 2. An artificial cap to fit over the stump of a carious or of a fractured tooth.

acrylic veneer c. A metal crown covered by a thin veneer of acrylic.

anatomical c. That part of the tooth which is covered by enamel, not all of which may be visible above the gum.

basket c. A form of three-quarter crown, with an acrylic facing, used as a semi-permanent restoration for a fractured incisor in a school-child.

bell c. A crown of a tooth in which the diameter, mesio-distally, is much greater at the occlusal surface than at the cervix.

cap c. A shell crown (q.v.).

clinical c. That part of the

natural tooth crown which projects above the gum surface.

collar c. An artificial crown attached to the tooth root by a metal band.

half-cap c. A form of crown covering all but the labial or buccal surface of a tooth, and attached by a metal band.

hood c. A half-cap crown covering the lingual, proximal and occlusal surfaces of a tooth.

jacket c. A porcelain or acrylic veneer crown which is placed over the prepared remains of a vital natural tooth.

open-face c. Half-cap crown (*q.v.*).

pivot c. An artificial crown attached by means of a metal post into the root canal of the natural tooth.

porcelain cusp c. A crown having porcelain and not metal on the occlusal surface.

porcelain-veneer c. A metal crown covered by a thin veneer of porcelain.

post c. Any artificial crown attached to the tooth root by means of a post or dowel; *also called* a pivot crown.

seamless c. A shell crown contoured from a metal cap, without soldering.

shell c. A crown consisting of a metal shell, contoured to fit over the crown of an existing natural tooth; *also called* a cap crown.

shoulder c. A crown which has been shaped at the base

to sit on a prepared root without a metal collar.

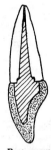

Post crown

split-dowel c. A removable crown attached to the tooth by means of a split-pin, which is fitted into a gold-lined root canel.

telescope c. A double metal crown, composed of two tubular or conical crowns, placed one over the other.

three-quarter c. A form of shell crown, retained by cement and slotted into the tooth, covering all but the labial or buccal surface; *also called* a Carmichael crown.

two-piece c. A crown made from a contoured metal band joined to a swaged cap.

verrucous c. A wart-like overgrowth of enamel on a tooth crown.

window c. An acrylic veneer gold crown, covering all but the labial or buccal surface of a tooth, and frequently used as a bridge abutment. For eponymous crowns *see* under the personal name by which the crown is known.

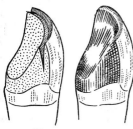

Three-quarter crown

crownwork (*krown'-werk*). 1. The construction or fitting of artificial crowns to the teeth. 2. The actual prosthesis, when in place in the mouth.

Crozat appliance (G. B. Crozat, 20th century American orthodontist). A removable orthodontic appliance consisting of a palatal arch wire joining retention clasps on the first molars which have a claw-like grip; used as a base for various types of attachment to provide tooth movement.

crucial (*kru'-shal*). 1. In the form of a cross. 2. Decisive.

crude (*krūd*). Raw, unrefined.

Cruveilhier's nerve (J. Cruveilhier, 1791-1874. French pathologist). An

occasional branch of the facial nerve.

Cryer's elevator (M. H. Cryer, 1840-1921. American surgeon). One of a pair of elevators for removing molar roots, one for the distal and one for the mesial, being reversible for opposite sides of the jaw.

cryocautery (*kri-o-kaw'-ter-i*). Cold cautery (*q.v.*).

cryoprobe (*kri-o-prob'*). An instrument used for cryosurgery.

cryosurgery (*kri-o-sur'-jer-i*). The use of extreme cold for surgical destruction of tissue.

crypt (*kript*). A pit or follicle. *dental c.* The bony space containing the developing tooth.

culture (*kul'-tyur*). 1. The growth of micro-organisms in an artificial medium. 2. A group of micro-organisms so grown.
mixed c. A culture containing several different species of micro-organism.
plate c. A bacterial culture grown on a glass plate, or in a Petri dish.
pure c. A culture containing only one species of micro-organism.
slant c. One grown on a slanting surface, to obtain a greater area for growth.
stab c. A culture made by inoculating the medium by means of a needle thrust deeply into it.

culture medium (*pl.* media). Any substance used to

cultivate bacteria; the principal media are broth, milk, blood serum, agar and potato.

cum (*kum*). Latin for *with*; used in prescription writing and abbreviated *c.*

cuneate (*kyu'-ne-āt*). Wedge-shaped.

cupreous (*kyu'-prĕ-us*). Relating to copper.

cure (*kyūr*). 1. To treat a disease or injury successfully. 2. Any method or drug used in treatment. 3. To harden materials such as those used for denture bases.

curettage (*kyu-ret-ahj*). 1. The removal of foreign matter from the walls of a bony cavity. 2. Also, in dentistry, the removal of material from root surfaces and periodontal pockets.

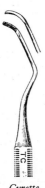

Curette

curette (*kyu-ret'*). An instrument used in curettage.

curled enamel. Enamel in which the prismatic rods are curled round.

curve of Spee (F. von Spee, 1855-1937. German embryologist). An imaginary curved line joining the buccal cusps of the posterior teeth.

cushion of Passavant. *See* Passavant's bar.

cusp (*kusp*). A pointed projection on the tooth crown.
supplemental *c.* Any abnormal or extra cusp on a tooth surface.

cusp angle. The angle of incline of the sides of a cusp made with a perpendicular line bisecting the cusp, measured mesiodistally or buccolingually.

cuspal (*kus'-pal*). Relating to a cusp.

cuspal interference. The contact of a cusp with an opposing tooth, preventing contact of other cusps.

cuspid (*kus'-pid*). 1. Having a cusp. 2. A canine tooth.

cuspidate (*kus'-pid-āt*). Pointed; having one or more sharp points or cusps.

cutaneous (*kyu-ta'-nĕ-us*). Relating to the skin.

cutaneous colli nerve. N. transversus colli. *See* Table of Nerves.

cuticle (*kyu'-tikl*). 1. The outer layer of the skin. 2. A layer covering the free surface of an epithelial cell.

acquired c. Acquired pellicle (*q.v.*).

acquired enamel c. Acquired pellicle (*q.v.*).

dental c. 1. Reduced enamel epithelium (*q.v.*). 2. Acquired pellicle (*q.v.*).

enamel c. 1. Primary enamel cuticle (*q.v.*). 2. Acquired pellicle (*q.v.*).

post-eruption c. Acquired pellicle (*q.v.*).

primary enamel c. An acellular layer of organic material attached to the surface of enamel; it is thought to be the final product of ameloblasts.

cuticula dentis (*kyu-tik'-yu-lă den'-tis*). Reduced enamel epithelium (*q.v.*).

cutis (*kyu'-tis*). The dermis, or skin.

cyanosis (*si-an-o'-sis*). Bluish discoloration of the skin and mucous membranes, often due to deficient oxygenation of the blood.

cyclopia (*si-klo'-pĭ-ă*). The condition of having only one eye.

cylinder (*sil'-in-der*). Any solid or hollow body having parallel sides and a circular cross-section in one direction.

cylindrical (*sil-in'-drik-al*). Shaped like a cylinder.

cymbocephalic (*sim-bo-sef-al'-ik*). Having a hollowed or boat-shaped skull.

cynodont (*si'-no-dont*). A canine tooth (*q.v.*).

cynodontism (*si-no-dont'-izm*). Having teeth with long roots and a small pulp

chamber entirely confined to the crown.

cyst (*sist*). A membranous sac containing fluid, gas, or soft matter.

adventitious c. A cyst which forms about a foreign body.

dental c. Any cyst affecting a tooth, or tooth-bearing structure.

dentigerous c. A cyst containing a tooth or part of a tooth, arising from the enamel organ.

dermoid c. A congenital cystic tumour containing hair follicles, teeth, and sweat or sebaceous glands.

eruption c. One occurring about the crown of an erupting tooth.

follicular c. Dentigerous cyst (*q.v.*).

multilocular c. Any cyst having many interconnected compartments.

radicular c. A cyst occurring about the root of a tooth, arising from a granuloma in that area.

retention c. One caused by the retention of glandular secretion.

sebaceous c. A cyst caused by the blocking of the duct of a sebaceous gland and the retention of its secretion.

sublingual c. A ranula (*q.v.*).

thyroglossal c. A cyst occurring in or arising from the thyroglossal duct.

traumatic c. One caused by some traumatic injury.

unilocular c. A cyst having only one cavity.

cystadenofibroma (*sist"-ad-en-o-fi-bro'-mă*). Adeno-fibroma (*q.v.*).

cystic (*sist'-ik*). Relating to a cyst; cyst-like.

cyto-. Prefix signifying *cell* or *cells*.

Czermak's lines (J. N. Czermak, 1828-73. Austrian physiologist). Rows of interglobular spaces, following the outline of the dentine of a tooth.

D

D Distal.

DB Distobuccal.

DBO Distobucco-occlusal.

DBP Distobuccopulpal.

DC Distocervical.

DG Distogingival.

DI Distoincisal.

DL Distolingual.

DLa Distolabial.

DLI Distolinguoincisal.

DLaI Distolabioincisal.

DLO Distolinguo-occlusal.

DLP Distolinguopulpal.

DLaP Distolabiopulpal.

dmf. The expression used to indicate the number of decayed, missing or filled teeth in the deciduous dentition.

DMF. The expression used to indicate the number of decayed, missing or filled teeth in the permanent dentition.

DO Disto-occlusal.

DP Distopulpal.

DPL Distopulpolingual

DPLa Distopulpolabial.

dacryon (*dak'-ri-on*). The point of juncture of the frontal, lacrimal and maxillary bones.

dakryon. See dacryon.

dam (*dam*). See rubber dam.

dappen dish. Trade name for a small decagonal glass stand, cupped at both ends, used to hold small quantities of medicaments during operative procedures on the teeth.

d'Arcet's metal. An alloy of tin, lead, and bismuth, which is used in dentistry.

dartrous (*dar'-trus*). Herpetic.

Daubenton's angle (L. J. M. Daubenton, 1716-1800. French physician). Occipital angle (*q.v.*).

Davis crown. A ready-made porcelain detachable post crown, having the post cemented into the artificial crown and into the tooth root.

de-. Prefix signifying *from, loss of, taken from*; it also indicates the reversal of a process, removal, or a negative effect.

De Salle's line (E. F. de Salle, 1796-1873. French physician). Nasal line (*q.v.*).

dead (*ded*). 1. Without life. 2. Without sensation.

debridement (*da-brēd'-mon*). The removal of dead tissue and foreign matter from a wound.

debris (*deb'-re*). 1. Any foreign matter attached to the surface of a tooth. 2. Any pieces of tooth substance removed by operation.

food d. Food remnants and bacteria loosely attached to the tooth, which can be removed by rinsing.

deca-. Prefix signifying *ten.*

decalcification (*de"-cal-sif-ik-a'-shun*). Loss or removal of the calcium salts in bone or calcified tissue.

decalcify (*de-kal'-sif-ī*). To remove calcium salts and so produce decalcification.

decay (*de-ka'*). 1. The progressive decomposition of organic matter. 2. The gradual decline in health, especially in old age. 3. Dental caries (*q.v.*).

deci-. Prefix signifying *one-tenth.*

deciduous (*de-sid'-yu-us*). Regularly or naturally shed; not permanent.

deciduous teeth. The primary dentition.

decussate (*de-kus'-āt*). To intersect or form an x-shaped crossing; used of nerve and muscle fibres.

decussation (*de-kus-a'-shun*). An intersection or x-shaped crossing of symmetrical parts; a chiasma.

dedentition (*de-den-tish'-un*). Loss of teeth, more especially due to atrophy of the sockets in old age.

deep (*dēp*). Some distance below the surface; as opposed to *superficial.*

deficiency disease. Any disease caused by absence or shortage of some element vital to bodily health.

deflect (*de-flekt'*). To alter the course or direction of anything.

deflection (*de-flek'-shun*). A turning to one side; altering the course or direction.

deformity (*de-form'-it-i*). Malformation of an organ or part.

degeneration (*de-jen-er-a'-shun*). Gradual deterioration of tissue, with loss of function and chemical change within the tissue.

calcareous d. Degeneration accompanied by deposit of calcareous material in the degenerate tissue.

degenerative disease. A process of general degeneration with no specific cause, commonly found in old age.

deglutition (*de-glu-tish'-un*). Swallowing.

deglutitive (*de-glu'-tit-iv*). Relating to deglutition.

deglutitory (*de-glu'-tit-or-ī*). Relating to deglutition.

degradation (*deg-rad-a'-shun*). The reduction of an organic chemical compound to one containing a smaller number of carbon atoms.

degustation (*de-gus-ta'-shun*). The function of tasting.

dehiscence (*de-his'-ens*). The development of an opening or split.

dehydration (*de-hi-dra'-shun*). 1. Loss or removal of water from the body, or from any tissues. 2. The condition resulting from this removal or loss.

deleterious (*de-let-e′-ri-us*). Harmful, injurious.

demi-. Prefix signifying *one half.*

demineralization (*de-min-er-al-i-za′-shun*). Loss or removal of minerals from the body.

demulcent (*de-mul′-sent*). 1. Bland, soothing, allaying irritation of inflamed surfaces, particularly of the mucous membrane. 2. Any soothing substance.

denervation (*de-ner-va′-shun*). Removal or resection of a nerve or nerves.

dens (*pl.* dentes). Latin for a tooth; used in anatomical nomenclature.

d. *acutus.* An incisor.

d. *adversus.* An incisor.

d. *angularis.* A canine.

d. *bicuspidatus.* A premolar.

d. *caninus.* A canine.

d. *cariosus.* A carious tooth.

d. *columellaris.* A molar.

d. *deciduus.* A deciduous tooth.

d. *excertus.* A tooth projecting in front of the dental arch.

d. *incisivus.* An incisor.

d. *lacteus.* A deciduous tooth.

d. *permanens.* A permanent tooth; a tooth of the second dentition.

d. *premolaris.* A premolar.

d. *primoris.* An incisor.

d. *sapientiae.* A third molar, or wisdom tooth.

d. *serotinus.* A third molar.

d. *tomici.* An incisor.

dens in dente. A condition in which a tooth-like structure is present within the pulp chamber of a tooth.

dentagra (*dent-ag′-ră*). 1. Tooth-ache. 2. A key or forceps for tooth extraction.

dental (*den′-tal*). Relating to the teeth and gums.

dental abscess. Any abscess connected with a tooth.

dental amalgam. An amalgam used for filling teeth; it usually contains silver, tin and mercury.

dental arch. The bow-shaped arrangement of the teeth in the mandible and the maxilla.

dental artery. British terminology for *alveolar* artery. *See* Table of Arteries—alveolaris.

dental arthritis. Inflammation affecting the periodontal membrane.

dental calculus. A deposit of calcium salts in an organic matrix attached to the teeth.

dental canals. Any of the canals in the maxilla or the mandible which afford passage to the vessels or nerves supplying the teeth.

dental caries. Localized decay and disintegration of tooth enamel, dentine, and cementum.

dental ceramics. The art of making porcelain teeth, crowns, or inlays.

dental chart. A diagrammatic representation of the tooth surfaces of the upper and lower jaws, on which may be recorded details of cavities, fillings, extractions, or other relevant information.

dental clutch. A metal casting of the dental arch, with space for the tooth crowns, which can be fitted over the teeth, leaving the occlusal surfaces free, and following the indentations of the teeth on both the lingual and buccal surfaces; it is used as an attachment for a facebow or other measuring instrument.

dental crest. Kölliker's dental crest (q.v.).

dental crest, Kölliker's. See Kölliker's dental crest.

dental crypt. The bony space containing the developing tooth.

dental cuticle. 1. Reduced enamel epithelium (q.v.). 2. Acquired pellicle (q.v.).

dental cyst. Any cyst affecting a tooth, or tooth-bearing structure.

dental engine. The apparatus which is used to drive instruments for cutting, drilling, and polishing the teeth; the interchangeable parts are held in an angled handpiece, and the driving power is supplied by some form of motor, generally electric.

dental epithelium, reduced. Reduced enamel epithelium (q.v.).

dental fistula. Alveolar fistula (q.v.).

dental floss; dental floss silk. Soft, waxed thread or tape, used to clear and to clean inter-proximal spaces.

dental forceps. Forceps used for the extraction of teeth.

dental formula. A formula devised to show the number and arrangement of teeth by means of letters and figures. In this formula I = incisor; C = canine; P = premolar; M = molar. The dental formula for the normal permanent dentition in man is I$\frac{2}{2}$ C$\frac{1}{1}$ P$\frac{2}{2}$ M$\frac{3}{3}$.

dental galvanism. The production of an electric current caused when two dissimilar metals used as restorations in the mouth come into contact; this can produce discomfort or even pain.

dental granuloma. A localized mass of granulation tissue on or near the root of a tooth.

dental index. The ratio of
$$\frac{\text{dental length} \times 100}{\text{length of cranial base}}$$

dental lamina. The ridge of thickened epithelium along the margin of the gum in the embryo, from which is formed the enamel organ.

dental length. The distance from the mesial surface of the first premolar to the distal surface of the last molar in the maxillary arch.

dental mirror. A small mirror designed for use in the mouth.

dental necrosis. Tooth decay.

dental nerve. In new terminology, branches of the alveolar nerve supplying the teeth. *Also* British terminology for *alveolar* nerve. *See* Table of Nerves.

dental notation. A form of symbols used to indicate the type and place of a tooth. The most commonly used notation is:—

for permanent teeth:

right   left

$$\frac{87654321 \mid 12345678}{87654321 \mid 12345678}$$

for deciduous teeth:

right   left

$$\frac{edcba \mid abcde}{edcba \mid abcde}$$

For example: the lower left lateral permanent incisor would be represented by $\overline{\mid 2}$ and the upper right central deciduous incisor by $\overline{a \mid}$.

dental orthopaedics. Orthodontics (*q.v.*).

dental perimeter. An instrument to measure the circumference of a tooth.

dental plaque. 1. A soft, concentrated mass, consisting of a large variety of bacteria, together with a certain amount of cellular debris, found adhering to the surfaces of the teeth when oral hygiene is neglected; it cannot be removed by rinsing. 2. Acquired pellicle (*q.v.*).

dental plate. A plate of metal, acrylic, or other material, shaped to fit the roof of the mouth, to which artificial teeth are attached.

dental plexus. A network of nerve fibres about the roots of the teeth; those of the maxilla are branches of the maxillary nerve and those of the mandible are branches of the inferior dental nerve.

dental prophylaxis. Preventive treatment for diseases of the teeth.

dental prosthesis. Partial or full dentures, crown or bridge, or any appliance to correct cleft palate.

dental pulp. The vascular and connective tissue, highly innervated, found at the core of a tooth.

dental ridge. Any elevation on a tooth, forming a cusp or a tooth margin.

dental sac. The vascular tissue enclosing the enamel organ.

dental senescence. The changes occurring in the mouth and in the teeth as a result of ageing.

dental splint. Any form of appliance or device used to fasten and immobilize the teeth.

dental ulcer. An ulcer on the oral mucosa produced by local trauma.

dentalgia (*dent-al'-ji-ă*). Tooth-ache.

dentaphone (*den'-tă-fōn*). A type of deaf-aid which transmits vibrations from the teeth to the auditory nerve.

dentarpaga (*dent-ar-pa'-gă*). An old instrument used in tooth extraction.

dentate (*dent'-āt*). Having teeth, or projections like teeth on a serrated edge.

dentate bur. A bur having the cutting edges set with teeth for very rapid cutting.

dentation (*dent-a'-shun*). The condition of having tooth-like projections or processes.

dentelation (*dent-el-a'-shun*). Dentation (*q.v.*).

dentia praecox (*den'-shǐ-ă prē'-koks*). Premature eruption of the deciduous teeth.

dentia tarda (*den'-shǐ-a tar'-dă*). Delayed eruption of the deciduous teeth.

dentiaskiascope (*dent"-ǐ-ǎ-skǐ'-as-kōp*). A dental x-ray apparatus.

dentibuccal (*dent-ǐ-buk'-al*). Relating to the teeth and the cheek.

denticle (*dent'-ikl*). 1. A small tooth or tooth-like process. 2. A pulp stone.

denticulate (*dent-ik'-yu-lāt*). Having tooth-like projections.

dentification (*dent-if-ik-a'-shun*). The process of tooth formation.

dentiform (*dent'-ǐ-form*). In the shape of a tooth.

dentifrice (*dent'-ǐf-ris*). Paste, powder or liquid used in cleaning the teeth.

dentigerous (*dent-ij'-er-us*). Containing or bearing teeth.

dentigerous cyst. A cyst containing a tooth or part of a tooth, arising from the enamel organ.

dentilabial (*dent-ǐ-la'-bǐ-al*). Relating to the teeth and the lips.

dentilave (*dent'-ǐ-lāv*). A mouth-wash.

dentilingual (*dent-ǐ-lin'-gwal*). Relating to the teeth and the tongue.

dentilinimentum (*dent"-ǐ-lin-im-ent'-um*). National Formulary name for drops prescribed for tooth-ache.

dentimeter (*dent'-ǐ-me-ter*). An instrument used to measure teeth.

dentin (*den'-tin*). See dentine.

dentinal (*den-te'-nal*). Relating to dentine.

dentinal canals. Dentinal tubules (*q.v.*).

dentinal fibres. Odontoblastic processes (*q.v.*).

dentinal sclerosis. Calcification of the dentinal tubules producing translucent areas and tissue changes in the tooth.

dentinal sheath. Neumann's sheath (*q.v.*).

dentinal tubule. One of the minute tubes in dentine, radiating from the pulp chamber to the amelo-dentinal junction and the cemento-dentinal junction.

dentinalgia (*dent-in-al'-jě-ă*). Pain or sensitiveness of the dentine.

dentine, dentin (*den'-tēn*). The calcified organic tissue forming the body of the tooth, surrounding the pulp chamber, and covered by enamel or cementum. *adventitious d.* Secondary dentine (*q.v.*).

hereditary opalescent d. Dentinogenesis imperfecta (*q.v.*).

mantle d. The thin, superficial outer layer of dentine.

secondary d. A new deposit of dentine laid down in the pulp chamber as a protection against caries or tooth damage.

vitreous d. A very hard type of dentine, having few dentinal tubules.

dentine bridge. A layer of dentine which reseals an exposed pulp or forms over the excised surface after pulpotomy.

dentinification (*dent-in-if-ik-a'-shun*). The formation of dentine; dentinogenesis.

dentinitis (*dent-in-i'-tis*). Inflammation of the dentinal tubules.

dentinoblast (*den-te'-no-blast*). One of the cells from which dentine is formed; an odontoblast.

dentinoblastoma (*dent"-in-o-blast-o-mă*). A benign tumour composed of dentine-forming cells.

dentinocemental (*den"-te-no-sem-en'-tal*). Relating to both the dentine and the cementum of a tooth.

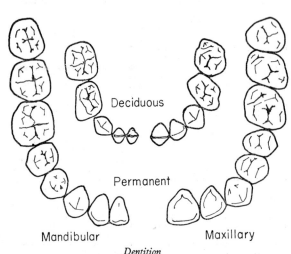

Dentition

dentinoenamel junction. Amelodentinal junction (q.v.).

dentinogenesis (*dent-e"-no-jen'-es-is*). The process of dentine formation.

dentinogenesis imperfecta. Defective calcification of dentine, characterized by an opalescent appearance of the teeth; it is an hereditary condition.

dentinogenic fibres. von Korff's fibres (q.v.).

dentinoid (*den'-tin-oyd*). 1. Resembling dentine. 2. A tumour composed of dentine.

dentinoma (*dent-in-o'-mă*). A tumour composed of dentine; an odontoma.

dentinosteoid (*dent-in-ost'-e-oyd*). A mixed tumour composed of dentine and bone tissue.

dentiparous (*dent-ip'-ar-us*). Relating to the formation of teeth.

dentiphone (*den'-ti-fōn*). Dentaphone (q.v.).

dentist (*dent'-ist*). Any person who practises dentistry, and is qualified to do so.

dentistry (*dent'-ist-ri*). That branch of medicine concerned with oral and dental diseases and their prevention and treatment, and with oral prostheses.

dentitia praecox (*den-tish'-i-ă pre'-koks*). Dentia praecox (q.v.).

dentitia tarda (*den-tish'-i-ă tar'-dă*). Dentia tarda (q.v.).

dentitio difficilis (*den-tish'-i-o dif-is'-il-is*). Teething troubles.

dentition (*den-tish'-un*). 1. The teeth in the jaws. 2. Also used occasionally to mean the eruption of the teeth.
permanent d. The second teeth, normally thirty-two: four incisors, two canines,

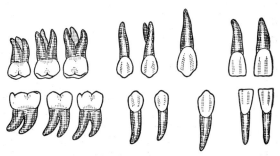

Dentition, permanent

four premolars, and six molars in each jaw.

primary d. The first, deciduous teeth, normally twenty, which are gradually shed.

dento-. Prefix signifying *teeth.*

dento-alveolar (*den″-to-al-ve′-o-lar*). Relating to the teeth and the alveolar process.

dento-alveolar abscess. An abscess affecting the tissues round the apex of a nonvital tooth root.

dentoalvoelitis (*den″-to-al-ve-ol-i′-tis*). Pyorrhoea alveolaris (*q.v.*).

dentocemental (*den′-to-sement′-al*). Dentinocemental (*q.v.*).

dento-facial (*den-to-fa′-shǐ-al*). Relating to that area of the face which contains and is supported by the teeth and gums.

dento-facial orthopaedics. Correction of dental and facial malformations.

dentography (*den-tog′-raf-ĭ*). A description of the teeth.

dentoid (*den′-toyd*). In the form of a tooth; tooth-like.

dentoidin (*den-toyd′-in*). The basic organic substance of a tooth.

dentolegal (*den″-to-le′-gal*). Relating to dental jurisprudence.

dentology (*dent-ol′-oj-ĭ*). Dentistry (*q.v.*).

dentoma (*dent-o′-mă*). A dentinal tumour; an odontoma.

dentomechanical (*den″-to-mek-an′-ik-al*). Relating to dental mechanics.

dentomental (*den″-to-men′-tal*). Relating to the teeth and the chin.

dentonasal (*den″-to-na′-zal*). Relating to the teeth and the nose.

dentonomy (*dent-on′-om-ĭ*). The classification of teeth.

dentosurgical (*den″-to-sur′-jik-al*). Relating to dental surgery.

dentotropic (*den″-to-tro′-pik*). Attracted to those tissues which compose the teeth.

dentulous (*dent′-yu-lus*). Having natural teeth present in the mouth; as opposed to *edentulous.*

dentural (*dent′-tyur-al*). Relating to a denture.

denture (*den′-tyur*). 1. A full set of natural teeth. 2. A set of artificial teeth.

artificial d. Any appliance designed to replace natural teeth.

continuous gum d. An obsolete form of denture constructed by fusing a porcelain base and teeth on to a platinum matrix.

full d. A denture which replaces all the teeth in either the upper or the lower jaw, or both.

immediate d. A denture constructed for insertion immediately after the removal of the natural teeth.

implant d. An artificial denture supported by a framework fastened to the alveolar process beneath the periosteum, and having protruding abutments.

partial d. A denture which replaces some of the natural teeth in one jaw.

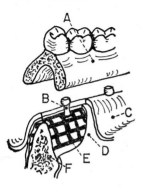

Implant denture

A Artificial denture.
B Supporting pillars.
C Gingiva.
D Periostium.
E Basket support.
F Alveolar bone.

skeleton d. A form of partial denture which is mainly tooth-borne, and which has connectors of the smallest size consistent with adequate strength, leaving the mucous membrane and the gingival margins exposed.

spoon d. A form of upper partial denture for the restoration of one or more anterior teeth, the teeth being attached to a plastic base plate which extends over the whole of the hard palate, but does not cover the gingival margins of the natural teeth.

denture, Every. *See* Every denture.

denture flange. The buccal, labial, or lingual vertical extension from the denture base into the oral cavity.

deossification (*de-os-if-ik-a'-shun*). The loss or removal of those materials which give bone its characteristics; the absorption of bony material.

depigmentation (*de-pigment-a'-shun*). The loss or removal of pigment.

deposit (*de-poz'-it*). 1. Sediment. 2. In dentistry, soft or hard material adhering to the tooth surface.

depression (*de-presh'-un*). 1. An indentation in a surface. 2. A general state of emotional dejection or unhappiness.

depressor muscles. *See* Table of Muscles.

dermal (*der'-mal*). Relating to the skin.

dermato-. Prefix signifying skin.

dermatostomatitis (*der"-mat-o-sto-mat-i'-tis*). Erythema multiforme with involvement of the conjunctiva and the oral tissues; Stevens-Johnson syndrome.

dermoid (*der'-moyd*). 1. Skin-like. 2. A dermoid cyst.

dermoid cyst. A congenital cystic tumour, containing

hair follicles, teeth, and sweat or sebaceous glands.

dermolabial (*der"-mo-la'-bĭ-al*). Relating to the skin and the lips.

descending cervical nerve. Ansa cervicalis (*q.v.*).

descending hypoglossal nerve. Ansa cervicalis (*q.v.*).

desiccation (*des-ik-a'-shun*). The process of drying.

desmoid (*des'-moyd*). 1. Resembling a ligament; fibrous. 2. A hard form of fibroma.

desquamation (*des-kwam-a'-shun*). Peeling off of the outer epithelial layer.

desquamative (*des-kwam'-at-iv*). Relating to desquamation.

detergent (*det-er'-jent*). Any drug used to cleanse or purify a wound, ulcer, etc.

detrital (*de-tri'-tal*). Relating to or composed of detritus.

detrition (*de-trish'-un*). Wearing away, as of teeth, by abrasion.

detritus (*det-ri'-tus*). 1. Any waste matter from disintegrated tissue. 2. In dentistry, waste matter adhering to a tooth surface or to disintegrated tooth substance.

detergent (*det-ur'-jent*). Relating to a detergent.

deuterocone (*dew'-ter-o-kōn*). The mesiobuccal cusp of a maxillary premolar in a mammal.

deuteroconid (*dew"-ter-o-kon'-id*). The mesiobuccal cusp of a mandibular premolar in a mammal.

deuteromere (*dew'-ter-o-mēr*). The lingual half of the enamel organ of a tooth.

developmental anomaly. An anomaly due to defective development.

developmental groove. One of the grooves in the enamel surface of a tooth, marking the divisions of primary formation.

deviation (*de-vi-a'-shun*). A turning away from a regular, normal course, position or standard.

devitalize (*de-vi'-tal-īz*). To destroy vitality; in dentistry, to destroy the vitality of the tooth pulp.

dexiotropic (*deks-ĭ-o-tro'-pik*). Relating to a clockwise spiral—i.e. one turning from left to right.

diagnosis (*di-ag-no'-sis*). The recognition of a disease or the location of an injury from observation of symptoms and signs.

diagnostic (*di-ag-nos'-tik*). Relating to diagnosis.

diaphanoscopy (*di-af-an-os'-kop-ĭ*). Transillumination (*q.v.*).

diaphragm (*di'-af-ram*). 1. In anatomy, a thin musculo-membranous partition or septum. 2. In dentistry, a thin metal plate adapted to form a cap over a tooth root and soldered to the collar of an artificial crown. *oral d.* The partition dividing the submandibular region from the sublingual, and formed by the hypoglossus and the mylohyoid muscles.

diaplasis (di-ă-pla'-sis). The reduction of a fracture or dislocation.

diaplastic (di-ă-plas'-tik). Relating to diaplasis.

diapyema (di"-ă-pi-e'-mă). An abscess (q.v.).

diapyesis (di-ă-pi-e'-sis). Suppuration (q.v.).

diarthrosis (di-arth-ro'-sis). A freely-movable joint.

diastema (di-as'-tem-ă). An abnormally wide space between two adjacent teeth.

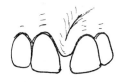

Diastema

diastematocheilia (di-as-tem"-at-o-ki'-li-ă). Congenital longitudinal fissure of the lip.

diastematoglossia (di-as-tem"-at-o-glos'-i-ă). Congenital longitudinal fissure of the tongue.

diastematognathia (di-as-tem"-at-o-na'-thi-ă). Congenital longitudinal fissure of the mandible.

diastole (di-as'-to-lă). The dilatation period in each heart beat, following the systole.

diastolic (di-as-tol'-ik). Relating to the diastole.

diathesis (di-ath'-es-is). An hereditary condition or combination of attributes predisposing a person to susceptibility to a certain disease or diseases.

diathetic (di-ath-et'-ik). Relating to diathesis.

diatoric (di-at-or'-ik). Referring to pinless teeth; artificial teeth which have pierced bases to allow rubber to flow in and so, when vulcanized, attach them to the base.

dicheilia (di-ki'-li-ă). Double lip (q.v.).

dichotomy (di-kot'-om-i). Division into two equal branches or parts.

die (di). A metal impression or mould from which casts or models can be made.

amalgam d. A model cast in amalgam from an impression and from which inlays or crowns may be fabricated.

die plate. A sheet of metal containing dies for forming cusps on a shell crown.

diet (di'-et). The nutritional intake of a person.

diffuse (dif-yūs'). Widespread, scattered.

digastric muscle. Raises and holds hyoid bone. *See* Table of Muscles—digastricus.

digestion (dij-est'-yun). The process whereby food is converted into materials for assimilation or absorption by the body.

diglossia (*di-glos'-ĭ-ă*). Double or bifid tongue; a developmental anomaly.

dilaceration (*di-las-er-a'-shun*). 1. Tearing apart. 2. In dentistry, a condition caused by damage or fracture of a tooth during development, resulting in distortion without interruption of the normal calcification.

dilatation (*di-la-ta'-shun*). The condition of being stretched, or enlarged beyond the normal size.

dilatator naris muscle. Assists in widening nostrils. *See* Table of Muscles.

diphtheria (*dif-the'-rĭ-ă*). An acute infectious disease characterized by the formation of patches of false membrane on mucous surfaces, especially of the throat and upper respiratory tract. *labial d.* A localized form of diphtheria in which membrane formation occurs on the outer edges of the lips; it has been noted as a complication of cheilosis.

diphyodont (*di-fi'-o-dont*). Having two successive sets of teeth, the first being deciduous, and giving place to the second, permanent dentition.

diplococcal (*dip-lo-kok'-al*). Relating to a diplococcus.

diplococcus (*dip-lo-kok'-us*). A form of micrococcus, which occurs attached in pairs.

Diplococcus (*dip-lo-kok'-us*). A genus of Lactobacteria-

ceae, parasitic and Grampositive, seen as elongated cells, growing in pairs or short chains.
D. pneumoniae. A species of *Diplococcus*, one of the causes of pneumonia, and of a variety of other infectious diseases; it is spherical, non-motile and Grampositive. *Also called* pneumococcus.

diploë (*dip'-lo-e*). The bony tissue between the tables of the cranial bones.

diploic (*dip-lo'-ik*). Relating to diploë.

diprotodont (*di-pro'-to-dont*). Having two incisors in the lower jaw.

direct retainer. An attachment or clasp on a partial denture which connects with the abutment tooth.

direct wiring. Immobilization of a jaw fracture by twisting wires round suitable teeth in both the upper and lower jaws and then joining the twisted ends of opposing upper and lower wires to help maintain the occlusion.

disc (*disk*). *In dentistry:* A round, solid ring of some material such as carborundum or emery, which can be revolved in the handpiece of a dental engine and is used for polishing, cutting, or grinding the teeth.
articular d. A fibrous plate between articulating bone surfaces in a joint.
suction d. A flexible disc attached to the fitting surface

of an upper denture in an attempt to improve its retention. This method is no longer used.

discharge (*dis-charj'*). An emission or secretion.

disclosing solution. A type of staining solution used to stain and disclose bacterial plaques or calculus on the teeth.

discoid (*dis'-koyd*). 1. In the shape of a disc. 2. In dentistry, an excavator having a disc-like blade. 3. A disc-shaped tablet.

discrete (*dis-krēt'*). Separate, composed of separate parts, not joined or blended; as, for example, some lesions.

disease (*diz-ēz'*). Any illness or abnormal state of health either of the whole body or of specific parts of organs, having characteristic symptoms. *See also* syndrome.
congenital d. A disease which is present at birth.
contagious d. A disease which is communicated by direct contact with an affected person, with any object with which such a person has been in contact, or with his secretions.
deficiency d. Any disease caused by absence or shortage of some element vital to bodily health.
degenerative d. A process of general degeneration with no specific cause, commonly found in old age.
infectious d. A disease caused by pathogenic organisms.

For eponymous diseases *see* under the personal name by which the disease is known.

disinfectant (*dis-in-fek'-tant*). Any agent which destroys pathogenic organisms.

disinfection (*dis-in-fek'-shun*). The destruction of pathogenic organisms and their products.

disintegration (*dis-in-teg-ra'-shun*). Decay or decomposition.

disk. *See* disc.

dislocation (*dis-lo-ka'-shun*). Displacement of any part from its normal position; commonly used of bones and joints.

disocclude (*dis-ok-lūd'*). To grind the occlusal surface of a tooth so that it does not ever occlude with the opposing tooth in the other jaw during mastication.

displacement (*dis-plās'-ment*). 1. Removal from the normal position. 2. In dentistry, the malposition of a tooth, or teeth, where the whole tooth has moved in the same direction, without tilting.

disseminated (*dis-sem'-in-a-ted*). Dispersed or scattered over a wide area.

distal (*dis'-tal*). Away from the midline; in dentistry, those surfaces farthest from the mid-line of the dental arch.

distal angle. *In dentistry*: Any angle formed by the junction of a distal surface of a tooth or cavity wall with any other tooth surface or cavity wall.

distal occlusion. A term denoting the position of a tooth which is distal to the normal position in occlusion.

distal wall. That wall of a tooth cavity which faces the distal surface of the tooth.

disto-. Prefix signifying *distal.*

disto-angular (*dis″-to-an′-gu-lar*). Relating to any distal angle.

distobuccal (*dis″-to-buk′-al*). 1. Relating to the distal and buccal surfaces of a tooth. 2. Relating to the distal and buccal walls of an occlusal cavity in a molar or premolar.
d. angle. The angle formed at the junction of these walls; a *line* angle.

distobucco-occlusal (*dis″-to-buk-o-ok-lu′-zal*). Relating to the distal, buccal and occlusal surfaces of a tooth.

distobuccopulpal (*dis″-to-buk″-o-pul′-pal*). Relating to the distal, buccal and pulpal walls in an occlusal cavity, or in the step portion of a proximo-occlusal cavity, in a molar or premolar.
d. angle. The angle formed at the junction of these walls; a *point* angle.

distocclusal (*dis″-tok-lu′-zal*). Disto-occlusal (*q.v.*).

distocclusion (*dis-tok-lu′-shun*). A form of malocclusion in which the teeth of the lower jaw are displaced distally in relation to those in the upper jaw.

distocervical (*dis″-to-ser-vi′-kal*). Distogingival (*q.v.*).

distogingival (*dis″-to-jin′-jiv-al*). Relating to the distal and gingival walls of a buccal or lingual cavity in a molar or premolar.
d. angle. The angle formed at the junction of these walls; a *line* angle.

disto-incisal (*dis″-to-in-si′-zal*). 1. Relating to the distal surface and the incisal edge of an anterior tooth. 2. Relating to the distal and incisal walls in a labial or lingual cavity.
d. angle. The angle formed at the junction of these walls; a *line* angle.

distolabial (*dis″-to-la′-bi-al*). 1. Relating to the distal and labial surfaces of a tooth. 2. Relating to the distal and labial walls in the step portion of a proximo-incisal cavity.
d. angle. The angle formed at the junction of these walls; a *line* angle.

distolabioincisal (*dis″-to-la″-bi-o-in-si′-zal*). Relating to the distal and labial surfaces and the incisal edge of an anterior tooth.

distolingual (*dis″-to-lin′-gwal*). 1. Relating to the distal and lingual surfaces of a tooth. 2. Relating to the distal and lingual walls of an occlusal cavity in a molar or premolar.
d. angle. The angle formed at the junction of these walls; a *line* angle.

distolinguoocclusal (*dis″-to-lin-gwok-lu′-zal*). Disto-linguo-occlusal (*q.v.*).

distolinguoincisal (*dis″-to-lin″-gwo-in-si′-zal*). Relating to the distal and lingual surfaces and the incisal edge of an anterior tooth.

distolinguo-occlusal (*dis″-to-lin-gwo-ok-lu′-zal*). Relating to the distal, lingual and occlusal surfaces of a tooth.

distolinguopulpal (*dis″-to-lin″-gwo-pul′-pal*). Relating to the distal, lingual and pulpal walls of an occlusal cavity, or in the step portion of a proximo-occlusal cavity in a molar or premolar.
d. angle. The angle formed at the junction of these walls; a *point* angle.

distomolar (*dis-to-mo′-lar*). A small supernumerary tooth which may erupt behind the molar teeth.

disto-occlusal (*dis″-to-ok-lu′-zal*). 1. Relating to the distal and occlusal surface of a tooth. 2. Relating to the distal and occlusal walls in a buccal or lingual cavity.
d. angle. The angle formed at the junction of these walls; a *line* angle.

distoplacement (*dis-to-plās′-ment*). Distal displacement of a tooth or teeth.

distopulpal (*dis″-to-pul′-pal*). Relating to the distal and pulpal walls of an occlusal cavity, or in the step portion of a proximo-occlusal cavity in a molar or premolar.
d. angle. The angle formed at the junction of these walls; a *line* angle.

distopulpolabial (*dis″-to-pul″-po-la′-bi-al*). Relating to the distal, pulpal and labial walls of a cavity in an incisor or a canine.
d. angle. The angle formed at the junction of these walls; a *point* angle.

distopulpolingual (*dis″-to-pul″-po-lin′-gwal*). Relating to the distal, pulpal and lingual walls of a tooth cavity.
d. angle. The angle formed at the junction of these walls; a *point* angle.

distortor oris muscle. M. zygomaticus minor. *See* Table of Muscles.

distoversion (*dis-to-ver′-shun*). The position of a tooth which is inclined away from the median line.

Dodge crown. A porcelain crown baked to a hollow metal cone and attached to the tooth by a wooden post.

dolicho-. Prefix signifying *long*.

dolichocephalic (*dol″-ik-o-sef-al′-ik*). Having an abnormally long skull.

dolichocranial (*dol″-ik-o-kra′-nĭ-al*.) Dolichocephalic (*q.v.*).

dolichoeuromesocephalic (*dol″-ik-o-yu″-ro-me″-so-sef-al′-ik*). Having an abnormally long skull which is also very broad in the temporal region.

dolichoeuro-opisthoce-phalic (*dol″-ik-o-yu″-ro-op-is″-tho-sef-al′-ik*). Having an abnormally long skull which is also very broad in the occipital region.

dolichoeuroprocephalic (*dol″-ik-o-yu″-ro-pros-ef-al′-ik*). Having an abnormally long skull which is also very broad in the frontal region.

dolichofacial (*dol″-ik-o-fa′-shi-al*). Having an abnormally long face.

dolicholeptocephalic (*dol″-ik-o-lep″-to-sef-al′-ik*). Having an abnormally long and narrow skull.

dolichoplatycephalic (*dol″-ik-o-plat″-i-sef-al′-ik*). Having an abnormally long and broad flat skull.

dolichoprosopic (*dol″-ik-o-pros-op′-ik*). Dolichofacial (*q.v.*).

dolichouranic (*dol″-ik-o-yur-an′-ik*). Having an abnormally long palate, with a palato-maxillary index of less than 110.

dolorimetry (*dol-or-im′-et-ri*). The measurement of pain.

dolorogenic (*dol-or-o-jen′-ik*). Pain-producing.

Donaldson broach (R. B. Donaldson, contemporary American dentist). A fine, barbed broach used particularly for removing the contents of pulp canals.

dormant (*dor′-mant*). 1. Inactive, quiescent. 2. Potential, concealed.

dorsal (*dor′-sal*). Relating to the dorsum.

dorsalis linguae artery. Supplies the dorsum of the tongue, tonsils and fauces. *See* Table of Arteries.

dorsalis nasi artery. Supplies the skin of the dorsum of the nose. *See* Table of Arteries.

dorsonasal (*dor″-so-na′-zal*). Relating to the bridge of the nose.

dorso-ventral (*dor″-so-ven′-tral*). From the front to the back.

dorsum (*dor′-sum*). The back of any organ.

dose (*dōs*). One measured portion of any medicine, which is to be taken at one time.

double lip. Superfluous tissue and mucous membrane occurring below the red margin of the lips.

dovetail (*duv′-tāl*). A flared cavity, like the spread of a dove's tail, serving as a lock in a metal or wooden joint; in dentistry it is applied to the flared cavity which serves to lock a filling or inlay in place in a tooth.

dowel (*dow′-el*). Post (*q.v.*).

drainage (*drān′-ej*). The gradual removal of fluid from a cavity or wound.

dressing (*dres′-ing*). 1. A medicament used to promote wound healing. 2. A covering for a wound used for protection or to assist healing. 3. In dentistry, a temporary filling or restoration.

drift (*drift*). The horizontal movement or displacement of a tooth.

drifting *of the teeth.* Movement of the teeth within the arch.

drill (*dril*). An instrument with spiral flukes used in a dental engine for boring or cutting holes in a tooth or in bone.

drop, enamel. Enameloma (*q.v.*).

dropsy (*drop'-si*). The abnormal accumulation of serous fluid in the tissues or in the body cavities.

drug (*drug*). Any medicinal substance. For drugs used in dentistry *see* Appendix.

dry abscess. An abscess which disperses without bursting or coming to a head.

dry socket. An acute inflammatory condition of the walls of a tooth socket following the extraction of a tooth; alveolalgia.

duct (*dukt*). A tube or canal serving as an outlet for secretion; used especially of glandular outlets.
nasolacrimal d. The membranous canal through which tears pass from the lacrimal sac to the nasal cavity.
sublingual d. One of the ducts of the sublingual gland; Bartholin's duct.
submaxillary d. Wharton's duct (*q.v.*).
thyroglossal d. A duct extending from the thyroid gland to the base of the tongue; found in the embryo and occasionally persisting into adult life.

For eponymous ducts *see* under the name of the person first describing the duct.

Dutch gold. An alloy of zinc and copper.

dwarfed enamel. Nanoid enamel (*q.v.*).

dwarfism (*dwarf'-izm*). The condition of being a dwarf; underdevelopment of the body.

dys-. Prefix signifying *difficult, painful.*

dysallilognathia (*dis''-al-il-o-na'-thi-ă*). The condition of having dissimilar, not matching, jaws.

dysfunction (*dis-funk'-shun*). Impairment or abnormality of function.

dysgnathic (*dis-na'-thik*). Relating to imperfectly developed and malrelated jaws.

dysjunction (*dis-junk'-shun*). Non-union.
craniofacial d. Le Fort fracture of the maxilla, Class III (*q.v.*).

dyslalia (*dis-la'-li-ă*). Impairment of speech due to some abnormality of the speech organs.

dysodontiasis (*dis-o-don-ti'-as-is*). Painful, difficult or delayed eruption of the teeth.

dysosteogenesis (*dis-os-te-o-jen'-es-is*). Dysostosis (*q.v.*).

dysostosis (*dis-os-to'-sis*). Congenital defective bone formation.
cleidocranial d. A rare form of dysostosis characterized by defective formation of the cranial bones and partial

or complete absence of the clavicles; eruption of the teeth is often affected, and there may be partial anodontia.

mandibulo-facial d. A rare congenital malformation of the face and jaws, characterized by hypoplasia of the facial bones, anti-mongoloid slanting of the lower eyelids, deformity of the pinna, macrostomia and a general fish-like facies.

dysphagia (*dis-fa'-ji-ă*). Difficulty in swallowing.

dysplasia (*dis-pla'-zi-ă*). Abnormal formation or development.

dyspnoea (*dis-pne'-ă*). Laboured breathing; shortness of breath.

dyspnoeic (*dis-pne'-ik*). Relating to or characterized by dyspnoea.

dystrophic (*dis'-trof-ik*). Relating to or affected by dystrophy.

dystrophy (*dis'-trof-ĭ*). Defective nutrition.

E

e-. Prefix signifying *from, out of, without.*

ext. Abbreviation for *extract.*

ear (*ĕr*). The organ of hearing.

Ebner's fibrils (V. von Ebner, 1842-1925. Austrian histologist). Connective tissue fibres pervading the dentinal matrix.

Ebner's glands (V. von Ebner, 1842-1925. Austrian histologist). Serous lingual glands.

ebur dentis. Dentine (*q.v.*).

eburnation (*e-bur-na'-shun*). An increase in hardness or density of tooth or bone structure following a pathologic change.

eburneous (*e-bur'-nĕ-us*). Like ivory.

eccentric (*ek-sen'-trik*). Situated away from a centre.

eccentric occlusion. The occlusion of the teeth with the mandible in any position other than that of rest.

ecchymosis (*ek-im-o'-sis*). A diffuse extravasation of blood into the tissues; also discoloration of the skin which this causes.

ecderon (*ek'-der-on*). The outer layer of the mucous membrane and the skin.

eclabium (*ek-la'-bi-um*). Eversion of a lip, or lips.

ecto-. Prefix signifying *outside,* or *on.*

ectoderm (*ek'-to-derm*). The outermost of the three primary germ layers of the embryo, from which are developed the epidermis, the external sense organs, and the oral and anal mucous membrane.

ectoloph (*ek'-to-lōf*). The outer ridge on an equine upper molar.

ectopic (*ek-top'-ik*). In an abnormal place or position.

ectosteal (*ek-tos'-tĕ-al*). Relating to, or situated on, the outside of a bone.

ectropion (*ek-tro'-pi-on*). Eversion (*q.v.*).

edema. *See* oedema.

edentate (*e-den'-tāt*). Edentulous (*q.v.*).

edentia (*e-den'-shĭ-ă*). Anodontia (*q.v.*).

edentulous (*e-dent'-yu-lus*). Having no teeth.

edge-to-edge bite. A form of malocclusion in which the anterior teeth occlude

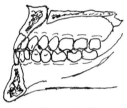

Edge-to-edge bite

along the incisal edges and do not overlap.

efferent (*ef'-er-ent*). Carrying or conveying away from a centre or from a part; as opposed to *afferent*.

efferent nerve. Any nerve carrying impulses from the centre to the periphery.

Ehrenritter's ganglion (J. Ehrenritter, d. 1790. Austrian anatomist). The superior ganglion of the glossopharyngeal nerve, in the jugular foramen.

eisanthema (*i-zan'-them-ă*). Enanthema (*q.v.*).

electro-. Prefix signifying *electricity*.

electrocautery (*el-ek''-tro-kav'-ter-ĭ*). 1. Cauterization by low voltage current producing burn-like tissue repair, but with no control over the extent or quality of tissue destruction. 2. The apparatus used for this purpose.

electrocision (*el-ek''-tro-sizh'-un*). The cutting of tissues by electrocautery or electrotome.

electrocoagulation (*el-ek''-tro-ko-ag-yu-la'-shun*). Biterminal application of damped high frequency alternating current dehydrating cells and coagulating their contents in a necrotic zone limited to the surface of the area to which it is applied; as, for example, in haemostasis.

electrodent (*el-ek'-tro-dent*). The negative electrode on a vitalometer (*q.v.*).

electrodesiccation (*el-ek''-tro-des-ik-a'-shun*). Deeply penetrating tissue dehydration produced by the insertion of electrodes into the tissue.

electroresection (*el-ek''-tro-re-sek'-shun*). Excision by electrosurgery.

electrosection (*el-ek''-tro-sek'-shun*). Biterminal application of undamped high frequency alternating current used with a surgical electrode moved along the tissue surface to create precise surgical incisions.

electrosurgery (*el-ek''-tro-sur'-jer-ĭ*). High frequency alternating current used for dehydration, coagulation and sectioning of tissues; able to be controlled in use.

elephantiasis gingivae (el-ef-ant-i'-as-is jin'-jiv-e). Abnormally large gums, a comparatively rare hereditary condition, with characteristic fibrosis of the gingivae; macrogingivae.

elevator (el'-ev-a-tor). An instrument used as a lever to remove sunken or embedded parts or particles; in dentistry, an instrument used to remove tooth roots.

Cryer's e. One of a pair of elevators for removing molar roots, one for the distal and one for the mesial, being reversible for opposite sides of the jaw.

screw e. An instrument which can be screwed into a retained root in order to draw it out.

Winter's e. An elevator for removing lower third molars.

elinguation (e-lin-gwa'-shun). Removal of the tongue.

elongation (e-long-a'-shun). 1. The process of becoming longer. 2. The condition of being lengthened.

emaciation (em-a-si-a'-shun). A wasted condition; the result of extreme loss of flesh.

emaculation (e-mak-yu-la'-shun). The removal of skin lesions and freckles, and more particularly of skin tumours.

emailloblast (em-al'-o-blast). Ameloblast (q.v.).

emailloid (em-a-a'-loyd). A tumour arising from the tooth enamel.

embed (em-bed'). In histology, to fix tissue in some rigid material, such as wax, in order to cut thin sections for microscope study.

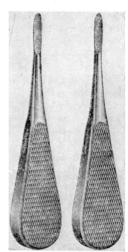

Elevator

embolism (em'-bol-izm). The sudden blockage of a blood vessel by a clot or other obstruction within the blood stream, causing failure of the circulation.

embolus (em'-bol-us). An obstruction or clot in the blood stream blocking a vessel and so restricting or stopping the circulation.

embrasure (*em-bra'-zhur*). The space on each side of the contact point, created by the rounding of the proximal surfaces away from each other.

buccal e. The space between molars or premolars, opening towards the cheek.

labial e. The space between incisors or canines, opening towards the lip.

lingual e. The space between any teeth, opening towards the tongue.

embryo (*em'-bri-o*). The fertilized ovum during the early stage of development; in man it is the foetus in the first three months of growth.

embryology (*em-bri-ol'-oj-i*). The science and study of the embryo and of its development.

embryonal cell. One of the developmental cells.

embryonic (*em-bri-on'-ik*). Relating to an embryo; in an early stage of development.

eminence (*em'-in-ens*). A prominent or projecting part, especially one on a bone surface.

canine e. The ridge on the anterior surface of the maxilla, occurring over the canine tooth.

hypobranchial e. A median swelling between the tongue and the laryngo-tracheal groove in the embryo, from which is developed the epiglottis and the aryepiglottic folds, and the posterior third of the tongue.

emollient (*em-ol'-i-ent*).
1. Soothing or softening.
2. Any agent used to soften or soothe the skin, or to soothe an irritated or inflamed internal surface.

emphragma salivare. Ranula (*q.v.*).

emphysema (*em"-fi-zem'-ă*). A distention caused by air in the interstices of the connective tissues, or of the alveolar tissue of the lungs.

empyema (*em-pi-e'-mă*). The accumulation of pus in a body cavity or hollow organ.

enamel (*en-am'-el*). Vitreous calcific tissue covering the dentine of the tooth crown.

curled e. Enamel in which the prismatic rods are curled round.

dwarfed e. Nanoid enamel (*q.v.*)

gnarled e. Enamel in which the prismatic rods are twisted in various directions.

mottled e. Hypoplasia and discoloration of the tooth enamel due to ingestion of excessive amounts of fluorine during the developmental period; chronic endemic (dental) fluorosis.

nanoid e. Enamel which is thinner than normal.

straight e. Enamel in which the prismatic rods run straight.

enamel cap. The enamel covering the top of a developing tooth papilla.

enamel capsule. Primary enamel cuticle (*q.v.*).

enamel cell. Ameloblast (*q.v.*).

enamel cord. A temporary structure in the developing tooth linking the enamel knot to the outer dental lamina.

enamel cuticle. 1. Primary enamel cuticle (q.v.). 2. Acquired pellicle (q.v.).

enamel cuticle, acquired. Acquired pellicle (q.v.).

enamel cuticle, primary. An acellular layer of organic material attached to the surface of enamel; it is thought to be the final product of ameloblasts.

enamel drop. Enameloma (q.v.).

enamel epithelium, reduced. A cellular layer, the remnants of the enamel organ, attached to the enamel surface of a tooth on eruption.

enamel epithelium, united. Reduced enamel epithelium (q.v.).

enamel fibre. Enamel prism (q.v.).

enamel hatchet. A type of chisel with a contra-angled shaft giving it a hatchet form.

enamel knot. An aggregation of epithelial cells at the base of the enamel organ, which have not yet been differentiated into stellate reticulum.

enamel lamellae. The flat, organic bands running transversely through the enamel of a tooth.

enamel organ. A proliferation of the dental lamina enclosing the dental papilla; it determines the shape of the tooth crown and forms the dental enamel.

enamel pearl. Enameloma (q.v.).

enamel prism. One of the prismatic rods of which tooth enamel is made up.

enamel pulp. The stellate reticulum (q.v.).

enamel rod. Enamel prism (q.v.).

enamel tufts. Bundles of poorly calcified enamel rods extending into the tooth enamel from the amelo-dentinal junction.

enameloblast (en-am″-el-o-blast). Ameloblast (q.v.).

enameloblastoma (en-am″-el-o-blast-o′-mǎ). Adamantinoma (q.v.).

enameloma (en-am-el-o′-mǎ). A benign tumour arising from embryonic enamel tissue.

enanthema, enanthem (en-an-the′-mǎ). An eruption occurring on a mucous surface, or on any surface within the body; as opposed to exanthema (q.v.).

encapsulated (en-kap′-su-la-ted). Enclosed in a capsule.

end to end bite. Edge-to-edge bite (q.v.).

Endamoeba (end-am-e′-bǎ). A genus of amoeba, including species parasitic to man. E. buccalis. Endamoeba gingivalis (q.v.). E. gingivalis. A species found about the gums and in the tartar on the teeth.

endemic (en-dem′-ik). Prevalent in a particular reigon.

endermic (*en-der-'mik*). Absorbed through the skin.

endermatic (*en-der-mat'-ik*). Endermic (q.v.).

endo-. Prefix signifying *within*.

endocarditis (*en-do-kar-di'-tis*). Inflammation of the endocardium, the lining of the interior of the heart, generally affecting the valves. *subacute bacterial e.* A type caused by *Streptococcus viridans*, and having a prolonged course.

endochondral (*en-do-kon'-dral*). Within a cartilage; developing in cartilage.

endocrine gland. Any one of the ductless glands—adrenal, thyroid, etc.—supplying internal secretions to the body directly through the blood stream.

endocrinodontia (*en-do-krin-o-don'-shi-ă*). The study of internal glandular secretion in relation to tooth development.

endododontics, endodontia (*en-do-don'-tiks*). The study and treatment of diseases affecting the tooth pulp and the root canal.

endodontitis (*en-do-don-ti'-tis*). Inflammation of the tooth pulp; *also called* pulpitis.

endogenous (*en-doj'-en-us*). Arising or developing within an organism.

endognathion (*en-do-na'-thi-on*). The hypothetical inner portion of the premaxilla.

endolymph (*en'-do-limf*). The liquid in the membranous labrynth of the ear.

endolymphatic (*en-do-lim-fat'-ik*). Relating to the endolymph.

endothelial (*en-do-the'-li-al*). Relating to, or derived from, the endothelium.

endothelioma (*en-do-the-li-o'-mă*). A tumour arising from the endothelial cells.

endothelium (*en-do-the'-li-um*). The membrane which lines the heart and blood vessels.

enervation (*en-er-va'-shun*). Removal of a nerve or of part of a nerve.

engine (*en'-jin*).
dental e. The apparatus which is used to drive instruments for cutting, drilling and polishing the teeth; the interchangeable parts are held in an angled handpiece, and the driving power is supplied by some form of motor.

engomphosis (*en-gom-fo'-sis*). Gomphosis (q.v.).

engorgement (*en-gorj'-ment*). 1. Excess of blood in any part of the body. 2. Localized congestion or distention.

enostosis (*en-os-to'-sis*). A localized morbid bone growth arising within the bone cavity.

Entamoeba. See Endamoeba.

Enterobacteriaceae (*en"-ter-o-bak-te-ri-a'-se-e*). A family of micro-organisms of the order Eubacteriales.

enthlasis (en'-thlas-is). A depressed and comminuted fracture of the skull.

ento-. Prefix signifying *inside, within*.

entocone (en'-to-kōn). The lingual posterior cusp of a maxillary molar.

entoconid (en-to-ko'-nid). The lingual posterior cusp of a mandibular molar.

entoglossal (en-to-glos'-al). Occurring within the tongue.

entomion (en-to'-mi-on). The point at the tip of the mastoid angle of the parietal bone where it crosses the parietal notch of the temporal bone.

entopic (en-top'-ik). Occurring in the normal position.

entostosis (ent-os-to'-sis). Enostosis (q.v.).

enucleate (e-nyu'-kle-āt). To remove an organ or part, or a circumscribed, space-filling lesion entire from its outer sheath or covering.

enula (en'-yu-lä). The inner aspect of the gums.

envelope (en'-vel-ōp). 1. Any outer covering. 2. A surrounding membrane or capsule.

epactal (e-pak'-tal). Supernumerary.

ephemeral (e-fem'-er-al). Of short duration, temporary.

epi-. Prefix signifying *upon* or *above*.

epiagnathus (ep-i-ag'-nath-us). One having a deficient upper jaw.

epicranial aponeurosis (ep-i-kra'-ni-al ap-o-nyu-ro'-sis). The galea aponeurotica (q.v.).

epicranius muscle. Muscular cover of the scalp. *See* Table of Muscles.

epidemic (ep-i-dem'-ik). 1. Affecting a large number of people within an area or a region. 2. A period during which some particular disease is so affecting many people.

epidemiology (ep-i-de-mi-ol'-oj-i). That branch of science concerned with the study of a disease or condition through its frequency and distribution.

epidermis (ep-i-der'-mis). Cuticle; the outer layer of the skin.

epidermoid (ep-i-der'-moyd). 1. Resembling the dermis. 2. An epidermoid carcinoma (q.v.).

epidermoid carcinoma. A form of carcinoma derived from the stratified squamous epithelium; it can be differentiated into various types.

epiglottis (ep-i-glot'-is). Fibrocartilage behind the base of the tongue covering the opening at the upper part of the larynx.

epimandibular (ep'-i-man-dib'-yu-lar). Upon the mandible.

epipharynx (ep-i-far'-inks). Nasopharynx (q.v.).

episcleral artery. Branch of the anterior ciliary, joining the greater arterial circle of the iris. *See* Table of Arteries—episcleralis.

epistaxis (*ep-ĭ-stak'-sĭs*). Nosebleed.

epistropheus (*ep-ĭ-stro'-fĕ-us*). The second cervical vertebra, the axis.

epithelial (*ep-ĭ-the'-lĭ-al*). Relating to the epithelium.

epithelial attachment. The epithelium at the base of the gingival crevice or periodontal pocket, lying in close proximity to the tooth surface and "attaching" the gingiva to the tooth. It is thought to originate from the cells of the reduced enamel epithelium.

epithelial attachment cells. Reduced enamel epithelium (*q.v.*).

epithelial cell. One of the cells which make up the epithelium.

epithelial pearls, Bohn's. Epstein's pearls (*q.v.*).

epithelioid (*ep-ĭ-the'-lĭ-oyd*). Resembling epithelium.

epithelioma (*ep-ĭ-the-lĭ-o'-mă*). Any tumour derived from the epithelium, or composed of epithelial cells.

epithelium (*ep-ĭ-the'-lĭ-um*). A thin cellular layer covering or lining the organs and tissues of the body.
inner zone e. Reduced enamel epithelium (*q.v.*).
reduced dental e. Reduced enamel epithelium (*q.v.*).
reduced enamel e. A cellular layer, the remnants of the enamel organ, attached to the enamel surface of a tooth on eruption.
united enamel e. Reduced enamel epithelium (*q.v.*).

epitympanic (*ep-ĭ-tim-pan'-ik*). Above the tympanum.

eponym (*ep'-on-im*). The name of an organ, syndrome, disease, etc., which contains or is derived from a proper name; *e.g.* Bartholin's duct.

eponymous (*ep-on'-im-us*). Relating to an eponym.

epostoma (*ep-os-to'-mă*). Exostosis (*q.v.*).

Epstein's pearls (A. Epstein, 1849-1918. Bohemian paediatrician). Small, slightly elevated yellowish-white masses seen on either side of the median line of the hard palate at birth.

epulis (*ep'-yu-lis*). Any tumour of the gums; more especially either a fibrous or a giant-cell tumour.
congenital e. A granular cell tumour which develops *in utero.*
fibrous e. An inflammatory pedunculated overgrowth of gum tissue; probably not a true tumour.
pregnancy e. A form of epulis developing during or as a result of pregnancy.

epulofibroma (*ep"-yu-lo-fi-bro'-mă*). A fibroma affecting the gums.

epuloid (*ep'-yu-loyd*). Resembling an epulis.

equation, Hanau's. See Hanau's equation.

equilibration (*ek-wil-ib-ra'-shun*). The maintenance or restoration of equilibrium.
occlusal e. The restoration of normal occlusion within the mouth by mechanical means.

equilibrium (*ek-wil-ib'-ri-um*). A state of equal balance or counteraction.

erode (*er-ōd'*). To wear away, producing erosion.

erosion (*er-o'-zhun*). The wearing away of a tooth surface due to chemical or abrasive action.

erosive (*er-o'-ziv*). 1. Relating to erosion. 2. Relating to a substance which tends to erode a surface.

eruption (*er-up'-shun*). 1. The act of appearing, or pushing through, as of teeth coming through the gums. 2. A visible skin lesion, occurring in disease.

eruption cyst. A cyst occurring about the crown of an erupting tooth.

eruptive (*er-up'-tiv*). Relating to or characterized by an eruption.

erythema (*er-ith-e'-mă*). Redness of the skin, either diffuse or patchy, caused by congestion of the subcutaneous capillaries.

erythema migrans linguae. Geographic tongue (*q.v.*).

erythrodontia (*er-ith-ro-don'-shi-ă*). The condition of having a reddish brown stain on the teeth.

erythroplasia of Queyrat. See Queyrat's erythroplasia.

eschar (*es'-kar*). A dry slough, the result of burning or contact with a corrosive agent.

escharotic (*es-kar-ot'-ik*). 1. Caustic or corrosive; producing an eschar. 2. A caustic or corrosive substance.

Esmarch's operation (J. F. A. Esmarch, 1823-1908. German surgeon). Surgical treatment of temporo-mandibular ankylosis by mandibular osteotomy.

esophagus. See oesophagus.

esosphenoiditis (*es'-o-sfe-noyd-i'-tis*). Osteomyelitis affecting the sphenoid bone.

esquillectomy (*es-kwil-ek'-tom-i*). The surgical removal of bone fragments after a fracture caused by a projectile.

ethmocranial (*eth-mo-kra'-ni-al*). Relating to the ethmoid bone and skull.

ethmofrontal (*eth-mo-fron'-tal*). Relating to the ethmoid and frontal bones.

ethmoid (*eth'-moyd*). 1. Sievelike; cribriform. 2. Relating to the ethmoid bone.

ethmoid artery. Supplies the dura mater, frontal and ethmoidal sinuses; two branches: anterior and posterior. See Table of Arteries—ethmoidalis.

ethmoid bone. A perforated bone forming the roof of the nasal fossae and part of the floor of the anterior fossa of the skull.

ethmoid canals. Canals between the ethmoid and frontal bones, through which pass the posterior ethmoid and the nasociliary nerves and the ethmoid vessels.

ethmoid foramen, anterior. A canal between the ethmoid and frontal bones, through which pass the nasal branch of the ophthalmic nerve and the anterior ethmoid vessels.

ethmoid nerve. Supplies the mucosa of the ethmoid sinuses and of the nasal cavity. *See* Table of Nerves —ethmoidalis.

ethmoid process. A projection from the upper border of the inferior nasal concha.

ethmoidal notch. The space between the orbital plates of the frontal bone, which, in an articulated skull, contains the cribriform plate of the ethmoid bone.

ethmoidal sinus. One of the many small intercommunicating cavities forming the labyrinth of the ethmoid bone, opening into the nasal cavity.

ethmolacrimal (*eth-mo-lak′-rim-al*). Relating to the ethmoid and the lacrimal bones.

ethmomaxillary (*eth″-mo-maks-il′-ar-i*). Relating to the ethmoid bone and the maxilla.

ethmopalatal (*eth″-mo-pal-a′-tal*). Relating to the ethmoid bone and the palate.

ethmosphenoidal (*eth-mo-sfe-noyd′-al*). Relating to the ethmoid and the sphenoid bones.

ethmovomerine (*eth-mo-vo′-mer-in*). Relating to the ethmoid bone and the vomer.

etiology. *See* aetiology.

Eubacteriales (*yu″-bak-te-ri-a′-lez*). True bacteria; an

order of the class Schizomycetes.

eugnathic (*yu-na′-thik*). Relating to well-developed jaws.

eurodontia (*yur-o-don′-shi-ă*). Old term for dental caries.

eurycephalic (*yu-ri-sef-al′-ik*). Having an abnormally wide skull.

eurycranial (*yu-ri-kra′-ni-al*). Eurycephalic (*q.v.*).

eurygnathic (*yur-ig-nath′-ik*). Having a broad jaw.

eurygnathism (*yur-ig′-nath-izm*). The condition of having an unusually broad jaw.

euryon (*yur′-i-on*). One of two points on the skull at either end of its greatest transverse diameter.

euryprosopic (*yu-ri-pros-o′-pik*). Having an abnormally wide face.

Eustachian tube. Pharyngotympanic tube (*q.v.*).

evagination (*e-vaj-in-a′-shun*). Protrusion from a sheath or outer covering.

evanescent (*ev-an-es′-ent*). Disappearing quickly; unstable.

Evans gold crown (G. Evans, fl. 1888. American dentist). An all-gold seamless crown contoured to the anatomical form of the natural tooth.

evaporation (*e-vap-or-a′-shun*). The conversion of a solid or a liquid substance into vapour.

eversion (*e-ver′-shun*). A turning outwards, or a state of being turned outwards.

Every denture (R. G. Every, contemporary New Zealand dental surgeon). An upper partial denture designed in such a way that, apart from the occlusion, the only contact made with the natural teeth is at their contact points; the denture base is extended to make contact with the distal surface of the most posterior tooth in the arch.

ex-. Prefix signifying *without, beyond, from, out of.*

exacerbation (*eks-as-er-ba'-shun*). An increase in the severity of a disease, or of any symptoms.

examination (*eks-am-in-a'-shun*). Investigation for diagnostic purposes.

exanthema, exanthem (*eks-an-the'-mă*). 1. A skin eruption. 2. Any eruptive fever.

exanthematous (*eks-an-the'-mat-us*). Relating to an exanthema.

excavation (*eks-kav-a'-shun*). 1. A hollow or cavity. 2. The process of cutting such a cavity. 3. In dentistry, the cavity prepared in a tooth, in which is placed a filling or inlay; also the process of preparing such a cavity.

excavator (*eks'-kav-a-tor*). A hand instrument used in dentistry for excavation and removal of caries.

excementosis (*eks-se-men-to'-sis*). Hypercementosis (*q.v.*).

excise (*eks-sīz'*). To cut out, or to remove by surgery.

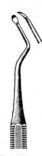

Excavator

excision (*eks-sĭ'-zhun*). Removal of any part by cutting.

excochleation (*eks″-kok-le-a'-shun*). The operation of curetting a cavity or scooping out foreign or diseased matter.

excoriation (*eks-kor-ĭ-a'-shun*). Superficial loss of surface skin.

excrete (*eks-krēt'*). To expel waste material from the body.

excretion (*eks-kre'-shun*). 1. The process by which waste matter is expelled from the body. 2. The matter thus expelled.

exelcymosis (*eks-el-sim-o'-sis*). Extraction (*q.v.*).

exesion (*esk-e'-zhun*). The gradual eating away of superficial tissue or of bone as in an ulcerative condition.

exfoliation (eks-fo-lĭ-a'-shun). A peeling off in layers or in scales.

exfoliative (eks-fo'-lĭ-at-iv). Relating to, or causing, exfoliation.

exfoliative cytology. The examination of cells shed from a body surface.

exfoliato areata linguae. Geographic tongue (q.v.).

exodontia (eks-o-don'-shi-ă). Tooth extraction.

exodontics (eks-o-don'-tiks). Exodontia (q.v.).

exodontist (eks-o-don'-tist). One who specializes in the extraction of teeth.

exodontosis (eks"-o-dont-o'-sis). Exostosis affecting the root of a tooth.

exogenous (eks-oj'-en-us). Arising or developing outside an organism.

exognathia (eks-o-na'-thĭ-ă). Prognathism (q.v.).

exognathion (eks-o-na'-thĭ-on). The maxillary alveolar process.

exolever (eks"-o-le'-ver). An elevator (q.v.).

exophthalmic goitre. A disease caused by hyperthyroidism, and characterized by enlarged thyroid glands and exophthalmos. *Also called* Graves' disease.

exophthalmos (eks-of-thal'-mos). Abnormal protrusion of the eyeball.

exorbitism (eks-or'-bit-izm). Exophthalmos (q.v.).

exostosis (eks-os-to'-sis). A bony tumour developing on the bone surface, or on a tooth root.

cementum e. Localized deposition of cementum.

exostotic (eks-os-tot'-ik). Relating to exostosis.

expansion (eks-pan'-shun). An increase in size, either of length, area, or volume.

expansion arch. An orthodontic appliance used to assist in the lateral movement of teeth.

expansion wire. An orthodontic appliance of wire, conforming to the dental arch, and used for anchorage in the movement of teeth.

explorer (eks-plor'-er). Any instrument used in diagnostic investigation.

exposure (eks-po'-zhur). The laying open; in dentistry, the removal of the protecting enamel and dentine from the pulp of a tooth by caries or trauma, thus laying it open to the mouth.

expulsive gingivitis. Osteoperiostitis affecting a tooth or teeth, gradually expelling them from their sockets.

extension bridge. A dental bridge having a free pontic attached at one end beyond the point of anchorage.

extension outline *of an impression.* The outline on the surface of a cast, including the entire area of the denture base.

external (eks-ter'-nal). Outside.

external auditory meatus. The external auditory canal from the concha to the tympanic membrane in the ear.

external fistula. One opening from a body cavity or abscess to the surface of the skin.

external nasal vein. The vein draining the side of the nose. *See* Table of Veins—nasalis externa.

external palatine vein. Drains the palatal region. *See* Table of Veins—palatina externa.

extirpation (eks-ter-pa'-shun). Complete eradication of a part.

extra-. Prefix signifying *outside*.

extrabuccal (eks"-tră-buk'-al). Outside the oral cavity.

extracoronal (eks"-tră-kor-o'-nal). Outside the tooth crown.

extraction (eks-trak'-shun). The process of pulling out or removing.

extractor (eks-trak'-tor). Any instrument used in dentistry for the extraction of teeth.

extragingival (eks"-tră-jin'-jiv-al). Outside the gums.

extra-oral (eks"-tră-or'-al). Outside the mouth.

extravasation (eks-trav-as-a'-shun). 1. The escape of fluid from a vessel into the surrounding tissues. 2. The fluid which escapes in this way.

extravascular (eks-tră-vas'-kyu-lar). Outside a vessel or vessels.

extrinsic (eks-trin'-sik). Having its origin outside and separate from a body, organ, or part; as opposed to *intrinsic.*

extrudocclusion (eks-trūd-ok-lu'-zhun). Extrusion (*q.v.*).

extrusion (eks-tru'-zhun). *In dentistry:* The condition of a tooth which has been pulled or pushed up slightly out of its socket.

exudate (eks'-u-dāt). The matter which passes out into the adjacent tissue through vessel walls in inflammation.

exudation (eks-u-da'-shun). The passage of matter into the adjacent tissues through vessel walls in inflammatory conditions.

exuviation (eks-u-vi-a'-shun). The shedding of any epidermal structure, such as the deciduous teeth.

eye (i). The organ of sight.

eye tooth. A maxillary canine.

eyelet wiring. A form of direct wiring in which the wires are doubled to form an eyelet and a tail; these are fastened round two teeth at a time and then linked between the jaws with connecting wires or rubber bands.

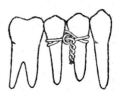

Eyelet wiring (double)

Eysson's bone (H. Eysson, 1620-90. Dutch physician). The ossa mentalia at the symphysis menti.

F

F. Abbreviation for *Fahrenheit.*

f. Abbreviation for *fiat*—let it be made; used in prescription writing.

F Chemical symbol for fluorine.

Fe Chemical symbol for iron.

f.h. Abbreviation for *fiat haustus*—make a draught; used in prescription writing.

fl. Abbreviation for *fluid.*

f.m. Abbreviation for *fiat mistura*—make a mixture; used in prescription writing.

f.p. Abbreviation for *fiat pilula*—make a pill; used in prescription writing.

ft. Abbreviation for *fiat*—let it be made; used in prescription writing.

ft. Abbreviation for *foot.*

face (*fās*). 1. The front of the head, from the forehead to the chin. 2. Any exterior surface or presenting aspect.

facebow (*fās'-bo*). 1. An instrument, used in dental prosthetics and designed originally by G. B. Snow, for determining the relationship of the teeth to the axis of movement of the mandible and transferring the bite-blocks to an articulator so that this movement may be reproduced in making the denture. 2. Any extra-oral wire arch or bow used in orthodontics to attach an internal appliance to an external anchorage.

faceometer (*fās-om'-et-er*). An instrument used for taking facial measurements.

facet (*fas'-et*). A small abraded area on a tooth surface.

facial (*fa'-shi-al*). Relating to the face.

facial anaesthesia. Loss of sensation in an area of the face as a result of trauma or of a pathological process affecting either the central nervous system or the sensory nerves supplying the area.

facial angle. In craniometry, the angle between a line joining the nasion and the prosthion and one passing through the orbital opening and the auricular point; it indicates the degree of protrusion of the chin.

facial artery. Branch of the external carotid supplying the pharynx, soft palate, submandibular glands, etc. *Also called* external maxillary. *See* Table of Arteries —facialis.

facial canal. A canal extending from the petrous portion of the temporal bone to the stylo-mastoid foramen, through which passes the facial nerve. *Also called* aqueduct of Fallopius.

facial hemiplegia. Paralysis affecting one side of the face only.

facial hiatus. Facial canal (*q.v.*).

facial index. The ratio of
$$\frac{facial\ length \times 100}{facial\ width}$$
which gives an indication of the shape and size of a face.

facial line. Camper's line (*q.v.*).

facial nerve. The 7th cranial nerve, supplying the muscles of facial expression, and also the posterior belly of the digastric muscle, the stapedius and the stylo-hyoid muscles. *See* Table of Nerves—facialis.

facial plane. The plane passing through the nasion and the pogonion and perpendicular to the sagittal plane.

facial surfaces of the teeth. The buccal and labial surfaces collectively.

facial triangle. The triangle formed by lines joining the alveolar and nasal points and the basion.

facial vein, posterior. V. retromandibularis. *See* Table of Veins.

facial veins. Those veins which drain the muscles and tissues of the face. *See* Table of Veins—facialis, and faciei.

facies (*fa'-she-ēz*). 1. A face, or the appearance of a face. 2. A surface.

facing (*fa'-sing*). A thin piece of porcelain trimmed to represent the outer surface of a tooth and to be re-inforced with gold or other backing, used to restore the full form of a tooth.

facio-. Prefix signifying *face*.

faciocervical (*fa''-shi-o-ser-vi'-kal*). Relating to the face and the neck.

faciolingual (*fa''-shi-o-lin'-gwal*). Relating to the face and the tongue.

faciolingual hemiplegia. Paralysis affecting one side of the face and the tongue.

facioplasty (*fa''-shi-o-plast'-i*). Plastic surgery operations on the face.

facioplegia (*fa''-shi-o-ple'-ji-ā*). Facial paralysis.

factitial (*fak-tish'-i-al*). Factitious (*q.v.*).

factitious (*fak-tish'-us*). Artificially or unintentionally produced.

Fahrenheit (*far'-en-hīt*) (G. D. Fahrenheit, 1686-1736. German physicist). Denoting a thermometric scale on which freezing point is 32° and boiling point 212°; this scale is used for clinical thermometers.

Fallopius, aqueduct of (G. Fallopius, 1523-62. Italian anatomist). Facial canal (*q.v.*).

falx cerebelli. A sickle-shaped process of the dura mater between the cerebellar hemispheres.

falx cerebri. A sickle-shaped vertical partition between the cerebral hemispheres.

familial (*fam-il'-i-al*). Relating to a family, or affecting several of its members.

family (*fam'-il-i*). In biological classification, the principal division of an order, which itself divides into genera.

fang (*fang*). 1. A sharp-pointed tooth, such as a canine or the tooth of a wild animal. 2. An old term for a tooth root.

Farabeuf's triangle (L. H. Farabeuf, 1841-1910. French surgeon). A triangle of the neck, formed by the internal jugular vein, the facial vein and the hypoglossal nerve.

fascia (*fash'-ĭ-ă*). 1. The layers of areolar tissue beneath the skin (superficial fascia). 2. The layers of areolar tissue investing the muscles, nerves and other organs (deep fascia).

fascial (*fash'-ĭ-al*). Relating to a fascia.

fauces (*faw'-sēz*) (*pl.*). The throat.
pillars of f. Curved muscular folds on either side of the pharyngeal opening, running from the palate to the base of the tongue and the pharynx; they enclose the tonsils. The *anterior* pillars are also known as the palatoglossal arch and the *posterior* as the palatopharyngeal arch.

Fauchard's disease (P. Fauchard, 1678-1761. French dental surgeon). Pyorrhoea alveolaris (*q.v.*).

faucial (*faw'-shĭ-al*). Relating to the fauces.

faucial reflex. Vomiting or gagging caused by irritation of the fauces.

faucial tonsil. Tonsil (*q.v.*).

febrile (*feb'-rīl*). Feverish.

Fede's disease (F. Fede, 1832-1913. Italian physician). Sublingual papillomatous ulceration, found especially in infants and caused by trauma from the lower incisors during suckling; *also called* Riga-Fede's disease.

Fergusson's operation (W. Fergusson, 1808-77. Scottish surgeon). 1. Excision of the maxilla for a malignant tumour. 2. An operation for the repair of harelip.

ferric (*fer'-ik*). Relating to iron as a trivalent metal.

ferrous (*fer'-us*). Relating to iron as a bivalent metal.

ferrule (*fer'-ul*). *In dentistry:* A metal band placed round the root or the crown of a tooth for strength.

festoon (*fes-tūn'*). The natural curved outline of the gums about the necks of the teeth.

fetid. *See* foetid.

fetus. *See* foetus.

fever (*fe'-ver*). 1. Abnormal increase in body temperature. 2. Any disease characterized by a high temperature, accompanied by other symptoms such as restlessness, delirium, rapid pulse.

fiat (*fi'-at*). Latin for *make* (imperative); used in prescription writing, and abbreviated *f.*, or *ft.*

fiber. *See* fibre.

fibre (*fi'-ber*). A threadlike structure found in organic tissue.

bone f's. Sharpey's fibres (*q.v.*).

dentinal f's. Odontoblastic processes (*q.v.*).

dentinogenic f's. von Korff's fibres (*q.v.*).

enamel f. Enamel prism (*q.v.*).

horizontal f's. Those fibres from the periodontal membrane which extend to the cementum of the tooth.

odontogenic f's. Those fibres which make up the connective tissue layer of the tooth matrix, surrounding the pulp.

For eponymous fibres *see* under the name of the person first describing them.

fibril (*fib'-ril*). A small fibre.

fibrilloblast (*fib'-ril-o-blast*). Odontoblast (*q.v.*).

fibrils, Ebner's. *See* Ebner's fibrils.

fibrin (*fi'-brin*). An insoluble fibrous protein formed by the action of thrombin on fibrinogen; it provides the network which retains corpuscles in the mechanism of blood clotting.

fibrinous (*fi'-brin-us*). Relating to fibrin.

fibroadamantinoblastoma (*fi''-bro-ad-am-ant''-in-o-blast-o'-mă*). A fibroma of ameloblastic origin.

fibroadenoma (*fi''-bro-ad-en-o'-mă*). Adenofibroma (*q.v.*). *Also called* f. xanthomatodes; foetal f.; pleomorphic f.

fibroblast (*fi'-bro-blast*). One of the germ cells from which connective tissue is formed.

fibrocartilage (*fi''-bro-kar'-til-āj*). Cartilage which also contains dense fibrous tissue.

fibroma (*fi-bro'-mă*). A tumour composed of fibrous tissue.

fibromatosis (*fi-bro-mat-o'-sis*). The development of multiple fibromas.

fibropapilloma (*fi''-bro-pap-il-o'-mă*). Adenofibroma (*q.v.*).

fibrosarcoma (*fi''-bro-sar-ko'-mă*). A malignant tumour derived from fibroblasts.

fibrosis (*fi-bro'-sis*). Fibrous degeneration; the abnormal formation of fibrous tissue.

fibrous (*fi'-brus*). Relating to a fibre or fibres; composed of fibres.

fibrous ankylosis. Stiffness due to fibrous adhesions or fibrosis in the joint.

fibrous epulis. An inflammatory pedunculated overgrowth of gum tissue; probably not a true tumour.

Filatov's spots (N. F. Filatov, 1847-1902. Russian pediatrician). Koplik's spots (*q.v.*).

file (*fil*). A hard steel tool with a roughened surface, for abrading or polishing.

filiform (*fil'-i-form*). Filamentous; threadlike.

filling (*fil'-ing*). 1. The operation of inserting material into a prepared cavity in a tooth. 2. The material used in this operation, when in place.

filtration (*fil-tra'-shun*). The separating out of a solid from a liquid by passing it through a filter.

finishing bur. A bur having a more finely cut head, used in finishing and burnishing restorations.

first arch syndrome. A congenital abnormality syndrome which includes cleft lip and palate, mandibulofacial dysostosis, hypertelorism, and deformities of the ear, all stemming from developmental deficiency in the first branchial arch.

fissural (*fis'-yur-al*). Relating to a fissure.

fissure (*fis'-yur*). A small groove or trough. In dentistry. used especially of the small grooves in the enamel surface of a tooth, caused by a fault in its structure.

lip f. Harelip (*q.v.*).

orbital f. inferior: A long cleft between the floor and lateral wall of the orbit, opening into the infratemporal fossa. *superior:* |An elongated cleft between the great and small wings of the sphenoid bone, giving passage to various blood vessels and nerves.

petrosquamous f. The narrow cleft between the petrous and squamous portions of the temporal bone.

petrotympanic f. The narrow opening posterior to the glenoid fossa, through which passes the chorda tympani nerve.

pterygoid f. The angular cleft between the pterygoid processes of the sphenoid bone.

pterygomaxillary f. A narrow cleft between the lateral pterygoid plate and the maxilla, through which passes the maxillary artery.

sphenoid f. Superior orbital fissure (*q.v.*).

sphenomaxillary f. Pterygomaxillary fissure (*q.v.*).

fissure, Glaserian. Petrotympanic fissure (*q.v.*).

fissure bur. A cylindrical dental bur used for preparing a cavity involving the occlusal fissures of a premolar or molar tooth.

fissure sealant. An impermeable material used to occlude the fissures of posterior teeth.

fistula (*fis'-tyu-lǎ*). An abnormal tract between two organs or an organ and the outer surface, often leading from a suppurating cavity.

alveolar f. One leading from a cavity of an alveolar abscess; an alveolar sinus.

antral f. A tract leading from an antral abscess or from a bone cavity.

blind f. One which has an opening at one end only; a sinus (*q.v.*, 4).

dental f. Alveolar fistula (*q.v.*).

external f. One which opens from a body cavity or abscess to the surface of the skin.

internal f. A fistula between two internal organs or cavities, with no opening to the outer surface.

labial f. A minute tract or congenital depression on the edge of the lower lip; a labial sinus.

fixation (*fiks-a'-shun*). The act of fastening in a rigid position.

external skeletal f. In surgery: A method of immobilizing the ends of a fractured bone by external metal pins or screw appliances, used especially for an edentulous mouth.

intramedullary f. In surgery: A method of uniting the ends of a fractured bone by means of a metal pin within the bone cavity.

fixed appliance. An orthodontic regulating appliance which is attached to the supporting teeth so that it cannot be removed by the wearer.

fixed bridge. A dental bridge which is fixed in place permanently to its abutments.

flagellar (*flaj-el'-ar*). Relating to or possessing flagella.

flagellum (*flaj-el'-um*) (*pl.* flagella). A thin, whiplike process, seen on certain micro-organisms.

flange (*flanj*). An external or internal rim, either for strength or as an attachment or guide to some other part.

denture f. The buccal, labial, or lingual vertical extension from the denture base into the oral cavity.

flange splint. A metal splint used in fracture of the mandible; it is cemented to several of the posterior mandibular teeth and has a high flange which rests on the buccal surfaces of the opposing maxillary teeth.

flap (*flap*). A partially detached layer of skin or tissue, either surgically produced, for access or repair, or accidentally formed.

flash (*flash*). Excess material squeezed out of a die during casting.

flask (*flask*). 1. Any glass or metal bottle with a narrow neck. 2. A metal box or frame containing plaster of Paris, in which dentures are enclosed and embedded for vulcanizing or curing.

flasking (*flask'-ing*). The process of packing a denture into a flask prior to vulcanizing it or curing it.

Fleischmann's bursa (F. L. Fleischmann, fl. 1841. German anatomist). An occasional sublingual bursa.

Fleischmann's follicle (F. L. Fleischmann, fl. 1841. German anatomist). An inconstant follicle on the floor of the mouth, near the edge of the genioglossus muscle.

flexible (*fleks'-ibl*). Not rigid; readily bendable without breaking.

floss, dental. Soft, waxed thread or tape, used to clear and to clean interproximal spaces.

Flower's index (Sir W. H. Flower, 1831-99. British physician). Dental index (*q.v.*).

fluoridation (*flu-or-id-a'-shun*). *See* water fluoridation.

fluoride (*flu'-or-īd*). A compound of fluorine with another element.

fluoridization (*flu-or-id-i-za'-shun*). The use of any fluoride, in any form, for the prevention of dental caries.

fluorine (*flu'-or-ēn*). A non-metallic element of the halogen group, having the chemical symbol F.

fluorosis (*flu-or-o'-sis*). 1. Fluorine poisoning. 2. A chronic condition resulting from prolonged ingestion of excessive amounts of fluorides and characterized by increased density of the skeletal bones, and hypoplasia and discoloration of the teeth.
chronic endemic (*dental*) *f.* Hypoplasia and discoloration of the tooth enamel due to ingestion of excessive amounts of fluorine during the developmental period; mottled enamel.

focal (*fo'-kal*). Relating to a focus.

focal sepsis. A local source of infection which may spread to cause systemic disease.

focus (*fo'-kus*) (*pl.* foci). The chief centre of activity or the point of convergence.

focus *of infection.* The chief centre of pathogenic activity from which the infection spreads to surrounding areas.

foetal (*fe'-tal*). Relating to a foetus.

foetal fibroadenoma. Adenofibroma (*q.v.*).

foetid (*fe'-tid*). Having an unpleasant or foul smell.

foetus, fetus (*fe'-tus*). The developing embryo in the womb, especially, in man, after the first three months of growth.

foil (*foyl*). Metal in a very thin sheet or ribbon, especially gold, tin, or platinum.

foil carrier. An instrument used to transfer strips of gold foil to a prepared tooth cavity.

follicle (*fol'-ikl*). A minute sac or gland.
dental f. The sac containing the unerupted tooth within the alveolar process.

follicle, Fleischmann's. See Fleischmann's follicle.

follicular (*fol-ik'-yu-lar*). Relating to or resembling a follicle.

follicular cyst. A dentigerous cyst (*q.v.*).

fontanel (*fon'-tan-el*). The membranous and cartilagenous structure present between the ossifying skull bones of a new-born infant.

food debris. Food remnants and bacteria loosely attached to the tooth, which can be removed by rinsing.

foramen (*for-a'-men*) (*pl.* foramina). A small hole in a bone, through which pass either blood vessels or nerves, or both.
alveolar f. One of the openings of the alveolar canals on the infratemporal surface of the maxilla, through which the posterior

superior alveolar nerves and vessels pass to the molar and premolar teeth. *Also called* posterior superior alveolar foramen.

anterior ethmoid f. A canal between the ethmoid and frontal bones, through which pass the nasal branch of the ophthalmic nerve and the anterior ethmoid vessels.

anterior palatine f. Incisive fossa *(q.v.).*

apical f. The small opening at the apex of the tooth by which the nerve and blood supply of the pulp enters.

caecal f. of the tongue. A depression above the root and dorsum of the tongue, the site of the former opening of the thyroglossal duct.

condylar f. Condylar canal *(q.v.).*

greater palatine f. The opening of the greater palatine canal into the hard palate, between the horizontal portion of the palatine bone and the adjacent maxilla.

incisive f. One of two to four openings of the incisive canal on the floor of the incisive fossa. *Lateral:* on the hard palate behind the incisors, transmitting branches of the greater palatine artery; *median:* in the midline of the hard palate, transmitting the nasopalatine nerves.

inferior dental f. Mandibular foramen *(q.v.).*

infraorbital f. The external opening in the maxilla

of the infraorbital canal, through which pass the infraorbital artery and nerve.

jugular f. The opening formed by the jugular notches of the temporal and occipital bones, through which pass a jugular vein and the ninth, tenth and eleventh cranial nerves.

lesser palatine f. One of the openings of the lesser palatine canals, on the anterior surface of the hard palate.

mandibular f. An oblong opening in the internal surface of the ramus, through which pass the inferior dental nerve and artery; *also called* the inferior dental foramen.

mastoid f. A small opening behind the mastoid process, through which pass an artery and a vein.

mental f. A large foramen in the mandible, below the second premolar, through which pass the mental branches of the inferior dental nerve, and their accompanying blood vessels.

nutrient f. One of the foramina in the maxilla and the mandible through which the nutrient canals pass.

posterior superior alveolar f. Alveolar foramen *(q.v.).*

sphenopalatine f. The space between the orbital and sphenoid processes of the palatine bone, opening into the nasal cavity.

stylo-mastoid f. An opening between the styloid and the mastoid processes, through which pass the stylomastoid artery and the facial nerve.

foramen caecum. Caecal foramen of the tongue (*q.v.*).

foramen lacerum. An interosseous foramen between the apex of the petrous bone and the attachment of the great wing of the sphenoid, through which the carotid artery passes.

foramen magnum. A large opening in the lower portion of the occipital bone, through which passes the medulla oblongata.

foramen ovale. 1. An opening in the great wing of the sphenoid bone, through which pass the inferior dental nerve and the small meningeal artery. 2. An opening between the auricles of the heart in the foetus.

foramen rotundum. A round opening in the great wing of the sphenoid bone, through which passes the maxillary branch of the trigeminal nerve.

foramen spinosum. An opening in the great wing of the sphenoid bone near to its posterior angle, through which passes the middle meningeal artery.

foramen zygomaticofaciale. The external opening on the surface of the zygomatic bone, through which the zygomatic nerve and vessels pass.

foramen zygomatico-orbitale. The canal through the zygomatic bone giving passage to the zygomatic branch of the maxillary nerve.

foramen zygomaticotemporale. The opening on the temporal surface of the zygomatic bone, through which passes the zygomaticotemporal nerve.

forceps (*for'-seps*). An instrument having two blades and handles, used for holding, compressing, or removing. *dental f.* Forceps used for the extraction of teeth.

Fordyce's spots (J. A. Fordyce, 1858-1925. American dermatologist). Small yellowish spots, of no pathological significance, occurring on the vermilion border and the inner surface of the lips and cheeks.

forebrain (*for'-brān*). Prosencephalon (*q.v.*).

formula (*for'-myu-lă*). 1. The chemical composition of a substance expressed by symbols. 2. A recipe or prescription for preparing a medicine. *dental f.* A formula devised to show the number and arrangement of teeth by means of letters and figures. In this formula I = incisor; C = canine; P = premolar; M = molar. The dental formula for normal permanent dentition in man is I $\frac{2}{2}$ C $\frac{1}{1}$ P $\frac{2}{2}$ M $\frac{3}{3}$. *instrument f.* Three figures representing three measurements: the width of the blade in 10ths of a millimetre; the length of the

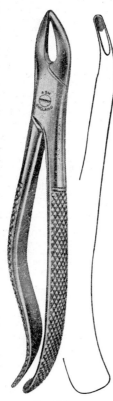

Dental forceps

blade in millimetres; and the angle of the shaft in centigrades.

formulary (*for'-myul-ar-ĭ*). A collection of recipes or formulae for making up medicines.

fossa (*fos'-ă*) (*pl.* fossae). A shallow, irregular depression in a surface.

canine f. A depression on the external surface of the maxilla, immediately distal to the canine tooth socket.

condylar f.; condyloid f. One of the two small depressions on the occipital bone, situated behind one of the condyles.

glenoid f. The depression in the squamous portion of the temporal bone below the zygomatic process, in which the condyle of the mandible rests.

incisive f. 1. A depression on the maxilla behind the incisors. 2. A depression on the mandible below the incisors, giving origin to the mentalis muscle. 3. A depression on the outer surface of the maxilla, giving origin to the depressor muscle of the nose.

infratemporal f. An irregular space on the skull, bounded by the zygoma and the ramus of the mandible, behind the maxilla.

jugular f. A depression in the petrous portion of the temporal bone, between the carotid canal and the stylo-mastoid foramen, for the jugular vein.

mandibular f. Glenoid fossa (q.v.).

mastoid f. A depression on the lateral surface of the temporal bone, for the lateral sinus.

palatine f. Incisive fossa (q.v., 1).

pterygoid f. A groove between the medial and lateral plates of the pterygoid process of the sphenoid bone.

pterygopalatine f. A small cleft between the pterygoid process of the sphenoid bone and the palatine bone and maxilla.

scaphoid f. A depression in the lower surface of the medial pterygoid plate of the sphenoid bone, from which arises the tensor veli palatini muscle.

sphenomaxillary f. Pterygopalatine fossa (q.v.).

sublingual f. A depression on the inner surface of the mandible, by the sublingual gland.

submaxillary f. A depression on the inner surface of the mandible, by the submaxillary gland.

suborbital f. Canine fossa (q.v.).

temporal f. The depression on the side of the cranium in which the temporal muscle lodges.

temporomandibular f. Glenoid fossa (q.v.).

zygomatic f. Infratemporal fossa (q.v.).

fossa, Bichat's. See Bichat's fossa.

Foster crown (F. W. Foster, fl. 1855. American dentist). A form of pivot tooth using a metal screw to secure it to the root canal.

Fournier's molars (J. A. Fournier, 1832-1914. French venereologist). Dome-shaped permanent first molars, with the cusps close together; seen in congenital syphilis. *Also called* mulberry molars.

fovea (fo'-vĕ-ă). A small pit, depression, or cup; used of depressions in the body, particularly the fovea centralis of the retina.

fovea pterygoidea mandibulae. A depression on the anterior side of the neck of the mandible, the site of insertion of the external pterygoid muscle.

fovea sublingualis mandibulae. Sublingual fossa (q.v.).

fovea submaxillaris mandibulae. Submaxillary fossa (q.v.).

foveate (fo'-ve-āt). 1. Pitted. 2. Relating to or characterized by the presence of fovea.

fracture (frak'-tchur). A break, or the act of breaking, in a bone or cartilage.

pyramidal f. Le Fort fracture, class II (q.v.).

fracture, Le Fort. See Le Fort fracture.

fracture bands, Angle's. See Angle's fracture bands.

fraenectomy (fren-ek'-tom-ĭ). Surgical excision of a fraenum.

fraenotomy (fren-ot'-om-ĭ). Surgical relief of tongue-tie by cutting the lingual fraenum.

fraenulum (*fre'-nyul-um*). A small fraenum.

fraenum (*fre'-num*). A membranous fold supporting or limiting the movement of an organ.

fraenum labiorum. The fold attaching the upper lip to the maxillary gums above the central incisors.

fraenum linguae. The fold attaching the under surface of the tongue to the floor of the mouth.

fragilitas ossium. A developmental bone disease in which the bones become abnormally brittle and fracture easily; osteogenesis imperfecta.

framework (*frām'-werk*). The metal skeleton of a denture or prosthesis on which the remaining portions are built up to produce a completed appliance.

Francheschetti syndrome (A. Francheschetti, b. 1896. Swiss ophthalmologist). Mandibulo-facial dysostosis (*q.v.*).

Frankfort plane. A plane determined by the position of the two poria and the left orbitale, used in anthropometry for orientating both living heads and skulls; adopted at the International Congress of Anthropologists, Frankfort-am-Main, 1884.

freeway space. The slight gap between the upper and lower teeth when the mandible is at rest.

frenulum, frenum. *See* fraenulum, fraenum.

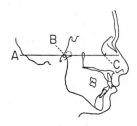

Frankfort plane

A Frankfort plane.
B Porion.
C Orbitale.

friable (*fri'-abl*). Easily crumbled.

friability (*fri-ab-il'-it-ĭ*). The quality of being easily crumbled.

Friteau's triangle (E. Friteau, b. 1867). A triangular area on the cheek having no branches of the facial nerve.

frog tongue. Ranula (*q.v.*).

frontal (*frun'-tal*). Relating to the forehead; in front.

frontal bone. One of the bones of the skull, forming the forehead.

frontal muscle. Raises eyebrows and draws forward scalp. *See* Table of Muscles —frontalis.

frontal nerve. Supplies the skin of the scalp. *See* Table of Nerves—frontalis.

frontal notch. A notch on the upper edge of the orbital bone, through which pass the frontal artery and nerve.

frontal process. A projection of the maxilla articulating with the frontal bone and forming part of the side of the nasal cavity and of the margin of the orbit.

frontal sinus. One of two cavities in the frontal bone, varying in size in different skulls, and found above the root of the nose.

frontomalar (*frun″-to-ma′-lar*). Relating to the frontal and the zygomatic (malar) bones.

frontomaxillary (*frun″-to-maks-il′-ar-i*). Relating to the frontal bone and the maxilla.

frontonasal (*frun″-to-na′-zal*). Relating to the frontal and the nasal bones.

frontonasal process. The front portion of bone in the head of an embryo which develops into the forehead and the bridge of the nose.

fronto-occipital (*frun″-to-ok-sip′-it-al*). Relating to the frontal and occipital bones.

frontoparietal (*frun″-to-par-i′-et-al*). Relating to the frontal and the parietal bones.

frontosphenoidal process. A thick ascending serrated process of the zygomatic bone articulating with the frontal bone and the great wing of the sphenoid.

frontotemporal (*frun″-to-tem″-por-al*). Relating to the

frontal and the temporal bones.

frontozygomatic (*frun″-to-zi-go-mat′-ik*). Relating to the frontal and zygomatic bones.

frugivorous (*frū-giv′-or-us*). Fruit-eating.

fulginous (*ful′-jin-us*). Of sooty or smoky appearance; used of a darkly coated tongue or mucous membrane.

fulguration (*ful-jur-a′-shun*). Superficial tissue dehydration produced by a surgical electrode held slightly away from the tissue, causing sparking.

full denture. A denture which replaces all the teeth in either the upper or lower jaws or in both.

fungal (*fun′-gal*). Relating to a fungus.

fungiform (*fun′-ji-form*). In the shape of a fungus.

fungoid (*fun′-goyd*). Resembling a fungus.

fungous (*fun′-gus*). Relating to a fungus.

fungus (*fun′-gus*) (*pl.* fungi). 1. A class of plant organisms which includes moulds, mushrooms, and toadstools. 2. A morbid growth of granulation tissue on the body.

fur (*fur*). A coating of epithelial scales and other matter found on the tongue in certain diseases or disorders.

furcal (*fur′-kal*). Forked.

furcation (*fur-ka′-shun*). The condition of being divided into prongs, or of being forked.

furnace (fur'-nas). An apparatus by means of which metals or minerals may be treated with continuous and intense heat.

muffle f. A type of oven used in dental ceramics, in which material may be heated without being directly exposed to the source of heat.

furred tongue. A tongue having the papillae coated, thus giving the mucous membrane a whitish, furry appearance.

furrow (fur'-o). A trench or groove.

mentolabial f. The groove just above the chin.

furuncle (fur'-un-kl). A boil (q.v.).

furunculosis (fur-un-kyu-lo'-sis). The condition marked by crops of boils.

fused teeth. Teeth, especially incisors, which have become joined together during development, and erupt as one large tooth.

fusible (fyu'-zibl). Capable of being melted.

fusiform (fyu'-zĭ-form). Spindle-shaped.

fusiform papilla. Any one of the slender spindle-shaped papillae on the anterior two-thirds of the dorsum of the tongue.

Fusiformis (fyu-si-form'-is). Fusobacterium (q.v.).

fusion (fyu'-zhun). *In dentistry:* The union of two tooth follicles to form one tooth; synodontia (q.v.).

Fusobacterium (fu"-so-bak-te'-ri-um). A genus of the Bacteriaceae family of bacteria, seen as slender spindle shapes, Gram-negative and anaerobic.

F. nucleatum. A species which has been found in deposits on teeth in a healthy mouth.

F. plautivincenti. A species found in ulcero-membranous stomatitis, and in other forms of gingivitis.

fusospirillary gingivitis. Acute ulcerative gingivitis (q.v.).

fusospirillosis (fyu''-so-spir-il-o'-sis). Acute ulcerative stomatitis (q.v.).

fusospirochaetal gingivitis. Acute ulcerative gingivitis (q.v.).

G

G Gingival.

g. Abbreviation for *gram*.

GA Gingivoaxial.

GBA Gingivobuccoaxial.

GLA Gingivolinguoaxial.

gm. Abbreviation for *gram*.

gutt. Abbreviation for *gutta*, or *guttæ*—a drop, or drops; used in prescription writing.

gag (gag). 1. To retch; to heave without vomiting. 2. A device to prevent the closure of the teeth during surgery, epileptic seizure, etc.

gag reflex. Pharyngeal reflex (q.v.).

galea aponeurotica (*gal'-ĕ-ă ap-o-nyur-ot'-ik-ă*). The aponeurosis connecting the separate parts of the occipitofrontal muscle.

Galen's bandage (Claudius Galen, c. 130-200 A.D. Greek physician and writer). A bandage used for head injuries in which each end is divided into three: the centre of the bandage is placed on the crown of the head, the two front strips fasten at the back of the neck, the two back strips fasten on the forehead, and the two side strips under the chin.

galvanism (*gal'-van-izm*). *dental g.* The production of an electric current caused when two dissimilar metals used as restorations in the mouth come into contact; this can produce discomfort and even pain.

galvanocautery (*gal"-van-o-kaw'-ter-ĭ*). Electrocautery (*q.v.*).

ganglion (*gan'-glĭ-on*) (*pl.* ganglia). 1. A knot or mass of nerve cells. 2. A tumour or swelling on an aponeurosis or on a tendon.
pterygopalatine g. Meckel's ganglion (*q.v.*).
sphenopalatine g. Meckel's ganglion (*q.v.*).
submaxillary g. A small ganglion on the hyoglossus muscle from which arises the nerve supply for the submaxillary and sublingual glands.
For eponymous ganglia *see* under the name of the person first describing the ganglion.

gangosa (*gan-go'-să*). Destructive ulceration affecting the nose and the hard palate; a late stage of yaws.

gangrene (*gan'-grēn*). Necrosis of tissue due to failure of the arterial blood supply, injury, or disease.

gangrenous (*gan'-gren-us*). Affected with gangrene.

gangrenous stomatitis. Noma; cancrum oris.

Garretson's bandage (J. E. Garretson, 1828-95. American dental surgeon). A bandage used to immobilize the lower jaw; it is taken from above the forehead, crossing at the neck and fastening under the chin.

Gasserian ganglion (J. L. Gasser, fl. 1757. Austrian anatomist). The ganglion of the trigeminal nerve, situated in a fossa on the anterior portion of the petrous part of the temporal bone.

Gates crown (W. H. Gates, fl. 1875. American dentist). Almost identical with the Bonwill crown (*q.v.*); also known as the Gates-Bonwill crown.

gauge (*gāj*). Any instrument used to obtain measurements.
bite g. An instrument designed to aid in the establishment of a correct bite in dentistry.
Boley g. A finely calibrated instrument used for intra-oral measurements.

geisoma (*gi-so'-mă*). The supra-orbital prominence; the eyebrow ridge on the skull.

geison (*gi'-son*). Geisoma (*q.v.*).

gel (*jel*). A colloid existing as a semisolid or gelatinous mass.

irreversible g. One converted from a sol, but which cannot be reconverted.

gelation (*jel-a'-shun*). 1. The process of change of a colloid from a sol to a gel. 2. Freezing.

geminate (*jem'-in-āt*). Twin; found in pairs.

gemination (*jem-in-a'-shun*). The development of twins or pairs. In dentistry, the development of the equivalent of two teeth from one follicle, having only one pulp chamber and a groove or depression down the centre to mark the division.

oliphyodontic g. A condition in which a deciduous tooth is fused to a permanent one.

genal (*je'-nal*). Relating to the cheek.

general (*jen'-er-al*). Affecting the body as a whole, or many parts; as opposed to *local*.

general anaesthesia. Anaesthesia of the whole body.

generic (*jen-er'-ik*). Relating to one genus.

genial (*je'-ni-al*). Relating to the chin.

genial angle. The angle formed between the ramus and the body of the mandible.

genial tubercle. One of two elevations on either side of the mental protuberance on the mandible.

genio-. Prefix signifying *chin.*

genioglossal (*je''-ni-o-glos'-al*). Relating to the chin and the tongue.

genioglossus (*je''-ni-o-glos'-us*). The muscle on the under side of the tongue, which protrudes and depresses the tongue. *See* Table of Muscles.

geniohyoid muscle (*je''-ni-o-hi'-oyd*). The muscle which raises and draws forward the hyoid bone, with the jaw fixed. *See* Table of Muscles—geniohyoideus.

genion (*je'-ni-on*). 1. The chin. 2. In craniometry, the apex of the mental protuberance.

genioplasty (*je-ni-o-plast'-i*). Plastic surgery on the chin.

genus (*je'-nus*) (*pl.* genera). In biological classification, the principal subdivision of a family, and itself dividing into *species*.

geny-. Prefix signifying *jaw.*

genyantralgia (*jen-i-ant-ral'-ji-ă*). Pain affecting the maxillary sinus (or antrum).

genyantritis (*jen-i-ant-ri'-tis*). Inflammation of the maxillary sinus (or antrum).

genyantrum (*jen-i-an'-trum*). The maxillary sinus (or antrum) (*q.v.*).

genycheiloplasty (*jen''-i-ki''-lo-plast'-i*). Plastic surgery of both the cheek and the lip.

genyplasty (*jen'-ĭ-plast-ĭ*). Plastic surgery of the mandible.

geographic tongue. A tongue having scaly patches, resembling maps, on the dorsal surface.

geotrichosis (*je-o-trik-o'-sis*). Any infection caused by a species of *Geotrichum*.

Geotrichum (*je-ot'-rik-um*). A genus of yeast-like fungi, associated with broncho-pulmonary and oral lesions.

geriodontics (*jer-i-o-don'-tiks*). Gerodontics (*q.v.*).

germ (*jerm*). 1. Any micro-organism, especially a pathogenic species. 2. A spore or seed. 3. The primitive embryo, or any part of it which will develop into a separate organ or part.
tooth g. The enamel organ, dental papilla and sac; the rudiments of the developing tooth.

germicidal (*jerm-is-i'-dal*). Germ-destroying.

germicide (*jerm'-is-īd*). Any agent used to kill germs.

germinal (*jer'-min-al*). Relating to germs.

gerodontia (*jer-o-don'-shĭa*); **gerodontics** (*jer-o-don'-tiks*). Dentistry which is concerned with old people.

gerodontic (*jer-o-don'-tik*). 1. Relating to gerodontics. 2. Relating to the effects of age on dental tissues.

giant cell. A large, multinuclear cell, such as an osteoclast.

Gibson bandage (K. C. Gibson, 1849-1925. American dentist). A bandage for immobilizing the jaw and retaining the bone fragments in fracture of the mandible.

Gilmer splint (T. L. Gilmer, 1849-1931. American oral surgeon). Immobilization of a fractured mandible and restoration of normal occlusion by means of silver wire fastening upper to lower teeth.

gingiva (*jin'-jiv-ă*) (*pl.* gingivae). The gum tissue and mucous membrane surrounding the tooth and alveolar process.

gingival (*jin'-jiv-al*). 1. Relating to the gingiva. 2. Relating to that wall of a tooth cavity which faces the gingival tooth surface.

gingival abscess. An abscess occurring in a periodontal pocket and affecting the gingiva round the cementum of a tooth.

gingival crest. Gingival margin (*q.v.*).

gingival crevice. The space lying between the inner aspect of the free gingiva and the tooth enamel or cementum, depending on the level of the epithelial attachment.

gingival line. Gingival margin (*q.v.*).

gingival margin. The unattached edge of the gingiva at the necks of the teeth.

gingival margin trimmer. A type of chisel designed for

bevelling gingival enamel margins.

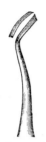

Gingival margin trimmer

gingival nerves. Nerves which supply the gingivae. *See* Table of Nerves—gingivalis.

gingival papillae. The gingiva in the interproximal spaces; *also called* interdental papillae.

gingival pocket. Periodontal pocket (*q.v.*).

gingival septum. Gingival papillae (*q.v.*).

gingival sulcus. Gingival crevice (*q.v.*).

gingivalgia (*jin-jiv-al'-ji-ă*). Neuralgic pain affecting the gums.

gingivectomy (*jin-jiv-ek'-tom-ĭ*). Surgical excision of the gum or of a gum lesion.

gingivitis (*jin-jiv-i'-tis*). Inflammation of the gingiva. Often used, inaccurately, to denote any form of gingival disease.

acute ulcerative g. An acute ulcerative condition of the gingivae in which the predominant micro-organisms are a mixture of Fusiformis fusiformis and Borrelia vincentii; *also called* Vincent's infection.

expulsive g. Osteoperiostitis affecting a tooth or teeth, gradually expelling them from their sockets.

fusospirillary g., fusospirochaetal g. Acute ulcerative gingivitis (*q.v.*).

necrotizing ulcerative g. Acute ulcerative gingivitis (*q.v.*).

phagadenic g. Acute ulcerative gingivitis (*q.v.*).

Plaut-Vincent g. Acute ulcerative gingivitis (*q.v.*).

pregnancy g. Gingivitis which is thought to be caused by the endocrine changes occurring during pregnancy; marked by hypertrophy and haemorrhage of the gums, and occasionally by tumour-like swelling.

ulceromembranous g. Acute ulcerative gingivitis (*q.v.*).

gingivoaxial (*jin"-jiv-o-ak'-si-al*). Relating to the gingival and axial walls in the mesial or distal portion of a proximo-occlusal cavity. *g. angle.* The angle formed at the junction of these walls; a line angle.

gingivobuccoaxial (*jin"-jiv-o-buk"-o-ak"-si-al*). Relating to the gingival, buccal and axial walls in the mesial or distal portion of a proximo-occlusal cavity.

g. angle. The angle formed at the junction of these walls; a *point* angle.

gingivoglossitis (*jin"-jiv-o-glos-i'-tis*). Inflammation of both the gums and the tongue.

gingivolabial (*jin"-jiv-o-la'-bi-al*). Relating to the gums and the lips.

gingivolinguoaxial (*jin"-jiv-o-lin"-gwo-ak'-si-al*). Relating to the gingival, lingual and axial walls in the mesial or distal portion of a proximo-occlusal cavity.

g. angle. The angle formed at the junction of these walls; a *point* angle.

gingivopericementitis (*jin"-jiv-o-per-i-se-men-ti'-tis*). Pyorrhoea alveolaris (*q.v.*).

gingivoplasty (*jin"-jiv-o-plast'-i*). Any method of eliminating periodontal pockets while preserving the natural outline of the gingivae as far as possible.

gingivosis (*jin-jiv-o'-sis*). Any degenerative condition affecting the gingivae.

gingivostomatitis (*jin"-jiv-o-sto-mat-i'-tis*). Gingivitis (*q.v.*).

ginglymoarthrodial (*jin"-glim-o-arth-ro'-di-al*). Relating to a joint which is partly ginglymoid and partly arthrodial.

ginglymoid (*jin'-gli-moyd*). Resembling a ginglymus, or hinged joint.

ginglymus (*jin'-gli-mus*). A hinged joint, allowing only a back and forward movement.

glabella (*glab-el'-ă*). The smooth prominence between the eyebrows.

glabrous (*gla'-brus*). Smooth and hairless.

gland (*gland*). An organ which produces secretion.

buccal g's. The mixed salivary glands of the buccal mucosa.

endocrine g. Any one of the ductless glands — adrenal, thyroid, etc.—supplying internal secretions through the blood stream.

mandibular g. Submandibular gland (*q.v.*).

mixed g. A salivary gland which produces both serous and mucous secretion.

molar g's. Mixed glands near the openings of the parotid ducts.

mucous g. One of the glands which form and secrete mucus.

parotid g. One of a pair of salivary glands lying below the ear, between the ramus and the mastoid process.

salivary g. Any one of three pairs of saliva-secreting glands in the mouth, i.e. the parotid, the sublingual, and the submandibular or submaxillary glands.

sebaceous g. One of the glands which secrete sebum.

sublingual g. One of a pair of salivary glands forming a ridge on either side of the floor of the mouth, below the tongue.

submandibular g. One of a pair of salivary glands lying

on the inner edge of the mandible, in the region of the angle.

submaxillary g. Submandibular gland (q.v.).

thyroid g. A large ductless endocrine gland situated in front of the trachea, and consisting of two lateral lobes joined by an isthmus. It is made up of follicles lined with epithelium and secretes a colloid material. For eponymous glands *see* under the personal name by which the gland is known.

gland, Nuhn's. Blandin's gland (q.v.).

gland, Rivinus'. Sublingual gland (q.v.).

glands, Weber's. *See* Weber's glands.

glandular (*glan'-dyu-lar*). Relating to a gland.

Glaserian artery (J. H. Glaser, 1629-75. Swiss anatomist). A tympanica anterior. *See* Table of Arteries.

Glaserian fissure (J. H. Glaser, 1629-75. Swiss anatomist). Petrotympanic fissure (q.v.).

glaze (*glāz*). The shiny vitreous covering fused on to porcelain; in prosthetic dentistry this is used to give the effect of tooth enamel.

glenoid fossa. The depression in the squamous portion of the temporal bone below the zygomatic process, in which the condyle of the mandible rests.

globular (*glob'-yu-lar*). Relating to or resembling a globule.

globular process. One of the bulbous expansions at either angle of the nose in the embryo, later fusing to form the philtrum.

globulo-maxillary (*glob"-yu-lo-maks-il'-ar-ĭ*). Relating to the globular and the maxillary processes.

gloss-, glosso-. Prefix signifying *tongue*.

-glossa. Suffix signifying *tongue*.

glossagra (*glos-ag'-ră*). Pain affecting the tongue.

glossal (*glos'-al*). Relating to the tongue.

glossalgia (*glos-al'-jĭ-ă*). Pain in the tongue.

glossanthrax (*glos-an'-thraks*). Carbuncle, or anthrax, affecting the tongue.

glossauxesis (*glos-auks-e'-sis*). The condition of having a swollen tongue.

glossectomy (*glos-ek'-tom-ĭ*). Total or partial excision of the tongue.

glossitis (*glos-i'-tis*). Inflammation of the tongue.

glossitis, Hunter's. *See* Hunter's glossitis.

glossitis, Moeller's. *See* Moeller's glossitis.

glossocele (*glos'-o-sēl*). Swelling of the tongue, and subsequent protrusion.

glossocoma (*glos-ok'-o-mă*). Retraction of the tongue.

glossodesmus (*glos-o-dez'-mus*). The lingual fraenum (q.v.).

glossodynamometer (*glos'-o-di-nam-om'-et-er*). An instrument used to measure the ability of the tongue to resist pressure.

glossodynia (*glos-o-din'-i-ă*). Pain in the tongue.

glossodynia exfoliativa. Moeller's glossitis (*q.v.*).

glossoepiglottic (*glos''-o-ep-i-glot'-ik*). Relating to the tongue and the epiglottis.

glossoepiglottidean (*glos''-o-ep-i-glot-id'-ĕ-an*). Glossoepiglottic (*q.v.*).

glossograph (*glos'-o-graf*). An instrument used to trace tongue movements during mastication or speech.

glossohyal (*glos-o-hi'-al*). Relating to the tongue and the hyoid bone.

glossoid (*glos'-oyd*). Resembling a tongue.

glossolabial (*glo''-o-la'-bi-al*). Relating to the tongue and the lips.

glossology (*glos-ol'-oj-i*). 1. The science and study of the tongue and its diseases. 2. The definition and explanation of words.

glossolysis (*glos-ol'-is-is*). Paralysis of the tongue.

glossomantia (*glos-o-man'-ti-ă*). Prognosis of a disease based on the appearance of the tongue.

glossoncus (*glos-on'-kus*). Any swelling of the tongue.

glossopalatine (*glos-o-pal'-at-in*). Relating to the tongue and the palate.

glossopalatine arch. Palatoglossal arch (*q.v.*).

glossopalatine muscle. M. palatoglossus. *See* Table of Muscles.

glossopalatine nerve. N. intermedius. *See* Table of Nerves.

glossopathy (*glos-op'-ath-i*). Any disease of the tongue.

glossopexy (*glos'-o-peks-i*). An operation for the correction of glossoptosis by tying the base of the tongue to the front of the mandible with sutures, thus pulling the tongue well forward in the mouth.

glossopharyngeal (*glos-o-far-in'-jĕ-al*). Relating to the tongue and the pharynx.

glossopharyngeal muscle. Part of constrictor pharyngis superior. *See* Table of Muscles—glossopharyngeus.

glossopharyngeal nerve. The ninth cranial nerve, supplying the stylopharyngeus muscle and the parotid gland, and the mucosa of the tongue. *See* Table of Nerves—glossopharyngeus.

glossophytia (*glos-o-fi'-ti-ă*). Black tongue (*q.v.*).

glossoplasty (*glos'-o-plast-i*). Plastic surgery of the tongue.

glossoplegia (*glos-o-ple'-ji-ă*). Paralysis of the tongue.

glossoptosis (*glos-op-to'-sis*). Displacement of the tongue downwards.

glossopyrosis (*glos-o-pi-ro'-sis*). A burning sensation of the tongue.

glossorraphy (*glos-or'-af-i*). Suturing of the tongue.

glossoscopy (*glos-os'-kop-ĭ*). Diagnostic examination of the tongue.

glossospasm (*glos'-o-spazm*). Spasm of the muscles of the tongue.

glossosteresis (*glos''-o-ster-e'-sis*). Glossectomy (*q.v.*).

glossotomy (*glos-ot'-om-ĭ*). Incision of the tongue.

glossotrichia (*glos-o-trik'-ĭ-ă*). Hairy tongue (*q.v.*).

glottis (*glot'-is*). The opening between the vocal cords.

glycosialia (*glī''-ko-si-al'-ĭ-ă*). A condition in which sugar is present in the saliva.

glycosialorrhoea (*glī''-ko-si-al-or-e'-ă*). A condition in which there is excessive secretion of saliva containing sugar.

gnarled enamel. Enamel in which the prismatic rods are twisted in various directions.

gnathalgia (*nath-al'-jĭ-ă*). Neuralgic pain affecting the jaw.

gnathankylosis (*nath-an-ki-lo'-sis*). Ankylosis of the jaw.

gnathic (*nath'-ik*). Relating to the jaw.

gnathic index. The ratio of

$$\frac{\text{facial length} \times 100}{\text{length of cranial base}}$$

which gives an indication of the shape and size of a jaw.

gnathion (*na'-thĭ-on*). 1. In physical anthropology, the lowest point on the median line of the mandible. 2. In cephalometrics, the point at which the line bisecting the angle between the facial and mandibular planes crosses the outline of the mental symphysis as seen on a lateral skull radiograph.

gnathitis (*nath-i'-tis*). Inflammation of the jaws.

gnatho-. Prefix signifying *jaw*.

gnathodynamics (*na-tho-di-nam'-iks*). The study of the physical forces involved in mastication.

g n a t h o d y n a m o m e t e r (*nath''-o-di-nam-om'-et-er*). An instrument used to record the force exerted in closing the jaws.

gnathodynia (*nath-o-di'-nĭ-ă*). Pain in the jaw.

gnathology (*na-thol'-oj-ĭ*). The study of the masticatory mechanism.

gnathoplasty (*nath'-o-plast-ĭ*). Plastic surgery of the jaw or of the cheek.

gnathoplegia (*na-tho-ple'-jĭ-ă*). Paralysis of the muscles of the cheek.

gnathorrhagia (*na-thor-a'-jĭ-ă*). Bleeding of the buccal mucosa or from the jaws.

gnathoschisis (*nath-os'-kis-is*). Congenital cleft of the jaw, as in cleft palate.

gnathospasmus (*nath-o-spas'-mus*). Trismus (*q.v.*).

gnathostatics (*na-tho-stat'-iks*). A method of extra-oral orthodontic diagnosis based on the craniometric relationship of the teeth to the rest of the skull.

gnathostomatics (*na-tho-sto-mat'-iks*). The physiology of the jaws and the mouth.

Goethe's bone (J. W. von Goethe, 1749-1832. German

poet and anatomist). The intermaxillary bone.

goitre (*goy'-ter*). Enlargement of the thyroid gland.

exophthalmic g. A disease caused by hyperthyroidism, and characterized by enlarged thyroid glands and exophthalmos. *Also called* Graves' disease.

lingual g. A thyroid tumour at the upper end of the original thyroglossal duct, at the posterior end of the dorsum of the tongue.

gold (*gōld*). A soft, yellow metal, chemical symbol Au, used in dentistry for fillings and inlays.

Dutch g. An alloy of zinc and copper.

sponge g. Cohesive gold in the form of spongy crystals.

gold, Alexander. *See* Alexander gold.

gomphiasis (*gom-fi'-as-sis*). Looseness of the teeth.

gomphosis (*gom-fo'-sis*). Firm attachment of two bones, as of teeth in the jaws.

Gongylonema (*gon''-jil-o-ne'-mă*). A genus of nematode parasites found generally in domestic animals.

gongylonemiasis (*gon-jil-o-nem-i'-as-is*) *of the mouth:* Oral infestation with Gongylonema; occasionally found in man.

gonial angle (*go'-ni-al*). Gonion (*q.v.*).

goniocheiloschisis (*go''-ni-o-ki-los'-kis-is*). Macrostomia; a transverse facial cleft.

goniocraniometry (*go''-ni-o-kra-ni-om'-et-ri*). Measurement of the angles of the cranium.

goniometer (*go-ni-om'-et-er*). An instrument used for measuring angles.

gonion (*go'-ni-on*). 1. The outer tip of the angle of the mandible. 2. In cephalometrics, the point on the shadow of the angle of the mandible located by bisecting the angle between the condylar and mandibular planes.

Goslee tooth (H. J. Goslee, 1871-1930. American dentist). A porcelain tooth, attached to a metal base and readily interchangeable, used in cast bridge work.

gothic palate. An abnormally high, pointed palatal arch.

Gottlieb's cuticle (B. Gottlieb, 1885-1950. Austrian dentist). Gottlieb's epithelial attachment (*q.v.*).

Gottlieb's epithelial attachment (B. Gottlieb, 1885-1950. Austrian dentist). The epithelial tissue attaching the gum to the tooth.

gouge (*gowj*). A chisel with a hollowed or grooved blade for cutting or removing bone.

graft (*graft*) 1. A slip of tissue, such as skin, muscle or bone, used to repair a defect by implantation. 2. To attach such a slip of tissue in place.

Gram's method of staining (H. C. J. Gram, 1853-1938. Danish bacteriologist). A method for staining bacteria, first with aniline-gentian violet and then, after washing with alcohol, restaining with some other stain. Those bacteria which retain the first stain are called *Gram-positive*; those which decolourise with the use of alcohol are called *Gram-negative*.

granular (*gran'-yu-lar*). Composed of granules.

granular layer of Tomes. See Tomes' granular layer.

granule (*gran'-yul*). A minute particle or grain. 2. A small pill or pellet.

granuloma (*gran-yu-lo'-mă*). A tumour composed of granulation tissue.

apical g. A dental granuloma (*q.v.*) associated with the apical area of a tooth.

dental g. A localized mass of granulation tissue on or near the root of a tooth.

Graves' disease (R. J. Graves, 1797-1853. Irish physician). Exophthalmic goitre (*q.v.*).

grinding-in. The process of rectifying occlusal disharmony by grinding the occluding surfaces either of natural or artificial teeth.

groove (*grūv*). A long, narrow channel or trough in any surface.

alveolingual g. A groove between the lower jaw and the tongue.

developmental g. One of the grooves in the enamel surface of a tooth, marking the divisions of primary formation.

labial g. A groove in the embryonic labial lamina which develops into the vestibule of the oral cavity.

mylohyoid g. A groove on the medial surface of the mandible below the mylohyoid line, in which run the mylohyoid nerve and vessels.

nasopalatine g. A groove on the surface of the vomer in which lodge the nasopalatine nerve and vessels.

pterygopalatine g. 1. A groove on the ventral aspect of the pterygoid process of the sphenoid bone. 2. A groove on the vertical portion of the palatine bone.

gubernaculum dentis. The band of connective tissue attaching the dental sac of a permanent tooth to the surrounding gum.

Guérin's fracture (A. F. M. Guérin, 1816-95. French surgeon). Le Fort fracture of the maxilla, Class I (*q.v.*).

gum (*gŭm*). 1. Gingivae (*q.v.*). 2. Sticky secretion from certain trees.

gum rash. Strophulus (*q.v.*).

gumboil (*gum'-boyl*). Parulis (*q.v.*).

gumma (*gum-ă*). A tertiary syphilitic lesion in the form of a soft rubbery tumour composed of granulation-like tissue.

gummatous (*gum'-at-us*). Relating to a gumma.

Gunning splint (T. B. Gunning, 1813-89. American dentist). An interdental splint, like a solid double dental plate, used in fracture of the mandible.

gustation (*gus-ta'-shun*). The sense of taste, or the act of tasting.

gustatory (*gus-ta'-tor-ĭ*). Relating to the sense of taste.

gustatory artery. A. lingualis. *See* Table of Arteries.

gutta (*gut'-ă*) (*pl.* guttae). Latin for *a drop;* used in prescription writing, and abbreviated *gutt.*

gutta-percha (*gut"-a-per'-kă*). The dehydrated product of the juice of certain sapotaceous trees. It is a plastic substance, used in dentistry for temporary fillings, in root canal treatment, and so on.

guttural (*gut'-ur-al*). Relating to the throat.

Gysi's articulator (A. Gysi, fl. 1936. Swiss dentist). An apparatus, used in the construction of artificial dentures, with which all possible movements of the mandible and the condyles can be reproduced.

H

H Chemical symbol for hydrogen.

HCl Chemical symbol for hydrochloric acid.

h.d. Abbreviation for *hora decubitus*—at bedtime; used in prescription writing.

Hg Chemical symbol for mercury.

h.s. Abbreviation for *hora somni*—at bedtime; used in prescription writing.

haemangioendothelioma (*he-man"-ji-o-en-do-the-li-o'-mă*). A tumour arising from the vascular endothelium.

haemangioma (*he-man-ji-o'-mă*). A benign tumour arising from blood vessels.

haemangiopericytoma (*he-man"-ji-o-per-is-i-to'-mă*). A tumour arising from the cells surrounding the capillaries and small arteries.

haemato-, haemo-. Prefix signifying *blood.*

haematogenous (*he-mat-oj'-en-us*). 1. Blood-produced. 2. Blood-producing.

haematoma (*he-mat-o'-mă*). A swelling caused by the extravasation of blood into the tissues.

haemodia (*he-mo'-di-ă*). The condition of having abnormally sensitive teeth.

haemophilia (*he-mo-fil'-i-ă*). An hereditary defect of the blood-clotting mechanism, appearing in the male but transmitted through the female.

haemophiliac (*he-mo-fil'-i-ak*). A sufferer from haemophilia.

Haemophilus (*he-mof'-il-us*). A genus of the Parvobacteriaceae family, Gram-negative, parasitic, rod-shaped organisms.

haemoptysic (*he-mop'-tis-ik*). Relating to or characterized by haemoptysis.

haemoptysis (*he-mop'-tis-is*). The presence of blood in the sputum, caused by bleeding in the upper respiratory tract or the lungs.

haemorrhage (*hem'-or-āj*). Internal or external loss of blood due to injury or other damage to a blood vessel.

haemorrhagic (*hem-or-a'-jik*). Relating to or affected by haemorrhage.

haemorrhoid (*hem'-er-oyd*). *lingual h.* Swelling of the veins at the root of the tongue.

haemostasis (*he-mo-sta'-sis*). 1. The arrest of bleeding. 2. The checking of the blood circulation at any point.

haemostatic (*he-mo-stat'-ik*). 1. Relating to the arrest of bleeding. 2. An agent used in haemostasis.

hairy tongue. A tongue having hair-like papillae.

half-cap crown. A form of crown covering all but the labial or buccal surface of a tooth, and attached by a metal band.

halitosis (*hal-it-o'-sis*). Foetid-smelling breath.

Haller's ansa (A. von Haller, 1708-77. Swiss anatomist and surgeon). The loop formed below the stylomastoid foramen between the glossopharyngeal nerve and the lingual branch of the facial nerve.

hamartoma (*ham-ar-to'-mă*). A tumour-like mass of superfluous tissue, the result of faulty embryonal development of tissues or cells.

Hamilton's bandage (F. H. Hamilton, 1813-86. American surgeon). A special bandage consisting of straps of linen webbing attached to a leather thong.

Hammond splint. 1. An orthodontic splint used for repositioning a tooth or teeth. 2. A double arch wire fixed to the teeth and used to immobilize a jaw fracture.

hamular, hamulate (*ham'-yu-lar; ham'-yu-lāt*). 1. Shaped like a hook. 2. Relating to a hamulus.

hamular notch. Pterygomaxillary notch (*q.v.*).

hamular process. A hooklike descending process of the medial pterygoid plate.

hamulus (*ham'-yu-lus*). A hook-shaped process on a bone.

Hanau's equation. An algebraic formula used in the setting up of an anatomical articulator. It provides for the simulation of the Bennett movement by relating the angular rotation (V) of the condylar path about a vertical axis to its rotation (H) about a horizontal axis.

$$V = \frac{H}{8} + 12$$

where V is the deviation from the sagittal plane and H the deviation from the coronal plane, measured in degrees.

handpiece (*hand'-pēs*). The part of a dental engine

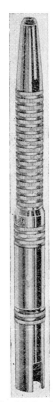

Straight handpiece

attached to the driving belt, and into which the various instruments may be fitted.

Hannover's intermediate membrane (A. Hannover, 1814-94. Danish anatomist). An acellular layer of material in a developing mammalian tooth separating developing cementum from root dentine and from the ameloblasts. In the fully formed root it is represented by an acellular layer lying between the dentine and the cementum—the stratum intermedium.

haphalgesia (*haf-al-je'-zi-ă*). A condition in which intense pain is felt from a slight touch.

haplodont (*hap'-lo-dont*). Having teeth with simple, smooth conical crowns and simple roots.

Hapsburg jaw. Mandibular prognathism, similar to the hereditary condition which affected the Hapsburg dynasty.

Hapsburg lip. The over-developed lower lip often accompanying Hapsburg jaw (*q.v.*).

hard palate. The bony, front portion of the roof of the mouth.

hard sore. Chancre (*q.v.*).

hare lip (*hār'-lip*). Congenital fissure of one or both sides of the upper lip.

harelip needle. A cannula which is introduced into the wound during an operation for harelip, and held in place by a figure-of-eight suture.

Hartley-Krause operation (F. Hartley, 1856-1913. American surgeon. F. V. Krause, 1857-1937. German surgeon). An operation for the relief of facial neuralgia by excision of the Gasserian ganglion. Devised, independently, by both Hartley and Krause.

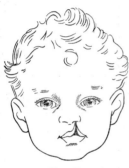

Hare lip

Hartman's solution (L. L. Hartman, 1893-1951. American dentist). A solution of thymol, sulphuric ether and ethyl alcohol used to desensitize dentine.

hatchet. A hand instrument with the blade running parallel to the handle, and bibevelled.

haustus (*how'-stus*). Latin for *a draught*; used in prescription writing, generally with *fiat*, abbreviated *f.h.* (fiat haustus).

Hawley retainer (C. A. Hawley, 20th century American dentist). A horseshoe shaped plate with clasps to the premolars and a labial wire from the lingual plate over the labial surface of the incisors; the most commonly used orthodontic removable retaining appliance.

head (*hed*). 1. The uppermost part of the body, containing the special sensory organs and the brain. 2. The upper end of a bone, especially of a long bone.

headcap (*hed'-kap*). 1. A webbing or plastic strapping harness which fits over the patient's head and is used to supply attachment for extra-oral traction in orthodontic treatment. 2. A plaster cap used with metal jaw splints in fracture of the jaw or of the facial bones.

Heath's operation (C. Heath, 1835-1905. English surgeon). An operation for ankylosis treated by dividing the ascending rami of the mandible with a saw; performed within the mouth.

hecto-, hect-. Prefix signifying *one hundred*.

helcoid (*hel'-koyd*). Ulcer-like.

helcosis (*hel-ko'-sis*). The condition of having ulcers; ulceration.

helix (*he'-liks*). *In anatomy:* The convex margin of the pinna of the ear.

hemangioma. *See* haemangioma.

hematoma. *See* haematoma.

hemi-. Prefix signifying *half*, or *one side* (right or left) of a body, organ, or part.

hemiageusia (*hem-ĭ-ag-u'-sĭ-ă*). Loss or absence of a sense of taste in one side of the tongue only; hemigeusia.

hemiatrophy (*hem-ĭ-at'-rof-ĭ*). Atrophy affecting one half of an organ or part, or one side of the body only.

hemifacial (*hem-ĭ-fa'-shĭ-al*). Relating to or affecting one side of the face only.

hemigeusia (*hem-ĭ-gu'-sĭ-a*). Loss or absence of a sense of taste to one side of the tongue; hemiageusia.

hemiglossal (*hem-ĭ-glos'-al*). Relating to or affecting one side of the tongue only.

hemiglossectomy (*hem-ĭ-glos-ekt'-om-ĭ*). Surgical removal of one side of the tongue.

hemiglossitis (*hem-ĭ-glos-i'-tis*). Inflammation affecting one side of the tongue only.

hemiglossoplegia (*hem"-ĭ-glos-o-ple'-jĭ-ă*). Paralysis affecting one side of the tongue only.

hemignathia (*hem-ĭ-na'-thĭ-ă*). The condition of having only half a jaw.

hemihypermetria (*hem"-ĭ-hi-per-met'-rĭ-ă*). Abnormal extension or protrusion of one half of a part.

hemihyperplasia (*hem"-ĭ-hi-per-pla'-zĭ-ă*). Hyperplasia affecting only one side or one half of an organ or part.

hemihypertrophy (*hem"-ĭ-hi-per'-trof-ĭ*). Hypertrophy affecting one side or one half of a body, an organ, or a part.

hemihypogeusia (*hem"-ĭ-hi-po-gu'-sĭ-ă*). Hemigeusia (*q.v.*).

hemilingual (*hem-ĭ-lin'-gwal*). Relating to or affecting one side of the tongue only.

hemimacroglossia (*hem"-ĭ-mak-ro-glos'-ĭ-ă*). Abnormal development and size of one side of the tongue.

hemimandibulectomy (*hem"-ĭ-man-dib-yu-lek'-tom-ĭ*). The surgical removal of one side of the mandible.

hemipalatolaryngoplegia (*hem"-ĭ-pal"-at-o-lar"-ing-o-ple'-jĭ-ă*). Paralysis affecting the muscles on one side of the soft palate and the larynx.

hemiplegia (*hem-ĭ-ple'-jĭ-ă*). Paralysis affecting one side of the body.
facial h. Paralysis affecting one side of the face only.
faciolingual h. Paralysis affecting one side of the face and the tongue.

hemo-. *See* haemo-.

herbivorous (*herb-iv'-or-us*). Grass- and herb-eating.

hereditary (*her-ed'-it-ar-ĭ*). Relating to heredity.

hereditary opalescent dentine. Dentinogenesis imperfecta (*q.v.*).

heredity (*her-ed'-it-ĭ*). The transmission of a characteristic from parent to child, or to later generations.

herpes (*her'-pēz*). An acute inflammatory skin infection, characterized by vesicles which appear in clusters.

herpes labialis (*her'-pēz labi-a'-lis*). Cold sores or blisters occurring on the lips.

herpes simplex (*her'-pēz sim'-pleks*). Herpes vesicles affecting the mucous membranes particularly, and developing on the borders of the lips and nostrils.

herpes zoster (*her'-pēz zos'-ter*). Herpes affecting the body, especially in areas supplied by certain nerves.

herpetic (*her-pet'-ik*). Relating to herpes.

Hertwig's sheath (W. A. O. Hertwig, 1849-1922. German anatomist). A continuation of the internal and external enamel epithelium at the lower rim of the enamel organ, which provides the inductive stimulus for root dentine formation and determines root morphology.

hetero-. Prefix signifying *different, other.*

heterocellular (*het"-er-o-sel'-yu-lar*). Formed of different types of cells.

heterodont (*het'-er-o-dont*). Having teeth which have different forms; as opposed to *homodont.*

heterogeneous (*het"-er-o-je'-nē-us*). Consisting of different substances; as opposed to *homogeneous.*

heterogenous (*het-er-oj'-en-us*). Derived from different species; as opposed to *homogenous.*

heteroplasia (*het"-er-o-pla'-zi-ă*). Formation of tissue either abnormal in structure or in position.

heterostomy (*het-er-ost'-om-ĭ*). The condition of having an asymmetrical mouth.

heterotopic (*het"-er-o-top'-ik*). Occurring in a place other than normal.

heterotrophic (*het"-er-o-tro'-fik*). Relating to organisms which require a complex source of carbon for nourishment and growth; as opposed to *autotrophic.*

hex-. Prefix signifying *six.*

hiatal (*hi-a'-tal*). Relating to a hiatus.

hiatus (*hi-a'-tus*). Any gap, opening or fissure.
buccal h. A transverse facial cleft.
h. of facial canal; facial h. Facial canal (*q.v.*).
maxillary h. The opening on the inner surface of the maxilla joining the nasal cavity and the maxillary antrum; hiatus semilunaris.

Highmore, antrum of (N. Highmore, 1613-85. English anatomist). Maxillary sinus (*q.v.*).

highmoritis (*hi-mor-i'-tis*). Inflammation of the antrum of Highmore, the maxillary sinus.

hilar (*hi'-lar*). Relating to a hilus.

hilus (*hi'-lus*). A pit or opening in an organ, generally where the vessels or ducts enter.

hinge-bow. A form of face-bow which is adjustable to permit of the location of the axis of rotation of the mandible.

Hirschfeld canal (I. Hirschfeld, b. 1881. American dentist). Nutrient canal (q.v.).

Hirschfeld's nerve (L. M. Hirschfeld, 1816-76. Polish anatomist). A lingual branch of the facial nerve which goes to form Haller's ansa.

hirudiniasis (hir-u-din-i'-as-is). Infestation of the mouth and the upper respiratory tract by leeches.

histo-. Prefix signifying tissue.

histochemistry (his"-to-kem'-is-tri). The chemistry of the body tissues and body fluids.

histogenesis (his"-to-jen'-es-is). The embryonic development of tissues.

histologic, histological (his-tol-oj'-ik-al). Relating to histology.

histological chemistry. Histochemistry (q.v.).

histology (his-tol'-oj-i). The anatomy and physiology of the tissues.

histopathological (his"-to-path-ol-oj'-ik-al). Relating to histopathology.

histopathology (his"-to-path-ol'-oj-i). The study of minute structural changes in diseased tissue; histological pathology.

hoe (ho). A form of chisel. *periodontal h.* An instrument used for removing calculus

and other deposits from the tooth surface.

hollow (hol'-o). 1. A depression or concavity. 2. Descriptive of an empty container.

hollow, Sebileau's. *See* Sebileau's hollow.

homalocephalus (hom"-al-o-sef'-al-us). A person having a flat head.

homaluranus (hom-al-yur-a'-nus). A person having an unusually flat palatal arch.

homo-. Prefix signifying same, like.

homodont (ho'-mo-dont). Having teeth all of the same form; as opposed to *heterodont*.

homogeneous (hom-o-je'-nĕ-us). Of one kind or species; as opposed to *heterogeneous*.

homogenous (hom-oj'-en-us). Derived from one species, and being therefore similar; as opposed to *heterogenous*.

homologous (ho-mol'-og-us). Having the same or corresponding structure or position, but not necessarily similar in function.

homology (ho-mol'-og-ĭ). The quality of being homologous.

hood
tooth h. The flap of mucosa which remains over the occlusal surface of an erupting posterior tooth.

hood crown. A half-cap crown covering the lingual, proximal and occlusal surfaces of a tooth.

hora decubitus (or'-ah da-ku'-bit-us). Latin for *at*

bedtime; used in prescription writing, and abbreviated *h.d.*

hora somni (*or'-ah som'-nĭ*). Latin for *at bedtime*; used in prescription writing, and abbreviated *h.s.*

horizontal overbite. Overjet (*q.v.*).

horizontal overlap. Overjet (*q.v.*).

hormion (*hor'-mĭ-on*). The point of attachment of the vomer and the sphenoid bone, between the alae of the vomer.

horn (*horn*). A pointed projection or protuberance.
pulp h. Horn-like projections of the pulp chamber into the crown of a tooth.

Hotchkiss's operation (L. W. Hotchkiss, 1859-1926. American surgeon). An operation for the removal of buccal carcinoma, involving the excision of a portion of the mandible and sometimes of the maxilla, and plastic repair of the cheek from the neck tissues.

How crown (W. S. How, fl. 1883. American dentist). A porcelain-faced crown attached by means of four pins bent round a post in the tooth root, the exposed parts being built up with amalgam.

Howland-Perry crown. An improved form of the Mack crown (*q.v.*), having better retention.

Howship's lacunae (J. Howship, 1781-1841. English surgeon). Absorption spaces

under the periosteum, semi-lunar hollows which are, or have been, occupied by osteoclasts.

Hullihan's acutenaculum (*ak-yu-ten-ak'-yu-lum*) (S. P. Hullihan, 1810-57. American dentist). A type of needle-holder used in cleft palate surgery.

humectant (*hyu-mek'-tant*). 1. Moistening. 2. Any moistening agent.

Humphry's operation (G. M. Humphry, 1820-96. English surgeon). An operation for excision of a mandibular condyle.

Hunter's glossitis (W. Hunter, 1861-1937. English physician). Ulcerative glossitis occurring in pernicious anaemia.

Hunter-Schreger bands. Schreger's lines *in enamel* (*q.v.*).

Hutchinson's incisors (Sir Jonathan Hutchinson, 1828-1913. English physician). Permanent incisors having narrow and notched incisal edges; found in congenital syphilis.

Hutchinson's incisor

hyaloid (*hi'-al-oyd*). Glass-like.

hydrargyrum (*hi-drar-ji'-rum*). Mercury (*q.v.*).

hydro-. Prefix signifying *water*.

hydrocolloid (*hi-dro-kol'-oyd*). A type of dental impression material; a viscous colloid sol which is converted to a rigid and insoluble gel; it may be reversible or irreversible.

hydrocyst (*hi'-dro-sist*). A cyst whose contents are of a watery nature.

hydro-flo technique (*hi'-dro-flo'*). A term originated by E. O. Thompson, American dentist, to designate a technique of cavity preparation in which the field of operation is constantly irrigated in a stream of warm water, and the water removed from the mouth by vacuum suction.

hydroglossa (*hi-dro-glos'-ă*). Ranula (*q.v.*).

hydropic (*hi-drop'-ik*). Relating to or affected with dropsy.

hydrostomia (*hi-dro-sto'-mi-ă*). A condition characterized by constant dribbling from the mouth.

hydrous (*hi'-drus*). Containing water.

hygiene (*hi'-jēn*). Principles and practice of general and personal cleanliness for the promotion of health and prevention of disease.
   oral h. Principles of hygiene as applied to the mouth, to ensure cleanliness of the teeth and promote healthy gingiva.

hygienic (*hi-je'-nik*). Relating to hygiene.

hygro-. Prefix signifying *moisture*.

hygroma (*hi-gro'-mă*). A swelling caused by fluid surrounding an inflamed bursa, or distending a sac or cyst.

hygrostomia (*hi-gro-sto'-mi-ă*). Chronic excessive salivation.

hyo-. Prefix used in anatomy to denote some relationship with the *hyoid* arch or bone.

hyobasioglossus (*hi''-o-ba''-si-o-glos'-us*). The basal portion of the hyoglossal muscle.

hyoglossal (*hi-o-glos'-al*). Relating to the hyoid bone and the tongue.

hyoglossus (*hi-o-glos'-us*). The muscle which draws down the sides of the tongue. *See* Table of Muscles.

hyoid artery. A. infrahyoidea and A. suprahyoidea. *See* Table of Arteries.

hyoid bone (*hi'-oyd*). U-shaped bone forming the arch between the larynx and the base of the tongue; it supports the tongue and provides attachment for some of the facial muscles.

hyomandibular (*hi''-o-man-dib'-yu-lar*). 1. Relating to the hyoid and mandibular arches in the embryo. 2. Relating to the cartilagenous portion of the hyoid arch in fish.

hypalgesia (hi-pal-je'-zǐ-ǎ). Reduced sensibility to pain.

hypanisognathism (hi-pan-is-og'-nath-izm). The condition of having the maxillary teeth broader than the mandibular teeth, causing a lack of correspondence between the jaws.

hypanisognathous (hi-pan-is-og'-nath-us). Relating to or characterized by hypanisognathism.

hyper-. Prefix signifying 1. *excessive, exaggerated;* 2. *above* (in anatomy or zoology).

hyperaemia (hi-per-e'-mǐ-ǎ). Excess of blood causing localized congestion.

hyperalgesia (hi"-per-al-je'-zǐ-ǎ). The condition of being excessively sensitive to pain.

hyperbrachycephalic (hi"-per-brak-ǐ-sef-al'-ik). Showing an extreme degree of brachycephaly, having an exceptionally broad head.

hypercementosis (hi"-per-se-ment-o'-sis). Over-development of cementum on tooth roots.

hyperdontia (hi-per-don'-shǐ-ǎ). The condition of having supernumerary teeth present in the mouth.

hyperdontogeny (hi"-per-dont-oj'-en-ǐ). Hyperodontogeny (q.v.).

hyperemia. *See* hyperaemia.

hyperfunction (hi-per-funk'-shun). Abnormal, excessive functioning.

hypergeusia (hi-per-gu'-sǐ-ǎ). Abnormally acute sense of taste.

hyperhidrosis (hi"-per-hi-dro'-sis). Excessive sweating.

hyperkeratosis linguae. Black tongue (q.v.).

hyperodontogeny (hi"-per-o-dont-oj'-en-ǐ). The condition of developing supernumerary teeth, or even a complete third dentition.

hyperorthognathous (hi"-per-or-thog'-nath-us). Relating to or characterized by hyperorthognathy.

hyperorthognathy (hi"-per-or-thog'-nath-ǐ). Excessive orthognathia (q.v.); having a very low gnathic index.

hyperostosis (hi"-per-os-to'-sis). Bone hypertrophy; exostosis.

hyperplasia (hi-per-pla'-zǐ-ǎ). Over-development of an organ or tissue, due to increased production of cells. *cementum h.* Localized deposition of cementum; cementosis.

hyperplastic (hi-per-plast'-ik). Relating to or affected by hyperplasia.

hyperptyalism (hi-per-ti'-al-izm). Hypersalivation (q.v.).

hypersalivation (hi"-per-sal-iv-a'-shun). A condition in which there is excessive secretion of saliva.

hypersialosis (hi"-per-si-al-o'-sis). Excessive salivary secretion.

hypertelorism (hi"-per-tel'-or-izm). 1. An abnormal distance between any two organs or parts. **2.** A craniofacial deformity characterized by enlargement of the sphenoid bone, great breadth across the bridge of the nose, and resulting width between the eyes; *also called* ocular hypertelorism.

hypertension (*hi-per-ten'-shun*). Exceptionally high tension, especially abnormally high blood pressure.

hypertensive (*hi-per-ten'-siv*). Relating to hypertension.

hyperthyroidism (*hi-per-thi'-royd-izm*). A condition caused by abnormal hyperfunction of the thyroid gland; exophthalmic goitre.

hypertrophic (*hi-per-tro'-fik*). Relating to or characterized by hypertrophy.

hypertrophy (*hi-per'-trof-i*). An abnormal increase in the size of an organ or part due to enlargement of its constituent cells.

hypnodontics (*hip-no-don'-tiks*). The application of hypnosis in dentistry.

hypnosis (*hip-no'-sis*). Sleep, or a trance state, especially one induced artificially by verbal suggestion or concentration upon some object.

hypnotic (*hip-not'-ik*). **1.** Relating to hypnosis. **2.** Inducing sleep.

hypnotism (*hip'-not-izm*). The process of inducing sleep or a trance.

hypo-. Prefix signifying **1.** *deficient, lacking;* **2.** *below* (in anatomy and zoology).

hypobranchial (*hi-po-bran'-ki-al*). Below the branchial arches.

hypobranchial eminence. A median swelling between the tongue and the laryngotracheal groove in the embryo, from which is developed the epiglottis and aryepiglottic folds, and the posterior third of the tongue.

hypocalcification (*hi"-po-kal-sif-ik-a'-shun*). Defective development resulting in an insufficient deposit of calcium salts in any normally calcified tissue.

hypocondylar (*hi-po-kon'-di-lar*). Below a condyle.

hypocone (*hi'-po-kŏn*). The disto-lingual cusp of a maxillary molar tooth.

hypoconid (*hi-po-ko'-nid*). The disto-buccal cusp on a mandibular molar tooth.

hypoconule (*hi-po-kon'-yul*). The fifth, distal cusp of a maxillary molar tooth.

hypoconulid (*hi-po-kon'-yu-lid*). The fifth, distal cusp of a mandibular molar tooth.

hypodermic (*hi-po-derm'-ik*). Under the skin.

hypodermic needle. A form of hollow needle used with a syringe for injections.

hypodontia (*hi-po-don'-shi-ă*). Under-development of the teeth.

hypofunction (*hi-po-funk'-shun*). Deficient or diminished function.

hypogeusia (*hi-po-gu'-si-ă*). Diminution of the sense of taste.

hypoglossal (*hi-po-glos'-al*). Underneath the tongue.

hypoglossal canal. The anterior condylar canal (*q.v.*).

hypoglossal nerve. The twelfth cranial nerve, supplying the muscles of the tongue. *See* Table of Nerves—hypoglossus.

hypoglossiadenitis (*hi"-po-glos-i-ad-en-i'-tis*). Inflammation of the sublingual glands.

hypoglossitis (*hi"-po-glos-i'-tis*). Inflammation of the sublingual tissues.

hypoglottis (*hi-po-glot'-is*). 1. The under part of the tongue. 2. Ranula (*q.v.*).

hypognathous (*hi-pog'-nath-us*). Having a protruding mandible.

hypomicrognathic (*hi"-po-mi-krog'-nath-ik*). Having an abnormally small lower jaw; extreme micrognathism.

hypomineralization (*hi"-po-min-er-al-i-za'-shun*). Deficiency of mineral salts in the body.

hypo-ostosis (*hi"-po-os-to'-sis*). Bone hypoplasia.

hypopharynx. (*hi-po-far'-inks*). The lower or laryngeal part of the pharynx; an obsolete term.

hypophyseal (*hi-pof-is'-e-al*). Relating to a hypophysis; more specifically, relating to the pituitary gland.

hypophysis (*hi-pof'-is-is*). An outgrowth, especially used of the pituitary body.

hypoplasia (*hi-po-pla'-zi-ă*). Under-development of an organ or tissue.

hypoplastic (*hi-po-plast'-ik*). Relating to hypoplasia.

hypoptyalism (*hi-po-ti'-al-izm*). Xerostomia (*q.v.*).

hyposalivation (*hi"-po-sal-iv-a'-shun*). Xerostomia (*q.v.*).

hyposiagonarthritis (*hi"-po-si-ag-on-ar-thri'-tis*). Inflammation affecting the temporomandibular joint.

hyposialadenitis (*hi"-po-si-al-ad-en-i'-tis*). Inflammation of the submandibular salivary glands.

hyposialosis (*hi"'-po-si-al-o'-sis*). Xerostomia (*q.v.*).

hypostomatous (*hi-po-sto'-mat-us*). A zoological term for those animals which have the mouth on the lower side.

hypostomia (*hi-po-sto'-mi-ă*). An extreme form of microstomia, the mouth being merely a slit opening into a pharyngeal sac.

hypostosis (*hi-pos-to'-sis*). Deficient bone development.

hypotension (*hi-po-ten'-shun*). Abnormally low tension, especially abnormally low blood pressure.

hypotensive (*hi-po-ten'-siv*). Relating to hypotension.

hypothyroidism (*hi-po-thi'-royd-izm*). Deficient thyroid secretion, or the condition which this produces.

hypotonic (*hi-po-ton'-ik*). Relating to hypotonicity.

hypotonicity (hi-po-ton-is'-it-i). Diminished or reduced tension or muscle tone.

hypsibrachycephalic (hip''-si-brak-i-sef-al'-ik). Having an exceptionally broad and high skull.

hypsicephalic (hip''-si-sef-al'-ik). Having an abnormally high skull.

hypsistaphylic (hip''-si-staf-il'-ik). Having a high, narrow palate.

hypsistenocephalic (hip''-sis-ten-o-sef-al'-ik). Having an abnormally high and narrow skull, with mandibular prognathism and prominent facial bones.

hypsocephalous (hip-so-sef'-al-us). Hypsicephalic (q.v.).

hypsodont (hip'-so-dont). Having teeth with long crowns and short roots.

I

I Chemical symbol for iodine.

I. Symbol for *permanent* incisor.

id. Abbreviation for *idem*—the same; used in prescription writing.

IL Incisolingual.

ILa Incisolabial.

in. Abbreviation for *inch*.

in d. Abbreviation for *in dies*—daily; used in prescription writing.

IP Incisopulpal.

-ic. Suffix signifying *relating to*.

ichor (i'-kor). The thin, watery discharge from a wound or ulcer.

ichorous (i'-kor-us). Relating to ichor.

ichthyosis linguae. Leukoplakia (q.v.).

idem (id'-em). Latin for *the same*; used in prescription writing and abbreviated *id*.

idio-. Prefix signifying *self*, *distinct*; in medicine it signifies *self-produced*.

idiopathic (id-i-o-path'-ik). Self-originated, primary, relating to idiopathy.

idiopathy (id-i-op'-ath-i). Any self-originated pathological condition.

idiosyncracy (id-i-o-sin'-kras-i). Reaction to a particular drug in therapeutic doses in a manner not necessarily related to its pharmacological properties.

imbalance (im-bal'-ans). Lack of equilibrium; unbalanced.

imbrication line. One of the grooves in the surface of tooth enamel, marking the edges of the lines of Retzius.

immature (im-at-yur'). Not fully developed; unripe.

immediate denture. A denture constructed for insertion immediately after the removal of the natural teeth.

immune (im-yūn'). Protected against or resistant to a specific disease.

immunity (im-yu'-nit-i). Natural or acquired resistance to specific diseases or poisons.

immunization (im-yu-ni-za'-shun). The process or the method of rendering immune.

immuno-. Prefix signifying *immune*.

immunology (im-yu-nol'-oj-ĭ). The study of immunity.

impacted (im-pak'-ted). Wedged in or confined.

impacted tooth. One so placed in the jaw that it cannot erupt.

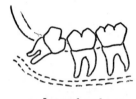

Impacted tooth

impaction (im-pak'-shun). The condition of being tightly wedged.

imperforate (im-per'-for-āt). Congenitally closed, applied to a structure which would normally be open.

imperforation (im-per-for-a'-shun). The condition of being congenitally closed, applied to a normally open structure.

impermeable (im-per'-me-abl). Not permitting a passage, especially of fluid.

impervious (im-per'-vĭ-us). Not affording a passage, particularly of fluid.

implant (im'-plant). 1. To graft, in plastic surgery. 2. The tissue used for a graft.

implant denture. An artificial denture supported by a framework fastened to the alveolar process beneath the periosteum, and having protruding abutments to which the denture is attached.

implantation (im-plant-a'-shun). 1. The operation of grafting. 2. The transfer of a sound tooth to replace one extracted, or to fill an artificial socket. 3. The placing of some foreign substance within the body tissues for restoration purposes.

impression (im-presh'-un). 1. Any dent or hollow in a soft substance. 2. A negative likeness or mould of an object obtained in a plastic substance from which a model may be cast—e.g. the impression obtained of the teeth and the mouth, prior to the construction of dentures.

impression compound. A plastic material used for taking dental impressions, and composed of fatty acids, shellac, glycerin, and some form of filler, such as talc or plaster of Paris. The actual composition of individual compounds is treated as a trade secret.

impression tray. A metal receptacle in which wax or plastic impression material is placed when taking mouth impressions.

in dies (in dē'-āz). Latin for *daily*; used in prescription writing, and abbreviated *in d.*

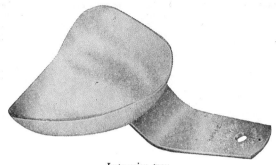

Impression tray

in vitro (*in vit'-ro*). Within glass; referring to observations made in a test-tube or culture dish, as opposed to *in vivo*.

in vivo (*in ve'-vo*). Within a living organism; as opposed to *in vitro*.

in-. Prefix signifying 1. *in, on, toward;* 2. *not.*

inankyloglossia (*in-an"-ki-lo-glos'-i-ă*). A condition in which the tongue is incapable of movement; tongue-tie.

inborn (*in'-born*). Formed or developed *in utero;* innate.

inception (*in-sep'-shun*). Beginning.

inch (*insh*). A unit of measurement of length, one-twelfth of a foot.

incidence (*in'-sid-ens*). The number of cases of a disease appearing in a given place over a given period of time.

incipient (*in-sip'-i-ent*). Beginning to develop, coming into existence.

incisal (*in-si'-zal*). Cutting.

incisal angle. In dentistry, any angle formed by the junction of an incisal edge, or cavity wall, in an anterior tooth, with any other tooth surface or cavity wall.

incisal edge *of a tooth.* The edge which cuts, the biting edge of an incisor or canine.

incisal rest. An extension or projection on a partial denture which rests on or engages with the incisal edge of an anterior tooth.

incisal wall. That wall of a tooth cavity facing the incisal edge of a tooth.

incision (*in-sizh'-un*). A wound or cut in body tissue, or the act of making such a cut.

incision (*in-siz'-ĭ-on*). The line of intersection between the median plane and the mandibular occlusal plane.

incisive (*in-si'-ziv*). 1. Capable of cutting. 2. Relating to the incisor teeth.

incisive canal. A canal in the maxilla leading from the incisive fossa to the floor of the nasal cavity.

incisive foramen. One of two to four openings of the incisive canal on the floor of the incisive fossa. *Lateral*: on the hard palate behind the incisors, transmitting branches of the greater palatine artery; *median*: in the midline of the hard palate, transmitting the nasopalatine nerves.

incisive fossa. 1. A depression on the maxilla behind the incisors. 2. A depression on the mandible below the incisors, giving origin to the mentalis muscle. 3. A depression on the outer surface of the maxilla, giving origin to the depressor muscle of the nose.

incisive papilla. The projection of the palatine mucosa overlying the incisive fossa at the anterior end of the palatine raphe.

incisivus labii inferioris. Part of the orbicularis oris muscle, extending from the area of the mandibular canine to the angle of the mouth.

incisivus labii superioris. Part of the orbicularis oris muscle, extending from the area of the maxillary canine to the angle of the mouth.

incisolabial (*in-si"-zo-la'-bi-al*). Relating to the incisal edge and the labial surface of an anterior tooth.

incisolingual (*in-si"-zo-lin'-gwal*). Relating to the incisal edge and the lingual surface of an anterior tooth.

incisoproximal (*in-si"-zo-proks'-im-al*). Relating to the incisal edge and either the distal or mesial surface of an anterior tooth.

incisor tooth (*in-si'-zor*). A cutting tooth in the centre of the dental arch. There are two incisors in each quadrant in both the deciduous and the permanent dentitions in man, one *central* and one *lateral*.

Incisor tooth

incisors, Hutchinson's. *See* Hutchinson's incisors.

inclination (*in-klin-a'-shun*). The tilt of a tooth away from the vertical, in any direction.

inclusion (*in-klu'-zhun*). *In dentistry*: The embedding of a tooth in the alveolar bone to such an extent that it cannot erupt.

increment (*in'-kre-ment*). The amount of increase within a given period.

incremental line. One of the lines which are said to show the laminar structure of dentine and enamel in a tooth.

incrustation (*in-krust-a'-shun*). The formation of a crust.

indentation (*in-dent-a'-shun*). 1. A dent, pit, or depression. 2. The condition of being serrated or notched.

index (*in'-deks*) (*pl.* indexes, or indices). 1. The forefinger. 2. A number or formula expressing the ratio between two dimensions of a part, used especially in craniometry.

alveolar i. Gnathic index (*q.v.*).

cephalic i. The ratio of

$$\frac{\text{cranial breadth} \times 100}{\text{cranial length}}$$

which gives an indication of the shape and size of a cranium.

cranial i. Cephalic index (*q.v.*).

dental i. The ratio of

$$\frac{\text{dental length} \times 100}{\text{length of cranial base}}$$

facial i. The ratio of

$$\frac{\text{facial length} \times 100}{\text{facial width}}$$

which gives an indication of the shape and size of a face.

gnathic i. The ratio of

$$\frac{\text{facial length} \times 100}{\text{length of cranial base}}$$

which gives an indication of the shape and size of a jaw.

palatal i. The ratio of

$$\frac{\text{palatal width} \times 100}{\text{palatal length}}$$

which gives an indication of the shape and size of a palate; *also called* palatine, or palatomaxillary, index.

index, Bodecker's. *See* Bodecker's index.

index, Flower's. Dental index (*q.v.*).

indigenous (*in-dij'-en-us*). Native, especially to a particular country or area.

indirect retainer. Part of a partial denture which acts indirectly on the opposite side of the fulcrum line from the direct retainers, to prevent displacement in free-end dentures.

indococcus (*in-do-kok'-us*). A form of micrococcus found in the mouth.

indolent (*in'-dol-ent*). Sluggish, or painless.

induced (*in-dyu'-sd*). 1. Brought on by an outside agency. 2. Artificially produced.

indurated (*in-dyur-a'-ted*). Hardened.

induration (*in-dyur-a'-shun*). 1. The state of being hard, or the process of becoming hard. 2. An area of hard tissue.

inert (*in-ert'*). Not active; having no action.

infancy ring. A line marking the arrested calcification of tooth enamel, formed at about 12 months.

infection (*in-fek'-shun*). The communication of disease by the invasion of body tissue by specific pathogenic micro-organisms.

infection, Vincent's. Acute ulcerative gingivitis (q.v.).

infectious (in-fek'-shus). Relating to or caused by infection.

infectious disease. A disease caused by pathogenic organisms.

infective (in-fek'-tiv). Infectious.

inferior (in-fe'-rĭ-or). Situated below; applied in anatomy to structures nearer the feet; as opposed to *superior*.

inferior sagittal sinus. A venous sinus joining the great cerebral vein to form the straight sinus. *See* Table of Veins—sinus sagittalis inferior.

inferolateral (in″-fer-o-lat′-er-al). Situated below and on one side.

inferomedian (in″-fer-o-me′-di-an). Situated below and in the middle.

inferoposterior (in″-fer-o-po-ste′-ri-or). Situated both below and behind.

infiltrate (in′-fil-trāt). 1. To pass into a cell or tissue or intercellular space, e.g. fluid, or cells. 2. The substance thus passed.

infiltration (in-fil-tra′-shun). 1. A process by which a substance or fluid enters a cell or tissue, or intercellular space; it may be either an abnormal amount of a substance normally present or some foreign

substance. 2. The condition produced by this process.

infiltration anaesthesia. Local anaesthesia of a limited area produced by the infiltration of an anaesthetic agent into the surrounding tissues.

inflammation (in-flam-a′-shun). The reaction of living tissue to injury; marked by redness, pain, heat and swelling, and by histological changes.

inflammatory (in-flam′-at-or-i). Relating to or characterized by inflammation.

inflation (in-fla′-shun). Distention with a gas, especially air.

infra-. Prefix signifying *beneath, within.*

infra-bony pocket. A form of true periodontal pocket in which the base of the pocket lies below the level of the alveolar bone.

infrabulge (in′-fră-bulj). *In prosthetic dentistry:* That part of the tooth crown below the clasp guide line.

infraclusion (in-fră-klu′-zhun). A form of malocclusion, in which the occluding surfaces of the teeth are below the normal occlusal plane.

infracondylism (in-fră-kon′-dil-izm). Deviation of the mandibular condyles in a downward direction.

infradentale (in″-fră-dent-a′-lĕ). The lowest point on the midline of the mandible on

inf   153   inj

the alveolar margin, between the central incisors.

infrahyoid (*in-fră-hi'-oyd*). Below the hyoid bone.

infrahyoid artery. Branch from the superior thyroid artery, supplying the thyrohyoid muscle. *See* Table of Arteries—infrahyoidea.

inframandibular (*in-fră-man-dib'-yu-lar*). Below the mandible.

inframaxillary (*in-fră-maks-il'-ar-i*). Below the jaw.

infra-occlusion (*in-fră-ok-lu'-zhun*). Infraclusion (*q.v.*).

infra-orbital (*in-fră-or'-bit-al*). Lying beneath the floor of the orbit.

infra-orbital artery. Branch of the maxillary artery, supplying the upper lip, side of the nose, lower eyelid and lacrimal sac. *See* Table of Arteries—infraorbitalis.

infra-orbital canal. One of the passages from the infra-orbital grooves to the infra-orbital foramen in the maxilla, through which pass the infra-orbital arteries and nerves.

infra-orbital foramen. The external opening in the maxilla of the infra-orbital canal, through which pass the infra-orbital artery and nerve.

infra-orbital process. A sharp pointed projection on the anterior surface of the zygomatic bone, articulating with the maxilla.

infraplacement (*in-fră-plās'-ment*). Downward displacement of a tooth.

infratemporal (*in-fră-tem'-por-al*). Below the temporal bone.

infratemporal fossa. An irregular space on the skull, bounded by the zygoma and the ramus of the mandible, behind the maxilla.

infratemporale (*in-fră-tem-por-a'-lē*). A craniometric point on the great wing of the sphenoid bone, below the temple.

infratrochlear nerve. Supplies the skin over the bridge of the nose. *See* Table of Nerves—infratrochlearis.

infraversion (*in-fră-ver'-shun*). A form of malocclusion in which the tooth is too short in relation to the normal occlusal plane.

ingestion (*in-jes'-chun*). The act of absorbing any substance, such as food, into the body.

Ingrassia's wing (G. F. Ingrassia, 1510-80. Italian anatomist). The lesser wing of the sphenoid bone.

inhalation anaesthesia. General anaesthesia induced by the inhaling of gaseous or volatile liquid anaesthetic agents.

inhale (*in-hāl'*). To draw breath into the lungs.

inial (*in'-e-al*). Relating to the inion.

inion (*in'-e-on*). The posterior occipital protuberance.

injection (*in-jek'-shun*). 1. The forcing, under pressure, of a liquid into some part or tissue of the body. 2. The liquid injected.

inlay (*in'-lā*). A type of tooth filling which is cast to fit the tooth cavity and cemented in position; inlays are usually of gold or porcelain.

inner zone epithelium. Reduced enamel epithelium (*q.v.*).

innervation (*in-er-va'-shun*). 1. The nerve supply or distribution of an organ or part. 2. The supply of nerve stimulus to a part.

innocent (*in'-os-ent*). Benign; not malignant.

innominate artery. Brachiocephalic trunk. *See* Table of Arteries—truncus brachiocephalicus.

innominate vein. V. brachiocephalica. *See* Table of Veins.

inoperable (*in-op'-er-abl*). Not able, or suitable, to be treated by surgery.

inorganic (*in-or-gan'-ik*). 1. Without organs. 2. Not of organic origin, or relating to substances not of organic origin. 3. In chemistry, relating to substances which do not contain carbon, with the exception of carbonates and cyanides.

inostosis (*in-os-to'-sis*). The process by which bony tissue is re-formed to replace tissue that has been destroyed.
cementum i. A pathological thickening of cementum developing inwards into the dentine.

insalivation (*in-sal-iv-a'-shun*). The moistening of food with saliva.

inscription (*in-skrip'-shun*). The main part of a prescription, containing the details of ingredients and quantities to be used.

insectivorous (*in-sekt-iv'-or-us*). Insect-eating.

insertion (*in-ser'-shun*). 1. The act of placing something in, of implanting. 2. The point of attachment of a muscle to the part which it moves.

insidious (*in-sid'-ĭ-us*). Unperceived, coming on gradually and stealthily.

inspection (*in-spek'-shun*). Examination by eye of the body or any of its parts.

inspissation (*in-spis-a'-shun*). The process of drying or thickening by evaporation of readily vaporizing parts.

instrument formula. Three figures representing three measurements: the width of the blade in tenths of a millimetre; the length of the blade in millimetres; and the angle of the shaft in centigrades.

instrumentation (*in-strum-ent-a'-shun*). The use of instruments in treatment.

intaglio (*in-tag'-li-ō*). Carving in hard material; used of carving on a dental model in the construction of a denture.

integument (*in-teg'-yu-ment*). The skin.

integumentary (*in-teg-yu-ment'-ar-i*). Relating to the integument, or skin.

inter-. Prefix signifying *between*, *within*.

interalveolar (*in-ter-al-ve-o'-lar*). Between alveoli.

interalveolar septum. The bony wall dividing two tooth sockets.

inter-articular (*in"-ter-ar-tik'-u-lar*). Within a joint; between articular surfaces.

intercavernous sinus. One of two sinuses joining the cavernous sinuses, and forming a ring round the pituitary fossa. *See* Table of Veins—sinus intercavernosus.

intercellular (*in-ter-sel'-yu-lar*). Between the cells in tissue.

intercondylar (*in-ter-kon'-di-lar*). Between condyles.

intercuspation (*in-ter-kus-pa'-shun*). The interlocking of the cusps on the posterior teeth of one jaw into the corresponding fissures in the teeth of the other jaw in occlusion.

interdental (*in-ter-den'-tal*). Between the teeth.

interdental canal. Nutrient canal (*q.v.*).

interdental papillae. The gingiva in the spaces between the mesial surface of one tooth and the distal surface of the one adjacent.

interdental septum. That portion of the alveolar process between adjoining tooth sockets.

interdental space. The space below the contact point between two adjacent teeth.

interdental splint. A type of splint used in fracture of the jaw, held in place by wires passed round the teeth.

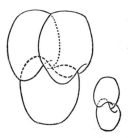

Intercuspation

interdental wiring. Immobilization of a jaw fracture by means of wires passed round several teeth on each side of the fracture.

interdentium (*in-ter-den'-shi-um*). The space between two adjacent teeth.

interdigitation (*in-ter-dij-it-a'-shun*). Intercuspation (*q.v.*).

interfrontal (*in-ter-frun'-tal*). Between the two halves of the frontal bone.

interglobular spaces (*in-ter-glob'-yu-lar*). Large spaces found in dentine close to the amelo-dentinal junction, caused by incomplete calcification.

intergonial (*in-ter-go'-ni-al*). Between the angles of the mandible, or gonia.

interior (*in-te'-ri-or*). Inside, situated within, an organ, part, or cavity.

interlabial (*in-ter-la'-bi-al*). Between the lips.

intermandibular suture. Symphysis menti (*q.v.*).

intermaxilla (*in-ter-maks-il'-ă*). The intermaxillary bone (*q.v.*).

intermaxillary (*in-ter-maks-il'-ar-i*). Between the maxillae.

intermaxillary bone. One of several small bones in the centre of the upper jaw in the foetus, which become fused in adult life; Goethe's bone.

intermaxillary wiring. Any form of wiring used for immobilizing jaw fractures which links the upper to the lower jaw.

intermediate (*in-ter-me'-di-at*). 1. Placed in between. 2. In dentistry, any non-conducting substance used to line a tooth cavity before it is filled either with gold or amalgam, to protect the pulp.

intermediate membrane, Hannover's. *See* Hannover's intermediate membrane.

intermedius nerve. Supplies the glands of the nose and mouth, and the taste-buds. *See* Table of Nerves.

intermittent (*in-ter-mit'-ent*). Occurring at intervals, with periods of cessation; as opposed to *continuous*.

internal (*in-ter'-nal*). Inside.

internal auditory meatus. The canal from the tympanic membrane through the petrous bone, giving passage to the facial and auditory nerves and the internal auditory artery.

internal fistula. A fistula between two internal organs or cavities, with no opening to the outer surface.

internarial (*in-ter-na'-ri-al*). Between the nostrils.

interocclusal (*in-ter-ok-lu'-zal*). Between the occlusal surfaces of opposing teeth.

interosseous (*in-ter-os'-e-us*). Occurring between bones.

interpolation (*in-ter"-pol-a'-shun*). Surgical tissue transplantation.

interproximal (*in-ter-proks'-im-al*). Between approximated surfaces.

interproximal space. Interdental space (*q.v.*).

interradicular (*in-ter-rad-ik'-yu-lar*). Situated between roots.

interradicular septum. The bony partition between the roots of a multi-rooted tooth.

interstitial (*in-ter-stish'-i-al*). Relating to or situated within the interspaces of a part or of tissue.

intertriginous (*in-ter-trij'-in-us*). Chafed; affected by chafing of the skin.

intervascular (*in-ter-vas'-kyu-lar*). Situated between vessels.

intra-. Prefix signifying *within*.

intra-alveolar septum. A bony partition within the tooth socket.

intra-arterial (*in"-tră-ar-te'-ri-al*). Within an artery.

intra-articular (*in"-tră-ar-tik'-yu-lar*). Within a joint.

intrabuccal (*in-tră-buk'-al*). Within the cheek, or within the oral cavity.

intracellular (*in-tră-sel'-yu-lar*). Occurring within a cell or cells.

intracoronal (*in-tră-kor-o'-nal*). Within the tooth crown.

intracranial (*in-tră-kra'-ni-al*). Within the cranium.

intralingual(*in-tră-lin'-gwal*). Within the tongue.

intramedullary (*in-tră-med-ul'-ar-ĭ*). Within the bone marrow.

intramedullary fixation. *In surgery:* a method of uniting the ends of a fractured bone by means of a metal pin within the bone marrow cavity.

intramembranous (*in-tră-mem'-bran-us*). Within a membrane.

intramuscular (*in-tră-mus'-kyu-lar*). Within a muscle or muscles.

intranarial (*in-tră-na'-rĭ-al*). Within the nostril.

intranasal (*in-tră-na'-zal*). Within the nose.

intra-oral (*in"-tră-or'-al*). Within the oral cavity.

intra-oral anaesthesia. Local anaesthesia produced by an injection into the oral tissues from within the mouth.

intra-oral pocket. In oral plastic surgery, a pocket created within the mouth, lined with a skin graft, which is used to support a prosthesis in restoration of facial contours caused by the loss or absence of a large portion of the mandible.

intra-osseous (*in"-tra-os'-ĕ-us*). Within a bone.

intra-osseous anaesthesia. Anaesthesia of a tooth produced by introducing the anaesthetic agent directly into the alveolar bone in the region of the tooth apex.

intrastitial (*in-tră-stish'-ĭ-al*). Within the tissue cells or tissue fibres.

intrathecal (*in-tră-the'-kal*). Within a sheath.

intratracheal (*in-tră-trak-e'-al*). Within the trachea.

intravascular (*in-tră-vas'-kyu-lar*). Within a vessel or vessels.

intravenous (*in-tră-ve'-nus*). Within or into a vein.

intravenous anaesthesia. General anaesthesia induced by the introduction of an anaesthetic agent into the blood stream by injection into a vein.

intraventricular (*in-tră-ven-trik'-yu-lar*). Within a ventricle.

intrinsic (*in-trin'-sik*). Situated within, or relating solely to one part; as opposed to *extrinsic*.

intrinsic nerve. Any nerve supplying impulses to the

muscles, glands, or mucous membranes of an organ or part.

intrusion (*in-tru'-zhun*). The condition of a tooth having been thrust down into its socket.

invaginate (*in-vaj'-in-āt*). To fold back one part of a tube or other tissue so that it is enclosed within another part of itself, as in a sheath.

inversion (*in-ver'-shun*). *Of a tooth:* the condition of a tooth which erupts with the root uppermost.

invest (*in-vest'*). To pack in investment material, in the construction of artificial dentures.

investment (*in-vest'-ment*). Any material used to enclose dentures or crowns preparatory to soldering, casting, or vulcanizing.

involucrum (*in-vol-u'-krum*). A sheath; particularly the new bone sheath which forms about a sequestrum.

involuntary muscle. Any muscle which contracts of itself, and is not under the control of the will.

involution (*in-vol-u'-shun*). A turning or rolling inwards. *buccal i.* The inward folding of the ectoderm in the embryo which forms the stomodeum.

iontophoresis (*i-on-to-for-e'-sis*). Therapeutic treatment by the electrical introduction of ions into the body tissues.

iron (*i'-ern*). A metallic element, hard, ductile, and malleable. Chemical symbol: Fe.

irradiation (*ir-ra-di-a'-shun*). Exposure to radiation; used of treatment with infra-red, ultra-violet, gamma, or *x*-rays.

irrigation (*ir-ig-a'-shun*). The process of washing out, as of a cavity with a stream of water.

irritant (*ir'-it-ant*). 1. Causing irritation. 2. An agent which causes irritation.

irritation (*ir-it-a'-shun*). 1. The act of stimulating. 2. A condition of over-excitement and hypersensitivity.

irritation point. In the testing of vital tooth pulp with an electric current, the average reading at which, on application of the current, a tingling sensation is felt, but before pain is produced.

iso-. Prefix signifying *same, equal.*

isocellular (*i-so-sel'-yu-lar*). Composed of equal-sized or similar cells.

isodont (*i'-so-dont*). Having teeth of the same shape and size.

isognathous (*i-sog'-nath-us*). Having jaws of the same size.

isomorphous (*i-so-mor'-fus*). Having the same form.

iter dentium. The passage through which a permanent tooth erupts.

-itis. Suffix signifying *disease, inflammation.*

ivory (*i'-vor-i*).   Dentine, especially the bone-like substance of the tusks of elephants, walrus, etc.

J

jacket crown.   A porcelain or acrylic veneer crown which is placed over the prepared remains of a vital natural tooth.

jackscrew (*jak'-skru*).   An old term for an orthodontic appliance which expanded the dental arch by means of a screw in a threaded socket.

Jackson crib (V. H. Jackson, 1850-1929. American dentist).   An orthodontic skeleton wire appliance, passing round both the buccal and lingual surfaces of all the teeth in one arch, and joined at intervals to keep it firmly in place. It is used as a foundation to which additions may be made to apply pressure to any given tooth or teeth.

Jacob's ulcer (A. Jacob, 1790-1874. Irish surgeon).   A rodent ulcer affecting the face and eyelid.

Jacobson's nerve (L. L. Jacobson, 1783-1843. Danish anatomist and physician).   The tympanic nerve (*q.v.*).

jaquette (*jak'-et*).   A root planing instrument, used for the removal of subgingival calculus, and for smoothing root surfaces by the removal of the surface layer of cementum.

jaw (*jaw*).   The mandibular or the maxillary facial process.
Hapsburg j.   Mandibular prognathism, the condition which affected the Hapsburg dynasty.
lower j. The mandible.
lumpy j.   Actinomycosis (*q.v.*).
parrot j. The facies produced by abnormal protrusion of the anterior teeth due to protrusion of the maxilla.

Jaws

phossy j.   Jaw necrosis caused by phosphorus poisoning.
pipe j. A painful jaw condition caused by constant carrying of a tobacco pipe in the mouth.
upper j.   The maxillae and the premaxilla.

wolf j. Bilateral cleft extending through the palate, jaw and lip.

jaw clonus reflex. Jaw jerk reflex (*q.v.*).

jaw jerk reflex. Clonic contraction of the muscles of mastication and upward jerking of the mandible, produced by a downward blow on the relaxed and open jaw. Observed in sclerosis of the lateral columns of the spine.

jaw prop. An appliance for holding the jaws open during an operation performed under a general anaesthetic.

jaw winking. Movement of the lower jaw causing an involuntary movement of the eyelids.

jaw-bone. The mandible.

Johnson band. A form of band which is adjusted with pliers to fit the tooth.

Johnson twin wire arch. An orthodontic archwire (*q.v.*) made up of two thin stainless steel wires in parallel, fastened to attachments on bands cemented to the teeth and used to correct misalignment of teeth within the dental arch.

joint (*joynt*). The place of connection between two bones, allowing for more or less movement; an articulation.
mandibular j. Temporomandibular joint (*q.v.*).
temporomandibular j. The joint between the mandible and the temporal bone; the articulating joint of the jaw.

Jourdain's disease (A. L. B. Jourdain, 1734-1816. French physician). Pyorrhoea alveolaris (*q.v.*).

jugal (*ju'-gal*). Relating to a jugum; especially relating to the zygomatic bone.

jugal bone. The malar or zygomatic bone.

jugal point. The craniometric point at the angle of the maxillary and masseteric edges of the zygomatic bone.

jugomaxillary (*ju″-go-maks-il'-ar-i*). Relating to the malar bone and the maxilla.

jugular (*jug'-yu-lar*). Relating to the neck.

jugular foramen. The opening formed by the jugular notches of the temporal and occipital bones, through which pass a jugular vein and the ninth, tenth and eleventh cranial nerves.

jugular fossa. A depression in the petrous portion of the temporal bone, between the carotid canal and the stylomastoid foramen, for the jugular vein.

jugular nerve. Communicating branch from the superior cervical ganglion to the vagus nerve. *See* Table of Nerves—jugularis.

jugular notch *of the occipital bone.* An indentation on the lower edge of the bone, which forms the posterior part of the jugular foramen.

jugular notch *of the temporal bone.* A small depression in the petrous portion of the bone, corresponding to the jugular notch in the occipital bone, with which it forms the jugular foramen.

jugular veins. The veins receiving blood from the veins of the brain, face and neck. *See* Table of Veins— jugularis.

jugum (*ju'-gum*). A yoke or yoke-like process; ridge connecting two points.

jumping the bite. The forcible movement forward of a retruded mandible to obtain normal occlusion.

junction (*junk'-shun*). The area of joining or meeting between two or more organs. *amelodentinal j.* The line marking the join between the enamel and the dentine. *cemento-enamel j.* The line where the cementum of the tooth joins the enamel of the crown; the cervix of the tooth. *dentinoenamel j.* Amelodentinal junction (*q.v.*). *mucogingival j.* The line at which the mucous membrane and the gingivae unite.

juxtangina (*jukst-an-ji'-nă*). Inflammation of the muscles of the pharynx.

K

K Chemical symbol for potassium.

karyokinesis (*kar"-i-o-kin-e'-sis*). Mitosis (*q.v.*).

kebocephaly (*keb-o-sef'-al-i*). *See* cebocephaly.

kelectome (*kel'-ek-tōm*). An instrument used to remove specimens of tissue from a tumour for examination.

keloid (*ke'-loyd*). A fibrous recurrent hyperplastic scar growth on the skin.

Kennedy bar (E. Kennedy, fl. 1932. American dentist). Continuous bar retainer (*q.v.*).

kephal-. *See* cephal-.

keratin (*ker'-at-in*). An insoluble protein which forms the basis of all horny tissue.

keratinize (*ker-at'-in-īz*). To become or to be made horny.

keratinous (*ker-at'-in-us*). 1. Relating to or containing keratin. 2. Horny.

keratogenesis (*ker-at-o-jen'-es-is*). The development of horny tissue.

keratogenous (*ker-at-oj'-en-us*). Promoting or causing the growth of horny material.

keratoglossus (*ker-at-o-glos'-us*). That part of the hyoglossus muscle arising from the greater horn of the hyoid bone.

keratolysis (*ker-at-ol'-is-is*). Exfoliation of the horny layer of the epidermis.

keratolytic (*ker-at-o-lit'-ik*). 1. Relating to keratolysis. 2. An agent causing keratolysis.

keratomycosis linguae. Black tongue (*q.v.*).

keratosis (*ker-at-o'-sis*). 1. A degenerative, horny growth of the skin. 2. A condition characterized by the presence of such growths.

keratosis labialis. A condition characterized by horny patches on the mucosa of the lips.

keratosis linguae. Leukoplakia linguae (q.v.).

key (kē). An old instrument used for extracting teeth; so called because of its resemblance to a door-key.

kinetic (ki-net'-ik). Relating to or producing motion.

Kingsley's splint (N. W. Kingsley, 1829-1913. American dentist). A vulcanized oral splint, made to a model of the fractured jaw with the fracture reduced, and having wires at each end extending outside the mouth to be attached to a headband.

knife (nīf). A cutting instrument, varying in size and shape, used in surgery and anatomy.

knitting (nit'-ing). The process of repair of a bone fracture.

knot (not). 1. A small solid mass of cells or of tissue. 2. The fastening of two ends of cord or suture by interlacing them so that they cannot easily come apart.
    enamel k. An aggregation of epithelial cells at the base of the enamel organ, which have not yet differentiated into stellate reticulum.

knurl (nurl). A small knob or protuberance, especially on instrument handles to ensure a firm grasp.

Kocher's operation (E. T. Kocher, 1841-1917. Swiss surgeon). An operation for excision of the tongue through an incision running from the mastoid process to the hyoid bone and to the symphysis of the mandible.

Kölliker's dental crest (R. A. von Kölliker, 1817-1905. Swiss anatomist). That portion of the maxillary ridge on which the incisor teeth develop.

kolyseptic (kol-i-sep'-tik). Checking septic processes.

Koplik's spots (H. Koplik, 1858-1927. American physician). Small, whitish spots on the mucous membrane of the mouth in the early stages of measles.

Korff's fibres. *See* von Korff's fibres.

koronion (kor-o'-ni-on). *See* coronion.

Koyter's muscle (V. Koyter, 1534-1600. Dutch anatomist). The corrugator supercilii muscle. *See* Table of Muscles.

Krause's operation (F. V. Krause, 1857-1937. German surgeon). Hartley-Krause operation (q.v.).

Krimer's operation (J. F. W. Krimer, 1795-1834. German surgeon). An operation for closure of a palatal fissure by means of wide mucoperiosteal flaps sutured at the median line.

Krompecher's tumour (E. Krompecher, 1870-1926. Hungarian pathologist). A rodent ulcer (q.v.).

Kuhnt's operation (H. Kuhnt, 1850-1925. German ophthalmologist). An operation for treatment of frontal sinus disease by the removal of the anterior wall and the curetting of the mucous membrane.

L

L Lingual.

l. Abbreviation for *litre*, or *left*.

La Labial.

LA Linguoaxial.

LaC Labiocervical.

LAC Linguoaxiocervical.

LaG Labiogingival.

LAG Linguoaxiogingival.

LaI Labioincisal.

LaL Labiolingual.

lb. Abbreviation for *libra*—a pound.

LC Linguocervical.

LD Linguodistal.

LG Linguogingival.

LI Linguoincisal.

LM Linguomesial.

LO Linguo-occlusal.

LP Linguopulpal.

labial (*la'-bi-al*). 1. Relating to the lips. 2. That surface of a tooth which is towards the lips.

labial angle. In dentistry, any angle formed by the junction of a labial tooth surface, or of a cavity wall, in an anterior tooth with any other tooth surface or cavity wall.

labial artery. Branch of the facial artery, supplying the lips and nasal septum; two branches: inferior and superior. *See* Table of Arteries—labialis.

labial bar. A metal connector conforming to the labial mandibular arch and joining two parts of a lower partial denture.

labial cavity. A cavity in the labial surface of a tooth; a Class V cavity.

labial commissure. The corners of the mouth, where the upper and lower lips join.

labial diphtheria. A localized form of diphtheria in which membrane formation occurs on the outer edges of the lips; it has been noted as a complication of cheilosis.

labial embrasure. The space between incisors or canines, opening towards the lip.

labial fistula. A minute tract or congenital depression on the edge of the lower lip; a labial sinus.

labial groove. A groove in the embryonic labial lamina which develops into the vestibule of the oral cavity.

labial nerves. Supply the skin of the lips and cheek. *See* Table of Nerves—labialis.

labial occlusion. A term to denote the position of an incisor or a canine when it is in front of the line of occlusion.

labial phimosis. Imperforation of the mouth.

labial wall. That wall of a tooth cavity which faces the labial surface of a tooth.

labio-. Prefix signifying *lips*.

labioalveolar (*la"-bi-o-al-ve-o'-lar*). Relating to the lips and the alveolar process.

labiocervical (*la"-bi-o-ser-vi'-kal*). Labiogingival (*q.v.*).

labiodental (*la"-bi-o-den'-tal*). Relating to the lips and the teeth.

labiodental sulcus. Vestibular lamina (*q.v.*).

labiogingival (*la"-bi-o-jin'-jiv-al*). Relating to the labial and gingival walls of a mesial, distal or proximo-incisal cavity in an incisor or a canine.
l. angle. The angle formed at the junction of these walls; a *line angle*.

labioglossolaryngeal (*la"-bi-o-glos"-o-lar-in'-je-al*). Relating to the lips, the tongue, and the larynx.

labioglossopharyngeal (*la"-bi-o-glos"-o-far-in'-je-al*). Relating to the lips, the tongue, and the pharynx.

labiogression (*la-bi-o-gresh'-un*). The condition of having the anterior teeth forward of their normal position in the dental arch.

labio-incisal (*la''-bi-o-in-si'-zal*). Relating to the labial surface and the incisal edge of an anterior tooth.

labiolingual (*la"-bi-o-lin'-gwal*). Relating to both the lips and the tongue.

labiolingual plane. Axiolabiolingual plane (*q.v.*).

labiomental (*la"-bi-o-men'-tal*). Relating to the lips and the chin.

labiomycosis (*la"-bi-o-mi-ko'-sis*). Any fungous disease of the lips.

labionasal (*la"-bi-o-na'-zal*). Relating to the lip and the nose.

labiopalatine (*la"-bi-o-pal'-at-in*). Relating to the lips and the palate.

labioplacement (*la"-bi-o-plas'-ment*). Displacement of a tooth labially.

labioplasty (*la'-bi-o-plast-i*). Cheiloplasty (*q.v.*).

labiotenaculum (*la"-bi-o-ten-ak'-yu-lum*). An instrument used for holding the lip during surgical procedures.

labioversion (*la-bi-o-ver'-shun*). The state of being labially displaced; used of a tooth.

labium (*la'-bi-um*) (*pl.* labia). A lip.

labium leporinum. Harelip (*q.v.*).

labrale (*lab-ra'-le*). A cephalometric soft tissue landmark representing the most prominent part on either lip; that of the upper lip is known as *labrale superior* and of the lower *labrale inferior*.

labyrinth (*lab'-ir-inth*). The inner ear.

labyrinthine artery. Supplies the internal ear. *See* Table of Arteries—labyrinthi.

laceration (*las-er-a'-shun*). 1. A tear or a wound made by tearing. 2. The act of tearing.

lacrimal artery. Supplies the cheek, eyelid, eye muscle, and lacrimal gland. *See* Table of Arteries—lacrimalis.

lacrimal bone. A very thin bone on the upper anterior portion of the orbit, articulating with ethmoid, frontal, and maxillary bones.

lacrimal nerve. Supplies the skin about the lateral commissure of the eye. *See* Table of Nerves—lacrimalis.

lacrimal notch. A notch on the inner edge of the orbital surface of the maxilla which receives the lacrimal bone.

Lactobacillus (*lak″-to-bas-il′-us*). A genus of the Lactobacteriaceae family of bacteria, Gram-positive rods, capable of producing lactic acid and carbon dioxide from carbohydrates.

Lactobacteriaceae (*lak″-to-bak-te-ri-a′-se-e*). A family of bacteria of the order Eubacteriales.

lacuna (*lak-u′-nă*) (*pl.* lacunae). A gap, space, or depression; a defect. In dental anatomy lacunae are spaces containing cementoblasts.

lacunae, Howship's. *See* Howship's lacunae.

laevocondylism (*le″-vo-kon′-dil-izm*). Deviation to the left of the mandibular condyles.

lagocheilus (*lag-o-ki′-lus*). Harelip (*q.v.*).

lagostoma (*lag-o-sto′-mă*). Harelip (*q.v.*).

Lain's disease (E. S. Lain, 1876-1970. American dermatologist). Burning of the tongue and the soft tissues of the mouth due to electrogalvanism caused by the use of dissimilar metals in dental restorations.

lambda (*lam′-dă*). The junction of the lambdoid and sagittal sutures, the site of the posterior fontanel.

lamella (*lam-el′-ă*) (*pl.* lamellae). A thin leaf or scale.
enamel l. One of the flat, organic bands running transversely through the enamel of a tooth.

lamellar (*lam-el′-ar*). Relating to a lamella.

lamina (*lam′-in-ă*) (*pl.* laminae). A thin, flat plate or layer.
dental l. The ridge of thickened epithelium along the margin of the gum in the embryo, from which is formed the enamel organ.
vestibular l. The oral ectoderm in the embryo which later divides to form the vestibule of the oral cavity.

lamina dentalis. Dental lamina (*q.v.*).

lamina dura. *In dentistry*: A thin layer of cortical bone lining the tooth socket, important on x-rays, where it shows up as a continuous thin white line.

laminated (*lam′-in-a-ted*). Composed of thin layers or laminae.

lamination (*lam-in-a′-shun*). The make-up of a structure composed of various thin layers of material.

lancet (*lan'-set*). A knife-like instrument used to cut soft tissues.

lancinating (*lan'-sin-a-ting*). Shooting, tearing or sharply cutting; used to describe pain.

Land's crown (C. H. Land, b. 1847. American dentist). A porcelain jacket crown.

laniary (*lan'-i-ar-i*). Dagger-like; used to describe a form of canine tooth.

lapis dentalis (*lap'-is den-ta'-lis*). Dental calculus (*q.v.*).

laryngeal (*lar-in'-jě-al*). Relating to the larynx.

laryngeal artery. Supplies the larynx; two branches: inferior and superior. *See* Table of Arteries—laryngea.

laryngeal nerves. Supply the larynx and cricothyroid. *See* Table of Nerves—laryngeus.

laryngeal reflex. Coughing caused by irritation of the larynx and fauces.

laryngo-. Prefix signifying *larynx*.

laryngopharyngitis sicca (*lar-ing"-o-far-in-ji'-tis sik'-ă*). Inflammation and dryness of the mucous membranes of the larynx and pharynx. Part of the syndrome complex known as *Sjörgen's syndrome.*

laryngospasm (*lar-ing'-o-spazm*). Spasmodic contraction of the larynx.

larynx (*lar'-inks*). The organ of voice production; a

musculo-cartilagenous structure situated between the trachea and the pharynx.

latent (*la'-tent*). Potential; concealed.

lateral (*lat'-er-al*). Relating to a side.

lateral nasal cartilage. One of the two wing-like expansions of the septal cartilage, attached to the nasal bones and to the maxillae.

lateral occlusion. The occlusion of the teeth with the mandible moved to one side or the other, not in centric occlusion.

lavage (*lav'-āj*). 1. The washing out or irrigation of some organ. 2. To wash out.

Lawrence crown (H. Lawrence, fl. 1849. American dentist). Identical with the Foster crown (*q.v.*).

Le Fort fracture (L. C. Le Fort, 1829-93. French surgeon). One of three main classes of fracture of the maxilla:
Class I: those affecting the alveolar process, the palate and the pterygoid processes, transversely.
Class II: a transverse fracture extending through the nasal bones, affecting the maxillary frontal process, the orbital plate, and descending through the maxillary antrum across to the pterygoid process; a pyramidal fracture.
Class III: those affecting the bridge of the nose and the orbit, the pyramidal processes of the maxilla and

zygoma remaining attached; craniofacial dysjunction.

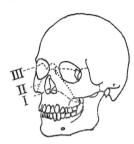

Le Fort fractures

lead (*led*). A soft, grey-blue metal, chemical symbol Pb, which has poisonous salts; it is much used in alloys.

lead line. A bluish line on the edge of the gums, seen in lead poisoning.

leeway space, Nance's. *See* Nance's leeway space.

leiomyoma (*li″-o-mi-o′-mă*). A myoma composed of smooth muscle fibres.

length.
dental l. The distance from the mesial surface of the first premolar to the distal surface of the last molar in the maxillary arch.

lenitive (*len′-it-iv*). Soothing, demulcent.

lenticel (*len′-ti-sel*). A small circular and biconvex (lens-shaped) gland, especially one found at the base of the tongue.

lentula (*len′-tyu-lă*). A flexible spiral instrument used to carry sealer into the root canal.

leontiasis ossea (*le-on-ti′-as-is os′-ĕ-ă*). Hypertrophy of the cranial bones, particularly the maxillae and the facial bones, giving the face a lion-like expression.

leotropic (*le-o-tro′-pik*). Relating to an anticlockwise spiral—i.e. one turning from right to left.

lepto-. Prefix signifying *small, fine, weak.*

leptocephalic (*lep-to-sef-al′-ik*). Having an abnormally small or narrow skull.

leptodontous (*lep-to-don′-tus*). Having abnormally slender teeth.

leptomicrognathus (*lep″-to-mi″-kro-na′-thus*). The condition of having a slight degree of micrognathia; having a slightly under-sized jaw.

leptoprosopic (*lep″-to-pros-o′-pik*). Having a narrow or thin face.

Leptospira (*lep-to-spi′-ră*). A genus of the Spirochaetaceae family of bacteria, able to survive in water.

leptostaphyline (*lep″-to-staf′-il-īn*). Having a narrow and high palate.

Leptothrix (*lep′-to-thriks*). A genus of micro-organisms of the Chlamydobacteriaceae, seen as unbranched filamentous organisms.

Leptotrichia (*lep-to-trik′-i-ă*). A genus of the Actinomycetaceae family, bacterial organisms seen as long tapering threads, unbranched.

L. buccalis. A non-pathogenic species to be found in the oral cavity.

L. placoides. A species to be found in a root canal.

lesion (*le'-zhun*). A wound or injury, or a patch of disease on the skin; a morbid change in tissue function.

leucaemia. *See* leukaemia.

leukaemia (*lu-ke'-mi-ä*). A fatal disease affecting the blood-forming organs, characterized by an increase of abnormal leucocytes in the blood and marked changes in the spleen, bone marrow, and lymphatic glands.

leuko-. Prefix signifying *colourless,* or *white.*

leukokeratosis mucosae oris. Leukoplakia (*q.v.*).

leukoma (*lu-ko'-mä*). 1. A whitish opacity of the cornea. 2. Leukoplakia (buccalis) (*q.v.*).

leukoplakia (*lu-ko-pla'-ki-ä*). A disease characterized by white thickened patches which develop on the tongue (*linguae*), the gums, and the buccal mucous membrane (*buccalis*); sometimes tends to malignancy.

levator menti muscle. M. mentalis. *See* Table of Muscles.

levator muscles. *See* Table of Muscles.

levator palati muscle. M. levator veli palatini. *See* Table of Muscles.

levocondylism. *See* laevocondylism.

lichen planus (*li'-ken pla'-nus*). An inflammatory skin infection characterized by a flat papular eruption; in the mouth the lesions may appear on the buccal mucosa, the tongue, or, more rarely, on the lips.

lichenoid (*li'-ken-oyd*). 1. Lichen-like. 2. A condition of the tongue found in the young and characterized by whitish spots surrounded by yellow rings.

ligament (*lig'-am-ent*). A tough band of fibrous tissue connecting bones or supporting vessels.

ligature (*lig'-at-yur*). 1. A cord or wire for tying vessels. 2. In orthodontics, a wire or thread used to fasten a tooth to an appliance or to another tooth. 3. The act of tying with a cord or thread.

limbus alveolaris. The free margin of the alveolar process.

line (*lin*). Any streak, long thin mark, edge, or boundary.

accretion l's. Retzius' lines (*q.v.*).

ala-tragal l. Camper's line (*q.v.*).

alveolar l. In craniometry, a line from the prosthion to the nasion.

alveolobasilar l. In craniometry, a line from the prosthion to the basion.

alveolonasal l. Alveolar line (*q.v.*).

basialveolar l. In craniometry, the line joining the basion and the alveolar point.

basinasal l. In craniometry, a line from the basion to the nasion.

blue l. Lead line (*q.v.*).

calcification l's. Retzius' lines (*q.v.*).

cervical l. The line formed at the junction of the enamel and the cementum of a tooth.

copper l. A greenish or a red line on the edge of the gums, seen in copper poisoning.

facial l. Camper's line (*q.v.*).

gingival l. Gingival margin (*q.v.*).

imbrication l. One of the grooves in the surface of tooth enamel, marking the edges of the lines of Retzius.

incremental l. One of the lines which are said to show the laminar structure of dentine and enamel in a tooth.

lead l. A bluish line on the edge of the gums, seen in lead poisoning.

mylohyoid l. A ridge on the inner surface of the mandible, running from the ascending ramus to the chin, to which the mylohyoid muscle and the superior constrictor pharyngis are attached.

nasal l. The line or furrow which runs on either side from the alae of the nose to the angles of the mouth.

nasobasilar l. Basinasal line (*q.v.*).

nasolabial l. A line joining the edge of the nose to the angle of the mouth on the same side.

neonatal l. An incremental line in the dentine and the enamel of a tooth formed *in utero*, marking the development of the tooth structure at the time of birth.

For eponymous lines *see* under the name of the person by which the line is known.

line angle. An angle formed at the junction of two tooth surfaces or two cavity walls. The name of the angle indicates the surfaces or walls between which it lies; *e.g.* axiodistal, buccogingival, mesiolingual.

line of occlusion. A term used by Angle to denote the line joining areas of contact of the teeth in normal occlusion.

linear (*lin'-ĕ-ar*). Relating to or resembling a line.

liner (*li'-ner*). Any material used on the inner surfaces of a cavity or container for protection or insulation.

cavity l. Material used in dentistry to protect and insulate the tooth tissues after the excavation of caries and before the placing of a restoration in a prepared cavity.

lingua (*lin'-gwă*). Tongue (*q.v.*).

lingua fraenata. Tongue-tie (*q.v.*).

lingua plicata. Fissure of the tongue.

lingua villosa nigra. Black tongue (*q.v.*).

lingual (*lin'-gwal*). Pertaining to the tongue.

lingual angle. In dentistry, any angle formed by the junction of a lingual tooth surface, or of a cavity wall, with any other tooth surface or cavity wall.

lingual arch. An orthodontic wire appliance conforming to the lingual aspect of the dental arch.

lingual artery. Supplies the sublingual gland, and the tongue, tonsils and epiglottis. *See* Table of Arteries—lingualis.

lingual bar. A metal bar fitted to the lingual arch of the lower jaw, and connecting two parts of a partial denture.

lingual embrasure. The space between any two teeth, opening towards the tongue.

lingual goitre. A thyroid tumour at the upper end of the original thyroglossal duct, at the posterior end of the dorsum of the tongue.

lingual haemorrhoid. Swelling of the veins at the root of the tongue.

lingual muscles, *inferior and superior:* M. longitudinalis inferior and M. longitudinalis superior.
transverse and vertical: M. transversus linguae and M. verticalis linguae. *See* Table of Muscles.

lingual nerve. Supplies the mucosa of the anterior portion of the tongue and the floor of the mouth. *See* Table of Nerves—lingualis.

lingual occlusion. A term for the position of a tooth behind the line of occlusion.

lingual papilla. Any one of the papillae on the dorsum of the tongue.

lingual plexus. A nerve plexus about the lingual artery.

lingual quinsy. *See* quinsy.

lingual raphe. The furrow along the midline of the dorsal surface of the tongue, corresponding to the fibrous septum which divides the tongue in two.

lingual rest. An extension or projection on a partial denture which rests on or engages with the lingual surface of an anterior tooth.

lingual septum. The median, vertical, fibrous partition of the tongue.

lingual sulcus, *medial:* A narrow and shallow groove on the dorsum of the tongue in the midline; *terminal:* A shallow groove on the posterior portion of the dorsum of the tongue, dividing it from the root of the tongue.

lingual tonsil. The collective term for the nodules, produced by the lingual follicles, and found on the pharyngeal portion of the dorsum of the tongue.

lingual wall. That wall of a

tooth cavity which faces the lingual surface of the tooth.

linguale (lin-gwa'-lĕ). The point at the upper end of the mandibular symphysis on the lingual surface.

linguiform (lin'-gwi-form). Tongue-shaped.

lingula mandibulae. The thin and sharp lower edge of the inferior dental foramen.

linguo-. Prefix signifying tongue.

linguoaxial (lin"-gwo-aks'-ĭ-al). Relating to the lingual and axial walls in the mesial or distal portion of a proximo-occlusal cavity.
l. angle. The angle formed at the junction of these walls; a *line* angle.

linguocclusal (lin"-gwok-lu'-zal). Linguo-occlusal (q.v.).

linguocervical (lin"-gwo-ser-vi'-kal). Linguogingival (q.v., 2).

linguocervical ridge. A ridge on the lingual surface of an anterior tooth near to the cervix.

linguoclination (lin-gwo-klin-a'-shun). Tilting of a tooth in a lingual direction.

linguodental (lin"-gwo-den'-tal). Relating to both the tongue and the teeth.

linguodistal (lin"-gwo-dis'-tal). 1. Distal and towards the tongue. 2. Relating to the lingual and distal surfaces of a tooth, or to the lingual and distal walls in the step portion of a proximo-occlusal cavity.

l. angle. The angle formed at the junction of these walls; a *line* angle.

linguofacial trunk. The common trunk by which the lingual and facial arteries frequently arise from the external carotid artery. *See* Table of Arteries—truncus linguofacialis.

linguogingival (lin"-gwo-jin'-jiv-al). 1. Relating to the tongue and the gums. 2. Relating to the lingual and gingival walls of a mesial, distal or proximo-incisal cavity, or of the mesial or distal walls in the step portion of a proximo-occlusal cavity.
l. angle. The angle formed at the junction of these walls; a *line* angle.

linguogingival ridge. Linguocervical ridge (q.v.).

linguoincisal (lin"-gwo-in-si'-zal). Relating to the lingual surface and the incisal edge of an anterior tooth.

linguomesial (lin"-gwo-me'-zi-al). Relating to the lingual and mesial surfaces of a tooth, or to the lingual and mesial walls in the step portion of a proximo-occlusal cavity.
l. angle. The angle formed at the junction of these walls; a *line* angle.

linguo-occlusal (lin"-gwo-ok-lu'-zal). Relating to the lingual and occlusal surfaces of a molar or premolar, or to a cavity affecting those surfaces.

linguopapillitis (*lin"-gwo-pap-il-i'-tis*). Inflammation and ulceration of the papillae of the tongue.

linguoplacement (*lin"-gwo-plās'-ment*). Displacement of a tooth lingually.

linguopulpal (*lin"-gwo-pul'-pal*). Relating to the lingual and pulpal walls of an occlusal cavity, or of the step portion of a proximo-occlusal cavity.
l. angle. The angle formed at the junction of these walls; a *line* angle.

linguoversion (*lin-gwo-ver'-shun*). The position of a tooth which is inclined inwards towards the tongue.

lip (*lip*). One of the fleshy outer edges of the mouth.
double l. Superfluous tissue and mucous membrane occurring below the red margin of the lip.
hare l. Congenital fissure affecting the upper lip.

lip, Hapsburg. See Hapsburg lip.

lip fissure. Hare lip (*q.v.*).

lip furrow band. Vestibular lamina (*q.v.*).

lipocyte (*lip'-o-sīt*). A fat cell.

lipofibroma (*lip-o-fi-bro'-mă*). A mixed tumour composed of both fatty and fibrous tissue.

lipoid (*lip'-oyd*). Resembling fat.

lipoma (*lip-o'-mă*). A benign tumour composed of fat cells.

lipomatoid (*lip-o'-mat-oyd*). Resembling a lipoma.

lipomatosis (*lip-o-mat-o'-sis*). Excessive localized accumulations of fat in the tissues.

lipomatous (*lip-o'-mat-us*). Relating to or resembling a lipoma.

lipomyoma (*lip-o-mi-o'-mă*). A mixed tumour composed of both fatty and muscular tissue.

liquefaction (*lik-wĕ-fak'-shun*). The change to a liquid state.

Liston's operation (R. Liston, 1794-1847. Scottish surgeon). An operation for excision of the maxilla.

lithiasis (*lith-i'-as-is*). Calculus-formation within the body.

litho-. Prefix signifying *calculus*.

livid (*liv'-id*). Of a leaden colour; black and blue; discoloured, as from congestion or contusion.

Lizar's operation (J. Lizar, c. 1787-1860. Scottish surgeon). An operation for the excision of the maxilla by a curved incision from the angle of the mouth to the zygoma.

load (*lōd*).
occlusal l. The force exerted on the posterior teeth during mastication.

lobe (*lōb*). 1. A rounded part or projection of an organ, marked off by fissures or constrictions. 2. A primary division in the formation of the tooth crown.

lobular (*lob'-yu-lar*). Relating to lobes or lobules.

lobulated (*lob'-yu-la-ted*). Composed of lobes or lobules.

lobule (*lob'-yūl*). A small lobe, or one of the divisions of a lobe.

local (*lo'-kal*). Restricted to or affecting one part or area only; as opposed to *general*.

local anaesthesia. Anaesthesia of a circumscribed area of the body.

lock (*lŏk*). The device used in orthodontics to fasten a wire appliance to the band on a tooth.
bite l. A device which can be attached to the bite rims of a denture to retain them in the same position out of the mouth as they occupied in it.

locked bite. Interlocking of the teeth in occlusion so that lateral movement of the mandible is restricted or prevented.

lockjaw (*lok'-jaw*). Tetanus (*q.v.*).

locular (*lok'-yu-lar*). Relating to or characterized by loculi.

loculus (*lok'-yu-lus*) (*pl.* loculi). A space or small cavity.

Logan crown (M. L. Logan, 1844-85. American dentist). A porcelain crown, having a concave base, and attached to the tooth by means of a platinum post baked into the porcelain.

long-handled instrument. One which has the handle, shank, and blade made from one piece of metal.

longissimus capitis muscle. Extends the vertebral column. *Also called* trachelomastoid. *See* Table of Muscles.

longissimus cervicalis muscle. Extends spinal column. *Also called* M. transversus colli. *See* Table of Muscles.

longitudinal muscle. Changes shape of tongue; two branches: inferior and superior. *Also called* lingual muscle. *See* Table of Muscles—longitudinalis.

longus cervicis muscle. M. longus colli. *See* Table of Muscles.

longus colli muscle. Flexes vertebral column. *Also called* M. longus cervicis. *See* Table of Muscles.

longus capitis muscle. Controls movement of head and neck. *See* Table of Muscles.

lophodont (*lof'-o-dont*). Having the crowns of the teeth in the form of ridges or crests.

loupe (*lūp*). A convex, magnifying lens.
binocular l's. A set of magnifying lenses mounted in spectacle frames.

Ludwig's angina (W. F. von Ludwig, 1790-1865. German surgeon). A rare but severe form of cellulitis affecting the floor of the mouth, and spreading to the pharynx.

lues (*lu'-ēz*). Syphilis (*q.v.*).

luetic (*lu-et'-ik*). Relating to syphilis.

lug (*lug*). A projection from a prosthetic appliance which fits into a prepared seat in an abutment and acts as support and retention.

Luken's band. A band having the clamps on the buccal side.

lumen (*lu'-men*). The space within the walls of a tube.

lumpy jaw. Actinomycosis (*q.v.*).

luxation (*luks-a'-shun*). 1. Dislocation (*q.v.*). 2. In dentistry, the separation of a tooth from its socket due to injury.

lycostoma (*li-ko-sto'-mă*). Cleft palate (*q.v.*).

lymph (*limf*). Clear fluid found in the lymphatic vessels and produced by the filtration of the liquid in blood through the capillary walls.

lymphangioma (*limf″-an-jĕ-o'-mă*). A tumour composed of newly-formed lymphatic vessels.

lymphatic (*limf-at'-ik*). 1. Relating to lymph. 2. One of the vessels containing lymph.

lymphoepithelioma (*limf″-o-ep-ith-e-lĭ-o'-mă*). A form of epidermoid carcinoma affecting the tonsils and pharynx; an anaplastic tumour containing lymphocytes and carcinomatous tissue.

lymphoid (*limf'-oyd*). Resembling lymph or lymphatic cells.

lymphoma (*limf-o'-mă*). A tumour composed of lymphoid tissue.

lymphomatoid (*limf-o'-mat-oyd*). Resembling a lymphoma.

lymphomatosis (*limf-o-mat-o'-sis*). The development of multiple lymphomas.

lymphomatous (*limf-o'-mat-us*). Resembling or relating to a lymphoma.

lymphosarcoma (*limf-o-sar-ko'-mă*). A malignant mesenchymal tumour with proliferation of lymphocytes.

Lyon forceps (J. A. Lyon, 1882-1955. American physician). Bone forceps with heavy toothed jaws, used especially in excision of maxillary bone.

lysozyme (*li'-so-zīm*). A basic protein, found in saliva, tears, etc.

M

m. Abbreviation for metre.

M. Abbreviation for 1. *permanent* molar; 2. *Misce*—mix; used in prescription writing.

MB Mesiobuccal.

MBO Mesiobucco-occlusal.

MBP Mesiobuccopulpal.

MC Mesiocervical.

MD Mesiodistal.

M. et sig. Abbreviation for *misce et signa*—mix and label; used in prescription writing.

M. ft. Abbreviation for *mistura fiat*—let a mixture be made; used in prescription writing.

MG Mesiogingival.

mg. Abbreviation for milligram.

MI Mesio-incisal.

MID Mesio-incisodistal.

mil. Abbrevation for millilitre.

mist. Abbreviation for *mistura*—a mixture; used in prescription writing.

ML Mesiolingual.

ml. Abbreviation for millilitre.

MLa Mesiolabial.

MLI Mesiolinguo-incisal.

MLaI Mesiolabio-incisal.

MLP Mesiolinguopulpal.

MLaP Mesiolabiopulpal.

mm. Abbreviation for millimetre.

MO Mesio-occlusal.

MOD Mesio-occlusodistal.

Mod. praesc. Abbreviation for *modo praescripto*—in the manner directed; used in prescription writing.

Mor. sol. Abbreviation for *more solito*—in the usual way; used in prescription writing.

MP Mesiopulpal.

maceration (*mas-er-a'-shun*). The softening of a substance by soaking in a liquid.

Mack crown (C. H. Mack, fl. 1872. American dentist). A hollow porcelain crown held in position by being cemented on to pins screwed into the root canal.

Mackenzie's syndrome (Sir S. Mackenzie, 1844-1909. English physician). Paralysis affecting the tongue, soft palate, and vocal fold on one side.

macro-. Prefix signifying enlargement.

macroblepharia (*mak"-ro-blef-a'-ri-ă*). The condition of having abnormally large eyelids.

macrocephalic (*mak-ro-sef-al'-ik*). Having an abnormally large head.

macrocheilia (*mak-ro-ki'-li-ă*). The condition of having abnormally large lips.

macrodontism (*mak-ro-dont'-izm*). The condition of having abnormally large teeth; megalodontia.

macrogingivae (*mak"-ro-jin'-jiv-ě*). Chronic hypertrophy of the gingivae, affecting the gingival margins and interdental papillae.

macroglossia (*mak-ro-glos'-i-ă*). Large, overdeveloped tongue.

macrognathic (*mak-ro-na'-thik*). Having an abnormally large jaw.

macrognathism (*mak-rog'-nath-izm*). The condition of having an excessively large jaw.

macrolabia (*mak-ro-la'-bĭ-ă*). Macrocheilia (*q.v.*).

macroplasia (*mak-ro-pla'-zi-ă*). Abnormal growth of tissue or of a part.

macroscopic (*mak-ro-skop'-ik*). Visible without the aid of a microscope.

macrosis (*mak-ro'-sis*). Excessive development.

macrostomia (*mak-ro-sto'-mi-ă*). The condition of having an abnormally large mouth.

macrotooth (*mak'-ro-tūth*). A tooth of abnormally large size.

mac 176 mal

macula (*mak'-yu-lă*) (*pl.* maculae). A circumscribed patch of discoloration on the skin.

macular (*mak'-yu-lar*). Relating to or characterized by maculae.

maculation (*mak-yu-la'-shun*). 1. The development of maculae. 2. The condition of being spotted.

macule. *See* macula.

maculopapular (*mak"-yu-lo-pap'-yu-lar*). Having the characteristics of both a macula and papule.

madescent (*mad-es'-ent*). Moist.

magenta tongue. Glossitis associated with ariboflavinosis, giving the tongue a magenta-coloured appearance.

Magill band (W. E. Magill, fl. 1871. American dentist). A plain band, cemented to the tooth and used in the fixation of an expansion arch or other orthodontic appliance.

Magitot's disease (E. Magitot, 1833-97. French dentist). Periodontoclasia (*q.v.*).

magma (*mag'-mă*). 1. A paste, or other amorphous pulpy mass. 2. In pharmacy, a suspension of a precipitate in water.

magnification (*mag-nif-ik-a'-shun*). Apparent increase in size especially by the use of lenses, as in a microscope.

makro-. *See* macro-.

mal-. Prefix signifying *faulty* or *impaired*.

mala (*ma'-lă*). The cheek.

malacia (*mal-a'-si-ă*). A morbid softening of the tissues or of other parts.

malacotic (*mal-ak-ot'-ik*). Relating to malacia; used particularly of the teeth.

malacotic tooth. A poorly formed tooth with a high susceptibility to dental caries.

malalignment (*mal-al-īn'-ment*). 1. Any condition in which the teeth are outside the line of the dental arch. 2. In the treatment of fractures, denotes a poor join between the two ends of the broken bone.

malar (*ma'-lar*). Relating to the cheek, or to the cheekbone.

malar bone. The cheekbone; the zygoma.

malar nerve. N. zygomaticofacialis. *See* Table of Nerves.

Malassez's rests. *See* rests of Malassez.

maldevelopment (*mal-devel'-op-ment*). Impaired or abnormal development.

maleruption (*mal"-er-up'-shun*). Eruption of a tooth out of its normal position.

malformation (*mal-for-ma'-shun*). Impaired formation, deformity.

malignant (*mal-ig'-nant*). Virulent, and becoming increasingly so; threatening life, as a malignant tumour.

malinterdigitation (*mal"-inter-dij-it-a'-shun*). Faulty occlusion of the teeth.

malleable (*mal'-ĕ-abl*). Able to be hammered out into

thin sheets, one of the properties of a metal.

mallet, automatic. An instrument used to condense gold or amalgam in restorations; the blow is produced either by hand operation, with a dental engine, or with compressed air.

malocclusion (*mal-ok-lu'-zhun*). Any deviation from the normal occlusion of the teeth, resulting in impaired function.

Angle's classification of malocclusion:

Class I. Relative position of the dental arches, mesiodistally, normal, with malocclusions usually confined to the anterior teeth.

Class II. Retrusion of the lower jaw, with distal occlusion of the lower teeth.

  Division 1, a. Narrow upper arch, with lengthened and prominent upper incisors, lack of nasal and lip function. Mouthbreathers.

  Division 1, b. Same as *a*, but with only one lateral half of the arch involved, the other being normal. Mouth-breathers.

  Division 2, a. Slight narrowing of the upper arch; bunching of the upper incisors, with overlapping and lingual inclination; normal lip and nasal function.

  Division 2, b. Same as *a*, but with only one lateral half of the arch involved, the other being normal;

normal lip and mouth function.

Class III, a. Protrusion of the lower jaw, with mesial occlusion of the lower teeth; lower incisors and cuspids lingually inclined. *b.* Same as *a*, but with only one lateral half of the arch involved, the other being normal.

skeletal classification. A classification based on the relationship between the deepest points in the incisor segment of the maxilla and of the mandible.

  Class I: basal bone of mandible is normal in relation to the maxilla.

  Class II: basal bone of mandible is post normal to the maxilla.

  Class III: basal bone of the mandible is pre-normal to the maxilla.

malomaxillary (*ma-lo-maks-il'-ar-i*). Relating to both the malar bone and the maxilla.

maloplasty (*ma'-lo-plast-i*). Plastic surgery of the cheek.

malposition (*mal-poz-ish'-un*). Any deviation from the normal position; used particularly of a tooth which is out of occlusion or out of the line of the arch.

malpractice (*mal-prak'-tis*). Improper or injurious treatment in medicine or dentistry.

malrelation (*mal"-rel-a'-shun*). Abnormal or faulty relation of two connected or contacting parts, as in mal-occlusion of the teeth.

malturned (*mal-turn'-d*). Abnormally turned, used of a tooth which is rotated on its long axis so that it is in an abnormal position.

mamelon (*mam'-el-on*). One of three rounded prominences on the incisal edge of a newly-erupted incisor.

mandible (*man'-dibl*). The bone of the lower jaw.

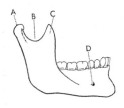

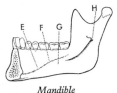

Mandible

A Condyle.
B Sigmoid notch.
C Coronoid process.
D Mental foramen.
E Sublingual fossa.
F Mylo-hyoid line.
G Submandibular fossa.
H Mandibular fossa.

mandibular (*man-dib'-yu-lar*). Relating to the mandible.

mandibular angle. The angle of the jaw; the external angle between the body of the mandible and the ramus, on either side.

mandibular arch. 1. The first branchial arch, from which the jaws and parts of the face develop. 2. The dental arch of the mandible.

mandibular canal. Inferior dental canal (*q.v.*).

mandibular foramen. An oblong opening in the internal surface of the ramus of the mandible, through which pass the inferior dental nerve and artery; *also called* the inferior dental foramen.

mandibular fossa. Glenoid fossa (*q.v.*).

mandibular gland. Submandibular gland (*q.v.*).

mandibular joint. Temporomandibular joint (*q.v.*).

mandibular nerve. *See* Table of Nerves—mandibularis.

mandibular notch. Sigmoid notch (*q.v.*).

mandibular plane. The plane passing through the lowest point of the lower border of the mandible in the region of the angle and through the mention, and perpendicular to the sagittal plane.

mandibular process. That part of the mandibular arch in the embryo from which the mandible develops.

mandibular reflex. Jaw jerk reflex (q.v.).

mandibulofacial (*man-dib″-yu-lo-fa′-shi-al*). Relating to both the mandible and the facial bones.

mandibulo-facial dysostosis. A rare congenital malformation of the face and jaws, characterized by hypoplasia of the facial bones, anti-mongoloid slanting of the lower eyelids, deformity of the pinna, macrostomia, and a general fish-like facies.

mandibuloglossus (*man-dib-yu-lo-glos′-us*). A variant portion of the genioglossus muscle, which extends to the side of the tongue from the posterior border of the mandible.

mandibulomarginalis (*man-dib″-yu-lo-mar-jin-a′-lis*). A variant portion of the platysma muscle, which extends forward over the angle of the mandible from the mastoid process.

mandibulopharyngeal (*man-dib″-yu-lo-far-in′-jĕ-al*). Relating to the mandible and the pharynx.

mandrel (*man′-drel*). A spindle or shaft for holding a tool for rotation; used with a dental engine to hold polishing discs, etc.

manducation (*man-dyu-ka′-shun*). Mastication (q.v.).

manducatory (*man-dyu-ka′-tor-ĭ*). Relating to mastication.

mane (*mah′-na*). Latin for *in the morning*; used in prescription writing and abbreviated *man.* or *m.*

manipulation (*man-ip-yu-la′-shun*). Skilful use of the hands, especially in treatment.

mantle dentine. The thin superficial outer layer of dentine.

manual (*man′-yu-al*). 1. Relating to the hand. 2. Performed by hand, as opposed to *mechanical*.

manudynamometer (*man″-yu-di-nam-om′-et-er*). An apparatus which measures the force of thrust of an instrument.

mappy tongue. Geographic tongue (q.v.).

marble bone disease. Osteopetrosis (q.v.).

margin (*mar′-jin*). 1. A border or edge. 2. *Of a cavity*, the edge of the cavity with the tooth surface.
gingival m. The unattached edge of the gingiva at the neck of a tooth.

marginal (*mar′-jin-al*). Relating to a margin.

marginal ridge. Any one of the ridges forming the outer margins on the occlusal surface of a molar or premolar, or the lingual surface of an incisor or canine.

marrow (*mă′-ro*). The soft tissue found in the canals and interstices of bones.

marsupialization (*mar-su″-pi-al-i-za′-shun*). An operation for the evacuation of a cyst and the suturing of its walls to the edges of the wound, the cavity closing by granulation. Used where complete extirpation is not possible.

masking (*mask'-ing*). An opaque covering for the metal portions of a restoration or prosthesis.

Mason's detachable crown (W. L. Mason, fl. 1896. American dentist). A crown having a removable porcelain facing on a post and collar base.

masseter (*mas'-et-er*). The muscle which raises the mandible in mastication. *See* Tables of Muscles.

masseteric (*mas-et-er'-ik*). Relating to the masseter muscle.

masseteric artery. Supplies the deep surface of the masseter muscle. *See* Table of Arteries—masseterica.

massodent (*mas'-o-dent*). An instrument used for massaging the gums.

mastication (*mas-tik-a'-shun*). The act of chewing.

masticatory (*mas-tik-a'-tor-ĭ*). Relating to mastication.

masticatory surface. The grinding surface of a molar or premolar.

mastoid (*mas'-toyd*). 1. A thick process of the temporal bone. 2. Relating to the mastoid process.

mastoid artery. Supplies the dura mater, lateral sinuses

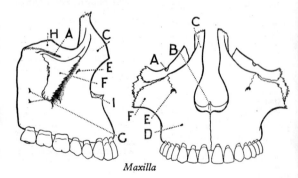

Maxilla

A Infra-orbital groove.
B Nasal crest.
C Frontal process.
D Canine eminence.
E Infraorbital foramen.

F Zygomatic process.
G Dental canals.
H Orbital surface.
I Piriform aperture.

and mastoid cells. *See* Table of Arteries—mastoidea.

mastoid foramen. A small opening behind the mastoid process, through which pass an artery and a vein.

mastoid fossa. A depression on the lateral surface of the temporal bone, for the lateral sinus.

materia alba (*mat-e'-rĭ-ă al'-ba*). 1. Food debris (*q.v.*). 2. Dental plaque (*q.v.*, 1).

materia medica (*mat-e'-rĭ-ă med'-ik-ă*). The science of drugs and their sources, preparations and uses.

matrix (*ma'-triks*). 1. Intercellular tissue. 2. A mould used in casting. 3. A thin band of metal used to provide a temporary tooth wall to support a filling.

amalgam m. A matrix (3) used to provide a temporary tooth wall to support and assist in the contouring of plastic fillings.

matrix band. Matrix (*q.v.*, 3).

maxilla (*maks-il'-ă*). One of the bones of the upper jaw.

maxillary (*maks-il'-ar-ĭ*). Relating to the maxilla.

maxillary angle. The angle formed at the point of contact of the central incisors by the intersection of lines from the ophryon and the most prominent point of the mandible.

maxillary antrum. Maxillary sinus (*q.v.*).

maxillary artery. Supplies the mandibular alveolar process, cheek muscles, etc.

Also called internal maxillary artery. *See* Table of Arteries—maxillaris.

external m.a. A. facialis.

maxillary canal. Superior dental canal (*q.v.*).

maxillary hiatus. The opening on the inner surface of the maxilla, joining the nasal cavity and the maxillary antrum; hiatus semilunaris.

maxillary nerve. *See* Table of Nerves—maxillaris.

maxillary plane. In cephalometrics, the plane, perpendicular to the sagittal plane, passing through the anterior and posterior nasal spines as seen on a lateral skull radiograph.

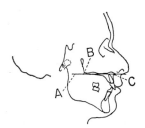

Maxillary plane

A Maxillary plane.
B Posterior nasal spine.
C Anterior nasal spine.

maxillary plexus. One of the nerve plexuses about the external and internal maxillary arteries.

maxillary process *in the embryo*. A protuberance from the mandibular arch in the embryo from which the maxilla, the zygomatic bone, and the upper cheek and lip region develop.

maxillary process *of the palatine bone*. A thin plate projecting forward from the anterior border of the palatine bone, closing the lower posterior end of the opening of the maxillary sinus.

maxillary process *of the zygomatic bone*. A blunt descending process of the zygomatic bone articulating with the maxilla.

maxillary protuberance. One of the eminences marking the embryonic rudiments of the jaws.

maxillary rampart. A ridge of epithelial cells found in the embryo in that part of the jaw which will develop into the alveolar border.

maxillary sinus. A large air sinus in the maxilla; also called the antrum of Highmore.

maxillary tubercle. A small rough prominence at the distal end of the maxillary alveolar process.

maxillate (*maks'-il-āt*). Possessing jaws.

maxillectomy (*maks-il-ekt'-om-ĭ*). Excision of the maxilla.

maxillitis (*maks-il-i'-tis*). Inflammation of the maxilla or of a maxillary gland.

maxillodental (*maks"-il-o-den'-tal*). Relating to the maxilla and the teeth.

maxillofacial (*maks"-il-o-fa'-shi-al*). Relating to the maxilla and other facial processes.

maxillofacial prosthesis. An artificial substitute for some facial structure which has been too severely damaged to be repaired by surgery.

maxillofrontale (*maks"-il-o-fron-ta'-lĕ*). The point at which the frontomaxillary suture meets the anterior lacrimal crest.

maxillojugal (*maks-il-o-ju'-gal*). Relating to the maxilla and the cheek.

maxillolabial (*maks"-il-o-la'-bi-al*). Relating to the maxilla and the lip.

maxillomandibular (*maks"-il-o-man-dib'-yu-lar*). Relating to both the maxilla and the mandible.

maxillopalatine (*maks"-il-o-pal'-at-īn*). Relating to the maxilla and the hard palate.

maxillopharyngeal (*maks"-il-o-far-in'-jĕ-al*). Relating to the maxilla and the pharynx.

maxilloturbinal (*maks"-il-o-tur'-bin-al*). The inferior nasal concha, or turbinate bone.

maximum (*maks'-im-um*). The greatest, or most, of anything; as opposed to *minimum*.

meatus (*me-a'-tus*). A passage, canal, or orifice.
auditory m., external: The external auditory canal from

the concha to the tympanic membrane in the ear. *internal:* The canal from the tympanic membrane through the petrous bone, giving passage to the facial and auditory nerves and the internal auditory artery.

meckelectomy (mek-el-ekt'-om-ĭ). Surgical removal of the sphenopalatine ganglion (Meckel's ganglion).

Meckel's cartilage (J. F. Meckel, *the younger,* 1781-1833. German surgeon). The cartilage forming the first branchial arch in the foetus.

Meckel's ganglion (J. F. Meckel, *the elder,* 1714-74. German anatomist). A ganglion in the pterygopalatine fossa, supplying sympathetic, facial and other nerves to the oral and nasal mucosa and the lacrimal glands.

mecocephalic (me"-ko-sef-al'-ik). Dolichocephalic (*q.v.*).

medial (me'-dĭ-al). Towards the midline; internal.

medial lingual sulcus. A narrow and shallow groove on the dorsum of the tongue in the midline.

median (me'-dĭ-an). Situated in the centre, or on the midline of the body.

medical (med'-ik-al). Relating to medicine.

medicament (med-ik'-ă-ment). Any medicinal substance.

medicinal (med-is'-in-al). 1. Relating to a medicine.

2. Possessing healing attributes.

medicine (med'-is-in). 1. The study and treatment of diseases, especially treatment without recourse to surgery. 2. Any drug used for the treatment of a disease.

medicodental (med"-ik-o-den'-tal). Relating to both medicine and dentistry.

medio-. Prefix signifying *middle.*

mediofrontal (me"-dĭ-o-frun'-tal). Relating to the middle of the forehead.

mediopalatine (med-i-o-pal'-at-in). Relating to the centre portion of the palate.

medium. See culture medium.

medulla (med-ul'-ă). Marrow (*q.v.*).

mega-. Prefix signifying *great, enlarged.*

megadont (meg'-ă-dont). A person with abnormally large teeth.

megadontia (meg-ă-don'-shĭ-ă). Megadontism (*q.v.*).

megadontic (meg-ă-don'-tik). Relating to megadontism.

megadontism (meg-ă-dont'-izm). The condition of having abnormally large teeth; macrodontism.

megagnathus (meg-ă-na'-thus). Having a large jaw; macrognathic.

megalo-. Prefix signifying *large,* especially *abnormally large.*

megalocephaly (meg"-al-o-sef'-al-ĭ). 1. The condition of having an abnormally large head.   2. Leontiasis ossea (q.v.).

megalodontia (*meg″-al-o-don′-shĭ′-ă*).   Macrodontism (q.v.).

megaloglossia (*meg″-al-o-glos′-ĭ-ă*).   A form of macroglossia (q.v.) due to hypertrophy of the tongue muscle.

megaprosopous (*meg″-ă-pro-so′-pus*).   Having an abnormally large face.

Méglin's palatine point (J. A. Méglin, 1756-1824. French physician).   The point at which the descending palatine nerve emerges from the palato-maxillary canal.

melanoamelobastoma (*mel″-an-o-am-e″-lo-blast-o′-mă*).   An amelobastoma which is also pigmented with melanin, giving it a dark discoloration.

melanoglossia (*mel″-an-o-glos′-ĭ-ă*).   Black tongue (q.v.).

melanoma (*mel-an-o′-mă*).   A malignant tumour composed of cells pigmented with melanin, and characterized by its black colour.

melanoplakia (*mel″-an-o-pla′-kĭ-ă*).   Patchy pigmentation of the oral mucous membrane, associated with stomatitis, jaundice, and other diseases.

melanotrichia linguae. Black tongue (q.v.).

melitis (*mel-i′-tis*).   Inflammation of the cheek.

melitoptyalism (*mel-it-op-ti′-al-izm*).   The condition in which the secretion of saliva contains glucose.

Melkersson's syndrome (E. Melkersson, contemporary Swedish physician).   A rare syndrome in which there is recurrent facial paralysis occurring with persistent facial swelling and lingua plicata.

melo-.   Prefix signifying cheek.

meloncus (*mel-on′-kus*).   Any tumour of the cheek.

meloplasty (*mel′-o-plast-ĭ*).   Plastic surgery of the cheek.

meloschisis (*mel-os′-kis-is*).   Macrostomia (q.v.).

Melotte's metal (G. W. Melotte, 1835-1915.   American dentist).   A soft alloy of bismuth, lead and tin, which is used in dentistry.

membrana adamantina. Reduced enamel epithelium (q.v.).

membrana eboris.   The membrane surrounding the tooth pulp, composed of the remains of odontoblasts.

membrane (*mem′-brān*).   A thin layer of tissue lining a cavity, covering a part, or separating two adjacent cavities.

buccopharyngeal m.   That area of the primitive embryo which later develops into the mouth and the pharynx.

mucous m.   The membrane containing mucous glands, which lines those passages and cavities of the body which communicate with the exterior.

periodontal m.   The layer of fibrous tissue surrounding

the root of the tooth, attached to the cementum, the alveolar bone and the free gingiva and supporting the tooth in its socket.

membrane, Hannover's intermediate. See Hannover's intermediate membrane.

membrane, Nasmyth's. See Nasmyth's membrane.

membranous (*mem'-bran-us*). Relating to or characteristic of a membrane.

meningeal artery. Branches from various arteries supplying the dura mater, cranium, and trigeminal ganglion. See Table of Arteries—meningea.

meningeal nerves. Supplying the meninges. See Table of Nerves—meningeus.

meniscus (*men-is'-kus*). A crescent-shaped inter-articular fibrocartilage.

mensa (*men'-să*). An old term for the occlusal surface of a molar tooth.

mental (*men'-tal*). 1. Relating to the mind. 2. Relating to the chin.

mental artery. Supplies the lower lip and chin. See Table of Arteries—mentalis.

mental foramen. A large foramen in the mandible below the second premolar, through which pass the mental branches of the inferior dental nerve and their accompanying blood vessels.

mental nerve. Supplies skin of chin and lower lip. See Table of Nerves—mentalis.

mental point. Gnathion (*q.v.*).

mental protuberance. The prominence at the angle of the mandible in the midline of the face.

mental spine. Mental tubercle (*q.v.*).

mental tubercle. One of two small projections of bone on the inner surface of the mandible on either side of the symphysis menti. *Also called* mental spine.

mentalis muscle. Protrudes lower lip and wrinkles skin of chin. *Also called* M. levator menti. *See* Table of Muscles.

mento-. Prefix signifying *chin*.

mentolabial (*men-to-la'-bi-al*). Relating to the chin and the lip.

mentolabial furrow. The transverse groove just above the chin.

mentolabialis (*men"-to-la-bi-a'-lis*). M. depressor labii inferioris. *See* Table of Muscles.

menton (*men'-ton*). The lowest point on the outline of the mental symphysis seen on a lateral skull radiograph which has been orientated with the Frankfort plane horizontal. It is equivalent to the anthropological point gnathion (*q.v.*, 1).

mentum (*men'-tum*). The chin.

mercurial (*mer-kyur'-ĭ-al*). Relating to mercury.

mercuric (*mer-kyur'-ik*). Relating to mercury as a bivalent element.

mercurous (*mer'-kyur-us*). Relating to mercury as a univalent element.

mercury (*mer'-kyur-ĭ*). A metallic element, a silver-white and shining fluid at normal temperatures. Chemical symbol: Hg. It is only soluble in nitric acid, and partially soluble in boiling hydrochloric acid. It combines both as a univalent and a bivalent element.

mero-. Prefix signifying *part*.

mesal (*me'-zal*). Relating to the median line or plane of the body.

mesaticephalus (*mes-at-ĭ-sef'-al-us*). Mesocephalic (*q.v.*).

mesenchyma (*mes-en'-kim-ă*). The embryonic connective tissue formed from the mesoderm.

mesenchymal (*mes-en'-kim-al*). Relating to, or derived from, the mesenchyma.

mesial (*me'-zĭ-al*). In the region of the mid-line. In dentistry, in the region of the mid-line of the dental arch.

mesial angle. In dentistry, any angle formed by the junction of a mesial surface of a tooth or cavity wall with any other tooth surface or cavity wall.

mesial occlusion. A term to denote the position of a tooth which is mesial of its normal position in occlusion.

mesial wall. That wall of a tooth cavity which faces the mesial surface of the tooth.

mesio-. Prefix signifying *towards the midline*, in dentistry.

mesio-angular (*me"-zĭ-o-an'-gyu-lar*). Relating to any mesial angle.

mesiobuccal (*me"-zĭ-o-buk'-al*). Relating to the mesial and buccal surfaces of a tooth, or the mesial and buccal walls of an occlusal cavity in a molar or pre-molar.
m. angle. The angle formed at the junction of these walls; *a line angle.*

mesiobuccocclusal (*me"-zĭ-o-buk'-ok-lu'-zal*). Mesiobucco-occlusal (*q.v.*).

mesiobucco-occlusal (*me"-zĭ-o-buk'-o-ok-lu'-zal*). Relating to the mesial, buccal and occlusal surfaces of a tooth.

mesiobuccopulpal (*me"-zĭ-o-buk'-o-pul'-pal*). Relating to the mesial, buccal and pulpal walls of an occlusal cavity, or in the step portion of a proximo-occlusal cavity in a molar or premolar.
m. angle. The angle formed at the junction of these walls; *a point angle.*

mesiocclusal (*me"-zĭ-o-ok-lu'-zal*). Mesio-occlusal (*q.v.*).

mesiocclusion (*me-zĭ-ok-lu'-zhun*). A form of malocclusion in which the mandibular teeth occlude anterior to the maxillary teeth.

mesiocclusodistal (*me"-zĭ-ok-lu"-zo-dis'-tal*). Mesio-occlusodistal (*q.v.*).

mesiocervical (*me"-zĭ-o-servi'-kal*). Mesiogingival (*q.v.*).

mesioclination (*mē''-zĭ-o-klin-a'-shun*). Mesial tilting of a tooth.

mesiodens (*mē'-zĭ-o-denz*). A supernumerary tooth, often unerupted, found in the upper jaw between the incisors.

mesiodistal (*mē''-zĭ-o-dis'-tal*). Relating to the mesial and distal surfaces of a tooth.

mesiodistal plane. Axiomesiodistal plane (*q.v.*).

mesiogingival (*mē''-zĭ-o-jin'-jiv-al*). Relating to the mesial and gingival walls of a buccal or lingual cavity in a molar or premolar.
m. angle. The angle formed at the junction of these walls; a *line* angle.

mesiogression (*me-zĭ-o-gresh'-un*). With the teeth forward of their normal position in the dental arch.

mesio-incisal (*mē''-zĭ-o-in-sī'-zal*). Relating to the mesial and incisal surfaces of an incisor or canine, or to a cavity affecting these surfaces.

mesio-incisodistal (*mē''-zĭ-o-in-sī''-zo-dis'-tal*). Relating to the mesial, incisal and distal surfaces of an incisor or canine, or to a cavity affecting those surfaces.

mesiolabial (*mē''-zĭ-o-la'-bĭ-al*). Relating to the mesial and labial surfaces of a tooth, or to the corresponding walls in the step portion of a proximo-incisal cavity.
m. angle. The angle formed at the junction of these walls; a *line* angle.

mesiolabioincisal (*mē''-zĭ-o-la''-bĭ-o-in-sī'-zal*). Relating to the mesial and labial surfaces and the incisal edge of an anterior tooth.

mesiolingual (*mē''-zĭ-o-lin'-gwal*). Relating to the mesial and lingual surfaces of a tooth, or to the mesial and lingual walls of an occlusal cavity in a molar or premolar.
m. angle. The angle formed at the junction of these walls; a *line* angle.

mesiolinguoocclusal (*mē''-zĭ-o-lin-gwok-lu'-zal*). Mesiolinguo-occlusal (*q.v.*).

mesiolinguoincisal (*mē''-zĭ-o-lin''-gwo-in-sī'-zal*). Relating to the mesial and lingual surfaces and the incisal edge of an anterior tooth.

mesiolinguo-occlusal (*mē''-zĭ-o-lin-gwo-ok-lu'-zal*). Relating to the mesial, lingual and occlusal surfaces of a tooth.

mesiolinguopulpal (*mē''-zĭ-o-lin''-gwo-pul'-pal*). Relating to the mesial, lingual and pulpal walls of an occlusal cavity, or in the step portion of a proximo-occlusal cavity.
m. angle. The angle formed at the junction of these walls; a *point* angle.

mesio-occlusal (*mē''-zĭ-o-ok-lu'-zal*). 1. Relating to the mesial and occlusal surfaces of a tooth, or to the mesial and occlusal walls of a buccal or lingual cavity in a molar or premolar.
m. angle. The angle formed at the junction of these walls; a *line* angle.

mesio-occlusodistal (*me''-zĭ-o-ok-lu''-zo-dis'-tal*). Relating to the mesial, occlusal and distal surfaces of a molar or premolar, or to a cavity affecting these surfaces.

mesiopulpal (*me''-zĭ-o-pul'-pal*). Relating to the mesial and pulpal walls of an occlusal cavity in a molar or premolar.
m. angle. The angle formed at the junction of these walls; a *line* angle.

mesiopulpolabial (*me''-zĭ-o-pul''-po-la'-bĭ-al*). Relating to the mesial, pulpal and labial walls of a cavity in an incisor or canine.
m. angle. The angle formed at the junction of these walls; a *point* angle.

mesiopulpolingual (*me''-zĭ-o-pul''-po-lin'-gwal*). Relating to the mesial, pulpal and lingual walls in the step portion of a proximo-incisal cavity.
m. angle. The angle formed at the junction of these walls; a *point* angle.

mesioversion (*me-zĭ-o-ver'-shun*). The position of a tooth which is inclined towards the median line.

mesoblast (*me'-zo-blast*). Mesoderm (*q.v.*).

mesocephalic (*me-zo-sef-al'-ik*). Having a cephalic index of between 76.0 and 80.9; having a head with a moderate relationship between its greatest length and breadth.

mesoconch (*me'-zo-konsh*). Having an orbit of medium height.

mesoconid (*me-zo-kon'-id*). The central distal cusp on a mandibular molar.

mesocranic (*me-zo-kra'-nik*). Mesocephalic (*q.v.*).

mesodens (*me'-zo-denz*). Mesiodens (*q.v.*).

mesoderm (*me'-zo-derm*). The middle germinal layer in the primitive embryo.

mesodont (*me'-zo-dont*). Having medium-sized teeth.

mesognathion (*me-zo-na'-thĭ-on*). The hypothetical lateral portion of the premaxilla.

mesognathous (*mes-og'-nath-us*). Having a gnathic index of between 98 and 103.

mesophryon (*me-zof'-rĭ-on*). The glabella (*q.v.*).

mesoprosopic (*me-zo-pros-o'-pik*). Having a medium-width face.

mesostaphyline (*me-zo-staf'-il-īn*). Meso-uranic (*q.v.*).

mesostyle (*me'-zo-stīl*). A small cusp or fold of enamel between the paracone and the metacone on the buccal surface of a maxillary molar.

meso-uranic (*me-zo-yur-an'-ik*). Having a palatal index of between 110 and 115.

mesuranic (*mes'-yur-an-ik*). Meso-uranic (*q.v.*).

metabolic (*met-ab-ol'-ik*). Relating to metabolism.

metabolism (*met-ab'-ol-izm*). The physical and chemical changes in the tissues by which a living body is maintained and energy generated.

metacone (*met'-a-kōn*). The distobuccal cusp of a maxillary molar.

metaconid (*met-ak-on'-id*). The mesiolingual cusp of a mandibular molar.

metaconule (*met-ak-on'-yul*). A small cusp between the metacone and the protocone on the maxillary teeth of animals.

metal (*met'-al*). Any element having the following properties: hardness, ductility, malleability, lustre, fusibility, good conduction of heat and electricity.
cliche m. A fusible alloy of tin, lead, antimony, and bismuth, used in dentistry.
queen's m. An alloy composed of tin and antimony.

metal, Babbitt's. *See* Babbitt's metal.

metal, d'Arcet's. *See* d'Arcet's metal.

metal, Melotte's. *See* Melotte's metal.

metallic (*met-al'-ik*). Relating to a metal.

metaplasia (*met-a-pla'-zĭ-ă*). The alteration of tissue from one form to another.

metaplasia *of pulp.* A degenerative condition in which the tooth pulp has lost its power to form dentine, and has become merely connective tissue.

metastasis (*met-as'-tas-is*). The transfer of a disease or of a tumour from a primary focus to other, unconnected, parts of the body, due to the transfer of the pathogenic organisms or of tumour cells.

metastatic (*met-as-tat'-ik*). Relating to metastasis.

metastyle (*met'-ă-stil*). A small cusp on the lingual side of a maxillary molar or premolar, just posterior to the metacone.

meter. *See* metre.

method, Callahan's. *See* Callahan's method.

metodontiasis (*met''-o-donti'-as-is*). 1. The permanent dentition. 2. Faulty tooth development or eruption.

metopic (*me-top'-ik*). Relating to the forehead.

metopic suture. The suture joining the two halves of the frontal bone; the frontal suture.

metopion (*met-o'-pĭ-on*). A craniometric point between the frontal eminences on the midline of the forehead.

metre (*me'-ter*). The basic unit of length in the metric system, about 39.3 inches.

metric system. The most commonly used system of weights and measures, based on multiples of ten and one hundred. The basic units are the metre (length), the gram (weight or mass), and the litre (capacity). Multiples of these basic units are designated by the prefixes deca- 10, hecto- 100, and kilo- 1000; fractional units are designated by corresponding prefixes deci- 1/10, centi- 1/100, and milli- 1/1000.

metriocephalic (*met''-rĭ-o-sef-al'-ik*). Having a skull of moderate convexity.

micro-. Prefix signifying 1. *small, extremely small;* 2. In medicine, *abnormally small.*

microbe (*mi'-krōb*). Any micro-organism, but used particularly of pathogenic bacteria.

microbiology (*mi-kro-bi-ol'-oj-ĭ*). The study of micro-organisms.

microcephalic (*mi-kro-sef-al'-ik*). Having an abnormally small head.

microcephaly (*mi-kro-sef'-al-ĭ*). The condition of having an abnormally small head.

microcheilia (*mi-kro-ki'-lĭ-ă*). The condition of having abnormally small lips.

Micrococcaceae (*mi''-kro-kok-a'-se-e*). A family of bacteria of the order Eubacteriales.

Micrococcus (*mi-kro-kok'-us*). A genus of the Micrococcaceae family of bacteria, Gram-positive, with the cells grouped in irregular clusters.

microdentism (*mi-kro-dent'-izm*). Microdontism (q.v.).

microdont (*mi'-kro-dont*). A person with abnormally small teeth.

microdontia (*mi-kro-don'-shĭ-ă*). Microdontism (q.v.).

microdontic (*mi-kro-don'-tik*). Relating to microdontism.

microdontism (*mi-kro-dont'-izm*). The condition of having abnormally small teeth.

microgenia (*mi-kro-je'-nĭ-ă*). The condition of having an abnormally small chin.

microglossia (*mi-kro-glos'-ĭ-ă*). The condition of having a small, under-developed tongue.

micrognathia (*mi-kro-na'-thĭ-ă*). Congenital hypoplasia of the mandible.

micromandible (*mi-kro-man'-dibl*). 1. An extremely small mandible. 2. The condition of having an extremely small mandible.

micromandibulare (*mi''-kro-man-dib-yu-lah'-rĕ*). Micromandible (q.v.)

micro-organism (*mi-kro-or'-gan-izm*). Any form of plant or animal organism which is visible only under the microscope.

microscope (*mi'-kro-skōp*). An instrument for magnifying minute objects.

microscopic (*mi-kro-skop'-ik*). Minute, visible only through a microscope.

microscopy (*mi-kros'-kop-ĭ*). Observation and examination with a microscope.

microstomia (*mi-kro-sto'-mĭ-ă*). The condition of having an abnormally small mouth.

microtia (*mi-kro'-shĭ-ă*). The condition of having an abnormally small external ear.

microtooth (*mi'-kro-tūth*). A tooth of abnormally small size.

migration (*mi-gra'-shun*) *of a tooth*. Gradual spontaneous movement of a tooth, seen in advanced periodontal diseases.

Mikulicz's disease (J. von Mikulicz - Radecki, 1850-1905. Polish surgeon). Chronic swelling of the lacrimal and salivary glands due to the replacement of glandular by lymphoid tissue.

milk teeth. Deciduous teeth (*q.v.*).

milli-. Prefix signifying *one-thousandth*.

milling-in. The process of perfecting the occlusion of dentures by rubbing them together, either in the mouth or in an articulator, with an abrasive between the occluding surfaces.

mimesis (*mim-e'-sis*). The imitation by one disease of another.

mineralization (*min-er-al-i-za'-shun*). The addition of minerals or mineral salts to the body.

Mirault's operation (G. Mirault, 1796-1879. French surgeon). 1. An operation for plastic repair of unilateral hare lip by means of a flap turned down at one side and attached on the opposite side. 2. An operation for excision of the tongue, in which the lingual arteries are tied off first.

mirror (*mir'-or*). A highly polished, reflective surface. *dental m.* A small mirror designed for use in the mouth. *mouth m.* Dental mirror (*q.v.*).

misce. Latin for *mix*; used in prescription writing and abbreviated *misc.*, or *m.*

miscible (*mis'-ibl*). Capable of being mixed.

mistura (*mis'-tur-ă*). Latin for *a mixture*; used in prescription writing, and abbreviated *mist.*, or *m.*

mitosis (*mi-to'-sis*). Indirect division of cells, the typical method of cell reproduction; karyokinesis.

mitotic (*mi-tot'-ik*). Relating to or characterized by mitosis.

mixture, Arkövy's. *See* Arkövy's mixture.

model (*mod'-el*). A reproduction in metal or plastics made from an impression of any object; a cast.

modiolus (*mod-ĭ-o'-lus*). A point near the corner of the mouth at which several of the facial muscles intersect.

modo praescripto. Latin for *in the manner directed*; used in prescription writing, and abbreviated *mod. praesc.*

Moeller's glossitis (J. O. L. Moeller, 1819-87. German surgeon). Chronic superficial inflammation and excoriation of the tongue, spreading to the palate and cheeks, and marked by smoothness and burning pain.

molar (*mo'-lar*). *See* molar tooth.

mulberry m's. Small, dome-shaped permanent first molars, with the cusps close together and affected by enamel hypoplasia; seen in congenital syphilis. *Also called* Moon's molars or Fournier's molars.

molar glands. A cluster of small mucous glands near the parotid duct on the buccopharyngeal fascia.

molar tooth. One of the back, grinding teeth. There are two in each quadrant in the deciduous dentition and three in each quadrant in the permanent dentition in man.

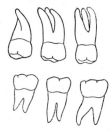

Molar teeth

molariform *(mo-lar'-ĭ-form).* In the shape of a molar.

molarion *(mo-lar'-ĭ-on).* The point of the most distal cusp on either side of the mandibular arch.

molars, Fournier's. Mulberry molars (*q.v.*).

molars, Moon's. Mulberry molars (*q.v.*).

mold. *See* mould.

mon-angle *(mon-an'-gl).* *Of an instrument:* Having only one angle in the shank.

Monilia *(mon-il'-ĭ-ă).* Candida (*q.v.*).

moniliasis *(mon-il-i'-as-is).* A condition resulting from infection by a species of *Candida* fungus, usually *C. albicans*, and affecting various parts of the body.
oral m. Infection of the mouth with *Candida albicans*; may be a precancerous condition when chronic.

mono-. Prefix signifying *one, single.*

monobloc *(mon'-o-blok).* Andresen appliance (*q.v.*).

monococcus *(mon-o-kok'-us).* A single coccus, one not united in pairs, chains or groups.

monodont *(mon'-o-dont).* Having only a single tooth.

mono-fluor phosphate. A chemical complex, containing fluoride, used in toothpaste and as a topical application for the prevention of dental caries.

monolocular *(mon-o-lok'-yu-lar).* Having only one cavity.

monomaxillary *(mon-o-maks-il'-ar-ĭ).* Relating to or affecting one jaw only.

monomer *(mon'-o-mer).* Any substance composed of single molecules.

mononuclear *(mon-o-nyu'-klĕ-ar).* Having only one nucleus.

monophyodont *(mon'-o-fi'-o-dont).* Having only one, permanent, set of teeth.

monoradicular (mon-o-rad-ik'-yu-lar). Having only one root.

monostotic (mon-os-tot'-ik). Affecting only one bone.

Monson's curve. The curved plane on which lie the occlusal surfaces of the posterior teeth.

Moon's molars (H. Moon, 1845-92. English surgeon). Mulberry molars (q.v.).

Moorehead's retractor (F. B. Moorehead, 1875-1947. American oral surgeon). A type of instrument for drawing back the edges of wounds, used in dental surgery.

Morand's foramen (S. F. Morand, 1697-1773. French surgeon). The caecal foramen of the tongue (q.v.).

morbid (mor'-bid). Relating to or affected with disease.

morbus gallicus. Syphilis (q.v.).

mordacious (mor-da'-shus). Biting, caustic, or pungent.

mordant (mor'-dant). Any substance used to fix dyes or stains.

more solito. Latin for *in the usual way*; used in prescription writing, and abbreviated *mor. sol.*

morphologic, morphological (mor-fol-oj'-ik-al). Relating to morphology.

morphology (mor-fol'-oj-i). The study of the forms and structure of living organisms.

Morrison crown (W. N. Morrison, 1842-1896. American dentist). A gold shell crown, formed by an axial band with a swaged occlusal cap; *also called* Beers' crown.

morsal (mor'-sal). Occlusal; relating to the masticating surface of a molar or premolar.

mortar (mor'-tar). A bell- or urn-shaped vessel in which drugs are ground and crushed with a pestle.

motile (mo'-til). Capable of spontaneous movement.

motor nerve. Any of the nerves whose impulses produce movement in the organism.

mottled enamel. Hypoplasia and discoloration of the tooth enamel due to ingestion of excessive amounts of fluorine during the developmental period; chronic endemic (dental) fluorosis.

mottling (mot'-ling). The condition of a surface marked by spots or patches of a different colour or of a different shade.

mould (mold). 1. The hollow shape in which something is cast or fashioned. 2. To model or cast an object in such a hollow shape. *acrylic m.* A stent used in oral plastic surgery to secure an intraoral skin graft.

mouth (mowth). 1. The oral cavity, containing the teeth and the tongue. 2. The entrance to any canal or body cavity. *tapir m.* A condition characterized by loose thickened lips, and caused by atrophy of the orbicularis oris muscle.

trench m. 1. Acute ulcerative gingivitis (*q.v.*). 2. Acute ulcerative stomatitis (*q.v.*).

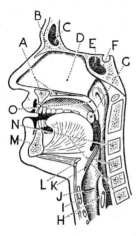

Mouth and oral cavity

A Maxilla.
B Frontal bone.
C Frontal sinus.
D Nasal septum.
E Sphenoid sinus.
F Sphenoid bone.
G Palatine tonsil.
H Cricoid cartilage.
I Thyroid cartilage.
J Vocal fold.
K Epiglottis.
L Hyoid bone.
M Mandible.
N Cervical vertebrae.
O Soft palate and uvula.

mouth mirror. Dental mirror (*q.v.*).

mouth-breathing. Habitual respiration through the mouth instead of through the nose.

muciferous (*myu-sif'-er-us*). Mucus-secreting.

mucilage (*myu'-sil-āj*). 1. A sticky paste used as a vehicle in pharmacy or as a demulcent. 2. A natural gum dissolved in plant juices, occurring in plants.

mucilagenous (*myu-sil-aj'-in-us*). Relating to or having the characteristics of mucilage.

mucin (*myu'-sin*). The chief constituent of mucus, a mixture of glycoproteins soluble in water but precipitated in alcohol or acids.

mucin plaque. Acquired pellicle (*q.v.*).

mucinous (*myu'-sin-us*). Relating to or characterized by mucin.

muco-. Prefix signifying *mucus*, or *mucous membrane*.

mucocele (*myu'-ko-sēl*). 1. Distention of an organ or vessel caused by an accumulation of mucus. 2. A mucous polypus.

mucocutaneous (*myu-ko-kyu-ta'-ne-us*). Relating to the mucous membrane and the skin.

mucodermal (*myu-ko-der'-mal*). Relating to the mucous membrane and the skin.

mucoepidermoid (*myu-ko-ep-i-der'-moyd*). Relating to the mucous membrane and the epidermis.

mucogingival (*myu-ko-jin'-jiv-al*). Relating to the mucous membrane and the gingivae.

mucogingival junction. The line at which the mucous membrane and the gingivae unite.

mucoid (*myu'-koyd*). Mucus-like.

mucomembranous (*myu"-ko-mem'-bran-us*). Relating to the mucous membrane.

mucoperiosteum (*myu"-ko-per-ĭ-os'-tĕ-um*). Periosteum having a mucous covering, as in the auditory apparatus.

mucopurulent (*myu-ko-pyu'-ru-lent*). Containing both mucus and pus.

mucormycosis (*myu"-kor-mi-ko'-sis*). A fungous disease starting in the nose and later invading the veins and the lymphatics.

mucosa (*myu-ko'-sä*). The mucous membrane.
alveolar m. The mucous membrane lining the vestibule of the mouth.

mucosal (*myu-ko'-sal*). Relating to the mucous membrane.

mucositis (*myu-ko-si'-tis*). Inflammation of the mucous membrane.

mucous (*myu'-kus*). Relating to mucus.

mucous gland. One of the glands which form and secrete mucus.

mucous membrane. The membrane containing mucous glands which lines those passages and cavities of the body which communicate with the exterior.

mucus (*myu'-kus*). The viscid secretion of the mucous glands, covering the mucous membrane.

muffle furnace. A type of oven used in dental ceramics, in which material may be heated without being directly exposed to the source of heat.

mulberry molars (*mul'-ber-ĭ*). Small, dome-shaped permanent first molars, with the cusps close together and affected by enamel hypoplasia; seen in congenital syphilis. *Also called* Moon's molars or Fournier's molars.

muller (*mul'-er*). A flat-bottomed pestle, used to grind drugs on a slab.

multi-. Prefix signifying *many*.

multicellular (*mul-tĭ-sel'-yu-lar*). Composed of numerous cells.

multicusped (*mul-tĭ-kus'-pd*). Multicuspidate (*q.v.*).

multicuspidate (*mul-tĭ-kus'-pid-āt*). Having several cusps, as on a posterior tooth.

multidentate (*mul-tĭ-den'-tāt*). Having many teeth, or many tooth-like projections.

multilocular (*mul-tĭ-lok'-yu-lar*). Containing many cells or small cavities.

multilocular cyst. Any cyst having many interconnected compartments.

multinuclear (*mul-tĭ-nyu'-klĕ-ar*). Having several nuclei.

multirooted (*mul-ti-ru'-ted*). Having several roots; used of molar teeth.

Mummery's fibres (J. H. Mummery, 1847-1926. English dentist). Nerve fibrils in developing dentine.

mummification (*mum-if-ik-a'-shun*) *of dental pulp.* Removal of previously devitalized pulp to the level of the pulp chamber floor, and the treatment of the radicular portion to render it inert.

muscle (*mus'-el*). A contractile organ by means of which movement is produced in an animal organism.

involuntary m. Any muscle which contracts of itself, and is not under the control of the will.

smooth m. Muscle consisting of spindle-shaped, unstriped fibres; involuntary muscle is usually of this type.

sphincter m. One which surrounds and closes a natural opening.

striated m. Muscle in which the fibres have cross-striations; voluntary muscle is usually of this type.

striped m. Striated muscle (*q.v.*).

unstriated m. Smooth muscle (*q.v.*).

unstriped m. Smooth muscle (*q.v.*).

voluntary m. Any muscle which is directly controlled by the will.

For muscles of the head and neck *see* Table of Muscles.

muscle, Koyter's. M. corrugator supercilii. *See* Table of Muscles.

muscular (*mus'-kyu-lar*). Relating to or characterized by muscle.

musculature (*mus'-kyu-lat-yur*). The system of muscles in the body, or in any one part of it.

musculocutaneous (*mus''-kyu-lo-kyu-ta'-nē-us*). Relating to both muscle and skin.

musculodermic (*mus''-kyu-lo-der'-mik*). Musculocutaneous (*q.v.*).

musculomembranous (*mus''-kyu-lo-mem'-bran-us*). Relating to both muscle and membrane.

mush bite. Squash bite (*q.v.*).

Mycobacteriaceae (*mi''-bak-te-ri-a'-se-e*). A family of parasitic rod-shaped organisms of the order Actinomycetales.

Mycobacterium (*mi''-ko-bak-te'-ri-um*). A genus of the Mycobacteriaceae family of bacteria, seen as slender rods, sometimes branching; Gram-positive and aerobic.

mycodermatitis (*mi-ko-derm-at-i'-tis*). Inflammation affecting a mucous membrane.

mycosis (*mi-ko'-sis*). A disease caused by a fungus.

mycotic (*mi-kot'-ik*). Relating to any fungous disease or mycosis.

mycotic stomatitis. Thrush (*q.v.*).

mycteric (*mik-ter'-ik*). Relating to the nasal cavity.

myelogenic (*mi-el-o-jen'-ik*); **myelogenous** (*mi-el-oj'-en-us*). Produced by the bone-marrow cells.

myeloid (*mi'-el-oyd*). Relating to bone marrow.

myeloma (*mi-el-o'-mă*). A tumour arising from, and composed of bone marrow cells.

mylo-. Prefix signifying *molar*.

mylodus (*mi-lo'-dus*). An old term for a molar tooth.

myloglossus (*mi-lo-glos'-us*). 1. Part of the superior constrictor phyaryngis muscle, arising from the mylohyoid ridge on the mandible. 2. A slip of muscle joining the styloglossus. *See* Table of Muscles.

mylohyoid (*mi-lo-hi'-oyd*). Relating to the mandibular molars and the hyoid bone.

mylohyoid groove. A groove on the medial surface of the mandible below the mylohyoid line, in which run the mylohyoid nerve and vessels.

mylohyoid line. A ridge on the inner surface of the mandible, running from the ascending ramus to the chin, to which the mylohyoid muscle and the superior constrictor pharyngis are attached.

mylohyoid muscle. Assists in raising hyoid bone and depressing mandible during swallowing. *See* Table of Muscles—mylohyoideus.

mylohyoid nerve. Supplies the mylohyoid muscle and the anterior belly of the digastric muscle. *See* Table of Nerves—mylohyoideus.

mylohyoid ridge. The ridge on the internal surface of the mandible to which the mylohyoid muscle is attached.

mylopharyngeal (*mi"-lo-far-in'-jĕ-al*) **muscle.** Part of constrictor pharyngis superior. *See* Table of Muscles—mylopharyngeus.

myo-. Prefix signifying *muscle.*

myoblast (*mi'-o-blast*). One of the cells from which muscle fibres develop.

myoblastoma (*mi-o-blast-o'-mă*). A tumour composed of muscle tissue resembling primitive myoblasts.

myofascial (*mi"-o-fash'-ĭ-al*). Relating to the muscle fascia.

myoid (*mi'-oyd*). Muscle-like.

myology (*mi-ol'-oj-ĭ*). The study of muscle and muscles.

myoma (*mi-o'-mă*). A tumour derived from or composed of muscle tissue. If it is smooth muscle it is called a *leiomyoma*, and if it is striated muscle a *rhabdomyoma.*

myomatosis (*mi-o-mat-o'-sis*). The development of multiple myomas.

myomatous (*mi-o'-mat-us*). Relating to or resembling a myoma.

myxadenitis labialis (*miks-ad-en-i'-tis la-bi-a'-lis*). Cheilitis glandularis (*q.v.*).

myxo-. Prefix signifying *mucus, mucous, mucoid.*

myxochondroma (*miks-o-kon-dro'-mă*). A tumour

composed of both cartilage tissue and mucous tissue.

myxofibroadenoma (*miks"-o-fi"-bro-ad-en-o'-mă*). Adenofibroma (*q.v.*).

myxoid (*miks'-oyd*). Mucus-like.

myxoma (*miks-o'-mă*). A tumour composed of mucous connective tissue.

myxorrhoea (*miks-or-e'-ă*). A copious flow of mucus.

N

N Chemical symbol for nitrogen.

Na Chemical symbol for sodium.

N.A.D. Abbreviation for *no appreciable disease; nothing abnormal discovered*.

NaF Chemical symbol for sodium fluoride.

Ni Chemical symbol for nickel.

noct. Abbreviation for *nocte*—at night; used in prescription writing.

noct. maneq. Abbreviation for *nocte maneque*—at night and in the morning; used in prescription writing.

N.T.P. Abbreviation for *normal temperature and pressure*.

N.Y.D. Abbreviation for *not yet diagnosed*.

naevoxantho-endothelioma (*ne"-vo-zan''-tho-en-do-the-li-o'-mă*). A condition characterized by hard yellowish nodules which appear on the skin in infants; most commonly seen on the face and extremities.

naevus (*ne'-vus*). A birth mark.

Nance's leeway space. The difference between the space occupied by the deciduous canine and two molars and that occupied by the permanent canine and premolars on each side of the dental arch.

nanocephalous (*na-no-sef'-al-us*). Having an abnormally small head.

nanoid (*nan'-oyd*). Dwarf-like.

nanoid enamel. Enamel which is thinner than normal; *also called* dwarfed enamel.

nape (*nāp*). The back of the neck, the nuche.

narcosis (*nar-ko'-sis*). A state of profound unconsciousness or stupor, generally produced by a drug.

narcotic (*nar-kot'-ik*). 1. Relating to narcosis. 2. Any agent which produces narcosis and the relief of pain. 3. Any person who is addicted to narcotics.

naris (*na'-ris*) (*pl.* nares). A nostril.

nasal (*na'-zal*). Relating to the nose.

nasal arteries. Supply the nasal cavity and septum and the adjacent sinuses. *See* Table of Arteries—nasales.

nasal bone. One of the two small bones which make up the nasal bridge.

nasal capsule. The cartilagenous structure around the embryonic nasal cavity.

nasal crest *of the maxilla.* A ridge on the medial border of the maxillary palatal process, articulating with the vomer.

nasal crest *of the palatine bone.* A ridge on the medial border of the palatal bone, articulating with the vomer.

nasal line. The line or furrow which runs on either side from the alae of the nose to the angles of the mouth.

nasal muscle. M. compressor naris & M. dilatator naris. *See* Table of Muscles.

nasal nerves. Supply the skin and mucosa of the nose. *See* Table of Nerves—nasalis.

nasal notch. An uneven space between the internal angular processes of the frontal bone.

nasal point. Nasion (q.v.).

nasal process *of the maxilla.* Frontal process (q.v.).

nasal reflex. Bekhterev's reflex (q.v.).

nasal spine, anterior. A median spine of bone projecting from the maxillae and supporting the septal cartilage of the nose.

nasal spine, posterior. The spine at the lower, posterior end of the nasal crest of the palatine bone.

nasal vein, external. The vein draining the side of the nose. *See* Table of Veins—nasalis externa.

nasion (*na'-zĭ-on*). The mid-point of the fronto-nasal suture.

nasitis (*na-zi'-tis*). Inflammation of the nasal mucous membrane.

Nasmyth's membrane (A. Nasmyth, d. 1848. Scottish dental surgeon). 1. Primary enamel cuticle (q.v.). 2. Reduced enamel epithelium (q.v.). 3. Primary enamel cuticle and reduced enamel epithelium.

naso-. Prefix signifying *nose*.

naso-antral (*na-zo-an'-tral*). Relating to the nose and the maxillary antrum.

nasobasilar line. Basinasal line (q.v.).

nasobronchial (*na-zo-bron'-ki-al*). Relating to the nose and the bronchi.

nasobuccal (*na-zo-buk'-al*). Relating to the nose and the cheek.

nasobuccopharyngeal (*na''-zo-buk''-o-far-in'-jĕ-al*). Relating to the nose, the cheek and the pharynx.

nasociliary (*na-zo-sil'-ĭ-ar-ĭ*). Relating to the nose and the eye and eyebrow.

nasociliary nerve. Supplies the eyeball, eyelid, nose, and ethmoid and sphenoid sinuses. *See* Table of Nerves—nasociliaris.

nasofrontal (*na-zo-fron'-tal*). Relating to the nose and the frontal bone.

nasolabial (*na-zo-la'-bĭ-al*). Relating to the nose and the lip.

nasolabial line. A line joining the edge of the nose to the angle of the mouth on the same side.

nasolabialis (na"-zo-la-bi-a'-lis). A slip of muscle from M. orbicularis oris, attaching the upper lip to the nasal septum.

nasolacrimal (na-zo-lak'-rim-al). 1. Relating to the nasal and lacrimal bones. 2. Relating to the nose and the lacrimal apparatus.

nasolacrimal canal. The canal in which runs the nasolacrimal duct.

nasolacrimal duct. The membranous canal through which tears pass from the lacrimal sac to the nasal cavity.

nasomaxillary (na-zo-maks-il'-ar-i). Relating to the nasal processes and the maxilla.

nasomental (na-zo-men'-tal). Relating to the nose and the chin.

nasomental reflex. Contraction of the mentalis muscle causing elevation of the lower lip, as a result of a tap on the side of the nose with a percussion hammer.

naso-oral (na-zo-or'-al). Relating to the nose and the mouth.

nasopalatine (na-zo-pal'-at-in). Relating to the nose and the palatine processes.

nasopalatine artery. A. sphenopalatina. *See* Table of Arteries.

nasopalatine canal. One of the passages from the nasal cavity to the palate, normally occluded in man.

nasopalatine groove. A groove on the surface of the vomer in which lodge the nasopalatine nerve and vessels.

nasopalatine nerve. Supplies the mucosa of the hard palate and the nose. *See* Table of Nerves—nasopalatinus.

nasopalatine plexus. A plexus of the nasopalatine nerves in the incisive foramen.

nasopharyngeal (na-zo-far-in'-jě-al). 1. Relating to both the nose and the pharynx. 2. Relating to the nasopharynx.

nasopharynx (na-zo-far'-inks). That part of the pharynx which extends above the soft palate.

natural (nat'-yur-al). Not artificial, abnormal or pathologic.

nausea (naw'-se-ă). A feeling of sickness, or a tendency to vomit.

nauseous (naw'-sě-us). Relating to or producing nausea.

neck (nek). 1. That part of the body connecting the head and the upper part of the trunk. 2. Any narrowed or constricted portion at the junction of two parts. 3. The narrowed junction between the enamel and the cementum of a tooth; the tooth cervix.

necrobiosis (nek-ro-bi-o'-sis). Gradual deterioration of cells, leading finally to their death.

necrobiotic (*nek-ro-bi-ot'-ik*). Necrotic (*q.v.*).

necrosis (*nek-ro'-sis*). Death of a circumscribed area of tissue.
dental n. Tooth decay.

necrotic (*nek-rot'-ik*). Relating to or characterized by necrosis.

needle (*nēdl*). A sharp-pointed instrument, used to suture or to puncture tissue.
aspirating n. A long hollow needle used to withdraw fluid from a cavity.
harelip n. A cannula which is introduced into the wound during an operation for harelip, and held in place by a figure-of-eight suture.
hypodermic n. A form of hollow needle used with a syringe for injections.

nefrens (*nef'-rens*). Having no teeth; an obsolete term.

negative overbite. Anterior open-bite (*q.v.*).

Neisseria (*ni-se'-ri-ǎ*) (A. L. S. Neisser, 1855-1916. German physician). A genus of the Neisseriaceae family of bacteria, Gram-negative, parasitic, non-motile and anaerobic.
N. discoides. A species found in the oral cavity.

Neisseriaceae (*ni-ser-i-a'-se-e*). A family of bacteria of the order Eubacteriales.

neo-. Prefix signifying *new*.

neoblastic (*ne-o-blast'-ik*). Relating to, or arising from, new tissue.

neonatal (*ne-o-na'-tal*). Relating to the newborn.

neonatal line. An incremental line in the dentine and enamel of a deciduous tooth formed *in utero*, marking the development of the tooth structure at the time of birth.

neonatal ring. Neonatal line (*q.v.*).

neonatal tooth. A deciduous tooth present in the mouth at birth or erupting within a few days of birth.

neonate (*ne'-o-nāt*). A new-born infant.

neoplasm (*ne'-o-plazm*). An abnormal mass of tissue, the growth of which exceeds and is uncoordinated with that of the normal tissues, and persists in the same excessive manner after cessation of the stimuli which evoked the change (Willis). Synonymous with *tumour*.

neoplastic (*ne-o-plast'-ik*). Relating to or characteristic of a neoplasm.

nephro-. Prefix signifying *kidney*.

nepiology (*nep-i-ol'-oj-i*). That branch of pediatrics relating to infants and young children.

nerve (*nerv*). A cord-like bundle of fibres which transmits sensations or impulses for movement from one part of the body to another.
afferent n. Any nerve transmitting impulses from the periphery to the centre.
autonomic n. Any nerve of the autonomic nervous system.

cranial n. Any one of twelve pairs of peripheral nerves arising directly from the brain stem.

efferent n. Any nerve carrying impulses from the centre to the periphery.

intrinsic n. Any nerve supplying impulses to the muscles, glands, or mucous membranes of an organ or part.

motor n. Any of the nerves whose impulses produce movement in the organism.

peripheral n. Any nerve whose distribution is to the skin; loosely used of any branch of the central nervous system.

secretory n. Any efferent nerve whose stimulation increases activity in the gland to which it is distributed.

sensory n. An afferent nerve, transmitting sensations of pain, touch, etc., to the central nervous system from the periphery.

somatic n. One of the nerves supplying voluntary muscles, tendons, joints, skin, and parietal serous membranes.

sympathetic n. Any one of of the nerves of the sympathetic nervous system.

vasomotor n. Any nerve which controls the calibre of blood or lymph vessels; it may be a *vasodilator* or a *vasoconstrictor.*

nerve, Hirschfeld's. *See* Hirschfeld's nerve.

nerve, Jacobson's. Tympanic nerve (*q.v.*).

nerve, pharyngeal, Bock's. *See* Bock's pharyngeal nerve.

nerve of Arnold (F. Arnold, 1803–90. German anatomist). N. auricularis. *See* Table of Nerves.

nerve of Cotunnius (D. Cotugno (Cotunnius), 1736–1822. Italian anatomist). The nasopalatine nerve (*q.v.*).

nerve of Cruveilhier (J. Cruveilhier, 1791–1874. French pathologist). An occasional branch of the facial nerve.

nerve of Scarpa (A. Scarpa, 1747–1832. Italian anatomist and surgeon). The nasopalatine nerve (*q.v.*).

nerve of the pterygoid canal. Supplies the lacrimal gland and the glands of the nose and palate. *See* Table of Nerves—canalis pterygoidei.

nerve of Vidius (V. Vidius [G. Guido], d. 1569. Italian anatomist and physician). N. canalis pterygoidei. *See* Table of Nerves.

nervous (*ner'-vus*). 1. Relating to a nerve. 2. Relating to the condition of nervousness.

Neubauer's artery (J. E. Neubauer, 1742–77. German anatomist). A. thyroidea ima. *See* Table of Arteries.

Neumann's sheath (E. F. C. Neumann, 1834–1918. German pathologist). Partially calcified tissue lining the dentinal tubules.

neural (*nyu'-ral*). Relating to a nerve or nerves.

neuralgia (*nyu-ral'-ji-ă*). Pain affecting a nerve or nerve-ending.

neuralgic (*nyu-ral'-jik*). Relating to or affected with neuralgia.

neuro-. Prefix signifying *nerve*.

neurofibroma (*nyu-ro-fi-bro'-mă*). A tumour arising from the nerve-fibre cells.

neuroid (*nyu'-royd*). Nerve-like.

neurology (*nyu-rol'-oj-i*). The study of the nervous system and the treatment of its diseases.

neuroma (*nyu-ro'-mă*). A tumour arising from or composed of nerve cell tissue.

neuromuscular (*nyu-ro-mus'-kyu-lar*). Relating to both nerves and muscles.

neurospasm (*nyu-ro-spazm*). Spasmodic muscular twitching due to nerve spasm.

neutral (*nyu'-tral*). Neither acid nor alkali.

neutralize (*nyu'-tral-īz*). To make neutral or inert.

neutrocclusion (*nyu-trok-lu'-zhun*). Angle Class I malocclusion (*q.v.*).

nevus. See naevus.

newborn (*nyu'-born*). Recently born, applied to infants in their first two or three days of life.

nickel (*nik'-el*). A silver-white metal, chemical symbol Ni, with properties very similar to those of iron.

nidus (*ni'-dus*). A focal point of infection.

nigrities linguae. Black tongue (*q.v.*).

nitro-. Prefix signifying *nitrogen*, or *nitrogen dioxide*.

nitrogen (*ni'-tro-jen*). A colourless and odourless gas, existing free in the atmosphere; chemical symbol N. It is an important constituent element in all animal and vegetable matter.

nitrogenous (*ni-troj'-en-us*). Containing nitrogen.

nitrous (*ni'-trus*). 1. Relating to nitrogen as a tri-valent element. 2. Relating to nitrous oxide.

nitrous oxide. N_2O; a colourless gas used to produce temporary general anaesthesia in dentistry and for minor surgical operations.

nociceptive (*no-si-sep'-tiv*). Relating to any pain-producing stimulus, or to pain-receptor nerves.

nociceptive reflex. Any reflex produced by a painful stimulus.

nocte. Latin for *at night*; used in prescription writing, and abbreviated *noct*.

node (*nōd*). A swelling or knob of tissue.

nodular (*nod'-yu-lar*). Relating to a node.

nodule (*nod'-yul*). A small node.

nodules, Bohn's. Epstein's pearls (*q.v.*).

noma (*no'-mă*). Gangrene of the mouth, occurring in children, and starting on the mucous membrane of the cheek or the gum; cancrum oris.

non-anatomical teeth. Artificial teeth having occlusal surfaces designed functionally rather than carved to reproduce the anatomic forms.

noncarious (*non"-ka'-ri-us*). Not affected with dental caries.

noninfectious (*non-in-fek'-shus*). Not infectious, not disease-spreading.

nonluetic (*non-lu-et'-ik*). Not caused by syphilis.

non-malignant (*non-mal-ig'-nant*). Benign.

nonmetal (*non-met'-al*). Any chemical element which is not a metal, such as a gas.

nonocclusion (*non-ok-lu'-zhun*). That form of malocclusion in which there is no contact between the opposing teeth; open-bite.

norm (*nōz*). A fixed standard against which other, similar, things may be measured.

normal (*nor'-mal*). Relating to the norm; of the regular and ideal standard.

Norwegian appliance. Andresen appliance (*q.v.*).

nose (*nōz*). The organ of the sense of smell, and one of the organs of respiration.

nosebleed (*nōz'-blēd*). A haemorrhage from the blood vessels of the nose; epistaxis.

noso-. Prefix signifying disease.

nosode (*no'-zōd*). Any product of a disease which is used in treatment.

nosology (*no-zol'-oj-i*). The science of the classification of diseases.

nostrate (*nos'-trāt*). Prevalent in a particular region; endemic.

nostril (*nos'-tril*). One of the two external openings of the nose.

notation (*no-ta'-shun*). A set of symbols, which may be letters, numbers or other forms, used to indicate briefly either data or ideas. *dental n.* A form of symbols used to indicate the type and place of a tooth. The most commonly used notation is:- for permanent teeth:

right	left
87654321	12345678
87654321	12345678

for deciduous teeth:

right	left
edcba	abcde
edcba	abcde

For example: the lower left lateral permanent incisor would be represented by ⌐2 and the upper right central deciduous incisor by a⌐.

notch (*notch*). A deep depression or indentation, usually in the edge of a bone. *craniofacial n.* A notch in the bony partition between the nasal and orbital cavities. *ethmoidal n.* The space between the orbital plates of the frontal bone, which, in an articulated skull, contains the cribriform plate of the ethmoid bone.

frontal n. A notch on the upper edge of the orbital bone, through which pass the frontal artery and nerve.

hamular n. Pterygomaxillary notch (*q.v.*).

jugular n. of the occipital bone. An indentation on the lower edge of the bone which forms the posterior part of the jugular foramen.

jugular n. of the temporal bone. A small depression in the petrous portion of the bone, corresponding to the jugular notch of the occipital bone, with which it forms the jugular foramen.

lacrimal n. A notch on the inner edge of the orbital surface of the maxilla which receives the lacrimal bone.

mandibular n. Sigmoid notch (*q.v.*).

nasal n. An uneven space between the internal angular processes of the frontal bone.

parietal n. The notch which occurs in the angle between the squamous and mastoid processes of the temporal bone.

parotid n. An indentation between the mastoid process of the temporal bone and the ramus of the mandible.

postcondylar n. An indentation on the lower surface of the occipital bone, occurring between the condyle and the foramen magnum.

pterygomaxillary n. The notch at the junction of the maxilla with the pterygoid process of the sphenoid bone.

sigmoid n. The crescent-shaped border of the ramus, between the coronoid process and the condyle of the mandible.

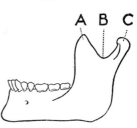

Sigmoid notch

A Coronoid process.
B Sigmoid notch.
C Condyle.

sphenopalatine n. A deep depression which divides the sphenoid and the orbital processes of the palatine bone.

noxious (*noks'-shus*). Poisonous, harmful, pernicious.

nuchal (*nyu'-kal*). Relating to the nape of the neck.

nuche (*nyu'-kě*). The nape of the neck.

nuclear (*nyu'-klě-ar*). Relating to a nucleus.

nucleated (*nyu'-kle-a-ted*). Possessing a nucleus or nuclei.

nucleus (*nyu'-klě-us*). 1. The vital differentiated protoplasm at the centre of a cell.

2. A group of nerve cells of similar function within the central nervous system.

Nuhn's gland (A. Nuhn, 1814-89. German anatomist). Blandin's gland (q.v.).

numbness (num'-nes). Partial or total loss of sensation; it may be pathologic or deliberately induced, as with a local or surface anaesthetic.

nutrient (nyu'-tri-ent). 1. Nourishing. 2. Any substance which nourishes.

nutrient canal. One of the tubular canals or grooves occurring in the alveolar bone structure of the maxilla and the mandible, through which pass anastomosing blood vessels.

nutrient foramen. One of the foramina in the maxilla and the mandible through which the nutrient canals pass.

nutriment (nyu'-tri-ment). Any nourishing substance.

nutrition (nyu-trish'-un). The process by which food is assimilated.

nycterine (nik'-ter-īn). Occurring at night.

nyctohemeral (nik"-to-hem'-er-al). Relating to or occurring both at night and during the day.

O

O Occlusal.

O Chemical symbol for oxygen.

OC Occlusocervical.

OG Occlusogingival.

Ol. Abbreviation for oleum—oil; used in prescription writing.

o.m. Abbreviation for omni mane—every morning; used in prescription writing.

omn. bih. Abbreviation for omni bihora—every two hours; used in prescription writing.

omn.h. Abbreviation for omni hora—every hour; used in prescription writing.

o.n. Abbreviation for omni nocte—every night; used in prescription writing.

oz. Abbreviation for ounce.

obelion (o-be'-li-on). The point of juncture of the sagittal suture and a line joining the parietal foramina.

obese (o-bēs'). Excessively fat, overweight, adipose.

oblique muscles. See Table of Muscles—obliquus.

oblique ridge. A ridge running obliquely across the occlusal surface of a maxillary molar.

obliteration (ob-lit-er-a'-shun). Complete removal or closure.

obtundent (ob-tun'-dent). Any drug which lessens or relieves pain.

obturator (ob'-tyur-a-tor). A plate, disc, or appliance used to fill or cover a cleft or an orifice; applied particularly to the prosthesis used in the treatment of cleft palate.

buccofacial o. An appliance used to close an opening through the cheek into the mouth.

occipital (*ok-sip'-it-al*). Relating to the occiput.

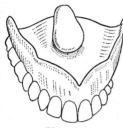

Obturator

occipital angle. The angle formed at the junction of lines connecting the lambda and the point of the external occipital protuberance with the point on the sagittal curvature of the occipital bone.

occipital artery. Supplies neck and scalp muscles. *See* Table of Arteries—occipitalis.

occipital bone. The bone forming the posterior part of the skull.

occipital muscle. Draws back scalp. *See* Table of Muscles—occipitalis.

occipital nerve. Supplies skin over scalp. *See* Table of Nerves—occipitalis.

occipital sinus. A variable anastomosing venous channel between the transverse and sigmoid sinuses. *See* Table of Veins—sinus occipitalis.

occipito-. Prefix signifying *occipital, occiput.*

occipitobasilar (*ok-sip''-it-o-bas-il'-ar*). Relating to the occiput and the base of the skull.

occipitobregmatic (*ok-sip''-it-o-breg-mat'-ik*). Relating to the occiput and the bregma.

occipitocervical (*ok-sip''-it-o-ser-vi'-kal*). Relating to the occiput and the neck.

occipitofacial (*ok-sip''-it-o-fa'-shi-al*). Relating to the occiput and the facial bones.

occipitofrontal (*ok-sip''-it-o-frun'-tal*). Relating to the occiput and the frontal bone.

occipitofrontal muscle. The scalp muscle. *See* Table of Muscles—occipitofrontalis.

occipitomental (*ok-sip''-it-o-men'-tal*). Relating to the occiput and the chin.

occipitotemporal (*ok-sip''-it-o-tem''-por-al*). Relating to the occiput and the temporal bones.

occiput (*ok'-sip-ut*). The back part of the skull.

occlude (*ok-lūd'*). To close or to shut. In dentistry, closure of the jaws to bring opposing teeth into contact.

occlusal (*ok-lu'-zal*). Relating to the occlusion of the teeth.

occlusal angle. Any angle formed by the junction of an occlusal tooth surface, or a cavity wall, in a posterior tooth, with any other tooth surface or cavity wall.

occlusal cavity. A cavity in the occlusal surface of a tooth; a Class I cavity.

occlusal equilibration. The restoration of normal occlusion within the mouth by mechanical means.

occlusal load. The force exerted on the posterior teeth during mastication.

occlusal pad. A pad of gingiva covering the occlusal surface of a tooth.

occlusal plane. The imaginary plane between the maxillary and mandibular teeth in occlusion; it is used in the construction of artificial dentures.

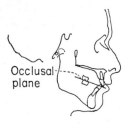

Occlusal plane

Occlusal plane

occlusal rest. A cast metal projection on a partial denture, extending over and resting upon the occlusal or other prepared surface of a natural tooth, and acting as an indirect retainer.

occlusal rim. A rim of wax mounted on a denture base; it is used in the recording of the relationships of the jaws.

occlusal surface. That surface of a tooth which comes into contact with a corresponding surface of another tooth in the opposing jaw in occlusion.

occlusal wall. That wall of a tooth cavity which faces the occlusal surface of the tooth.

occlusion (ok-lu'-zhun). The contact of the upper and lower teeth in any jaw position.

balanced o. 1. The ideal interdigitation of the teeth, in which there is no cuspal interference in lateral excursions of the mandible. 2. In prosthetic dentistry, the simultaneous contact of all occlusal areas to prevent the tipping or rotating of the denture base.

centric o. The relationship of the upper and lower dental arches when the teeth are brought into contact from centric relation (*q.v.*).

distal o. A term denoting the position of a tooth which is distal to the normal position in occlusion.

eccentric o. The occlusion of the teeth with the mandible in any position other than that of rest.

labial o. A term to denote the position of an incisor or a canine which is in front of the line of occlusion.

lateral o. The occlusion of the teeth with the mandible moved to one side or the other, not in centric occlusion.

lingual o. A term for the

position of a tooth behind the line of occlusion.

mesial o. A term to denote the position of a tooth which is mesial of its normal position in occlusion.

posterior o. The occlusion resulting when the mandibular teeth occlude posterior to their normal position in relation to the maxillary teeth.

protrusive o. The occlusion produced by a protruding mandible.

retrusive o. The occlusion produced by a receding mandible.

traumatic o. Any form of malocclusion which causes damage to the teeth or to the periodontal tissues.

occlusive (*ok-lu'-siv*). Relating to occlusion.

occlusocervical (*ok-lu"-zo-ser-vi'-kal*). Relating to the occlusal surface and the neck of a tooth.

occlusometer (*ok-luz-om'-et-er*). Gnathodynamometer (*q.v.*).

occupational (*ok-yu-pa'-shun-al*). *Of a disease*: Caused by the patient's occupation; it may be organic or functional.

octo-. Prefix signifying *eight*.

ocular (*ok'-yu-lar*). Relating to the eye.

ocular hypertelorism. A craniofacial deformity characterized by enlargement of the sphenoid bone, great breadth across the bridge of the nose, and resulting width between the eyes.

oculo-. Prefix signifying *eye*.

oculomotor nerve. The third cranial nerve, supplying the muscles of the eye and upper eyelid. *See* Table of Nerves—oculomotorius.

odont-. Prefix signifying *teeth*, or *tooth*.

odontagra (*o-dont-ag'-ră*). Tooth-ache.

odontalgia (*o-dont-al'-ji-ă*). Tooth-ache.

phantom o. Tooth-ache felt in the socket from which a tooth has been extracted.

odontalgic (*o-dont-al'-jik*). Relating to or characterized by tooth-ache.

odontatrophia (*o-dont-at-ro'-fi-ă*). Atrophy of the teeth.

odontectomy (*o-dont-ekt'-om-ĭ*). Surgical excision for the removal of retained roots, unerupted or partially erupted teeth.

odonterism (*o-dont'-er-izm*). Teeth-chattering.

odontexesis (*o-dont-eks-e'-sis*). Cleaning the teeth, especially by means of a scraping instrument.

odonthaemodia (*o-donth-e-mo'-di-ă*). Excessive sensitivity in the teeth.

odontharpaga (*o-donth-ar-pa'-gă*). Tooth-ache.

odonthyalus (*o-donth-i'-al-us*). Tooth enamel; obsolete.

odontia (*o-don'-shĭ-ă*). Any dental abnormality.

odontia deformans. Any deformity of the teeth.

odontia incrustans. Dental calculus (*q.v.*).

odo

odontiasis (*o-dont-i'-as-is*). Eruption of the teeth; dentition.

odontiatria (*o-don-shǐ-at'-rǐ-ǎ*). Dental treatment.

odontic (*o-dont'-ik*). Relating to the teeth.

odontinoid (*o-dont'-in-oyd*). 1. Resembling a tooth. 2. A tumour containing tooth substance.

odontitis (*o-dont-i'-tis*). Inflammation of the tooth pulp; pulpitis.

odontoamelosarcoma (*o-dont'-o-am-e"-lo-sar-ko'-mǎ*). Ameloblastosarcoma (*q.v.*).

odontoatlantal (*o-dont"-o-at-lan'-tal*). Atlantoaxial (*q.v.*).

odontoblast (*o-dont'-o-blast*). 1. One of the germ cells from which dentine is formed. 2. One of the layers of cylindrical cells in the connective tissue surrounding the dental pulp.

odontoblastic processes. The branching processes of the odontoblasts which occur in the dentinal canals.

odontoblastoma (*o-dont'-o-blast-o'-mǎ*). A tumour composed of odontoblasts.

odontobothrion (*o-dont-o-both'-ri-on*). The socket of a tooth; obsolete term.

odontobothritis (*o-dont"-o-both-ri'-tis*). Inflammation of the tooth sockets; obsolete term.

odontocele (*o-dont'-o-sēl*). An alveolodental cyst.

odontoceramic (*o-dont"-o-ser-am'-ik*). Relating to porcelain teeth.

odontoceramotechny (*o-dont"-o-ser-am"-o-tek'-nǐ*). Dental ceramics (*q.v.*).

odontochalix (*o-dont-to-ka'-liks*). Cementum (*q.v.*).

odontochirurgical (*o-dont"-o-kir-ur'-jik-al*). Relating to dental surgery.

odontocia (*o-dont-o'-sǐ-ǎ*). A condition which is characterized by softening of the teeth.

odontoclamis (*o-dont-o-kla'-mis*). The condition in which an erupted tooth is hooded over by gingival tissue.

odontoclasis (*o-dont-o-kla'-sis*). 1. Fracture of a tooth. 2. The process of resorption of a tooth.

odontoclast (*o-dont'-o-klast*). One of the multinuclear cells, occurring between the deciduous and the permanent teeth, associated in the process of resorption of the deciduous roots and with pathological resorption of the permanent tooth roots; a form of osteoclast.

odontocnesis (*o-dont-ok-ne'-sis*). An itching sensation of the gums.

odontodynia (*o-dont"-o-din'-ǐ-ǎ*). Tooth-ache.

odontogenesis (*o-dont-to-jen'-es-is*). 1. Odontogeny (*q.v.*). 2. Dentinogenesis (*q.v.*).

odontogenesis imperfecta. Dentinogenesis imperfecta (*q.v.*).

odontogenic (*o-dont-o-jen'-ik*). Originating from a tooth or tooth germ.

odontogenic fibres. Those fibres which make up the connective tissue layer of the tooth matrix, surrounding the pulp.

odontogeny (*o-dont-oj'-en-i*). The origin and development of the teeth.

odontoglyph (*o-dont'-o-glif*). A dental scaler.

odontogram (*o-dont'-o-gram*). The record made by an odontograph.

odontograph (*o-dont'-o-graf*). An instrument for recording any unevenness on a tooth surface.

odontography (*o-dont-og'-raf-i*). 1. The description of tooth anatomy. 2. The use of an odontograph.

odontohyperaesthesia (*o-dont"-o-hi"-per-es-the'-zi-ă*). Hypersensitivity of a tooth.

odontoiatria (*o-dont-o-i-at'-ri-ă*). Treatment of the teeth.

odontoid (*o-dont'-oyd*). Resembling a tooth.

odontolith (*o-dont'-o-lith*). Dental calculus (*q.v.*).

odontolithiasis (*o-dont-o-lith-i'-as-is*). The condition of having deposits of calculus on the teeth.

odontologist (*o-dont-ol'-oj-ist*). Dentist.

odontology (*o-dont-ol'-oj-i*). Dentistry (*q.v.*).

odontoloxia (*o-dont-ol-ok'-si-ă*). Irregularity or slanting of the teeth.

odontolysis (*o-dont-ol'-is-is*). The absorption of calcified tooth substance.

odontome, odontoma (*o-dont'-ōm, o-dont-o'-mă*). A tumour derived from or composed of dental tissue. *composite o.* One made up of various elements of the tooth germ.

odontomere (*o-dont'-o-mēr*). One of the two halves of the enamel organ of a tooth, the buccal being the *protomere* and the lingual the *deuteromere.*

odontonecrosis (*o-dont"-o-nek-ro'-sis*). Gross dental caries.

odontoneuralgia (*o-dont"-o-nyu-ral'-ji-ă*). 1. Neuralgia caused by dental disease. 2. Neuralgic pain felt in the teeth.

odontonomy (*o-dont-on'-om-i*). Dental terminology.

odontonosology (*o-dont"-o-no-zol'-oj-i*). The study of tooth diseases.

odontoparallaxis (*o-dont"-o-par-al-aks'-is*). Irregularity in the position of the teeth.

odontopathy (*o-dont-op'-ath-i*). Any disease of the teeth.

odontoperisoteum (*o-dont"-o-per-i-os'-tě-um*). Periodontium (*q.v.*).

odontophobia (*o-dont-o-fo'-bi-ă*). Fear of teeth.

odontoplast (*o-dont'-o-plast*). Odontoblast (*q.v.*).

odontoplasty (*o-dont'-o-plast-i*). 1. Orthodontics (*q.v.*). 2. In periodontology, the modification of tooth contours to aid in the maintenance of healthy gingivae.

odontoplerosis (*o-dont-o-pler-o'-sis*). The operation of filling a tooth cavity.

odontoprisis (*o-dont"-o-pri'-sis*). Grinding the teeth; bruxism.

odontopsis (*o-dont-op'-sis*). Loss of the teeth.

odontoradiograph (*o-dont"-o-ra'-dĭ-o-graf*). A radiograph of the teeth or of a tooth.

odontorrhagia (*o-dont-or-ra'-jĭ-ă*). Bleeding after tooth extraction.

odontorthrosis (*o-dont-or-thro'-sis*). Orthodontics (*q.v.*).

odontoschisis (*o-dont-os'-kis-is*). Splitting of a tooth or of teeth.

odontoschism (*o-dont'-o-sizm*). A fissure or cleft in a tooth.

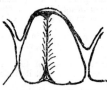

Odontoschism

odontoscope (*o-dont'-o-skōp*). 1. A dental mirror. 2. An instrument containing a magnifying lens, used to examine tooth surfaces.

odontoscopy (*o-dont-os'-kop-ĭ*). The recording of the occlusion in an individual mouth, used for identification.

odontoseisis (*o-dont-o-si'-sis*). Looseness of the teeth.

odontosis (*o-dont-o'-sis*). Dentition (*q.v.*).

odontosteophyte (*o-dont-os'-tĕ-o-fīt*). An osseous tumour occurring on a tooth.

odontosteresis (*o-dont-o-ster-e'-sis*). Loss of the teeth.

odontosynerismus (*o-dont"-o-sin-er-iz'-mus*). Teeth-chattering.

odontotechny (*o-dont-o-tek'-nĭ*). The practice of dentistry.

odontotheca (*o-dont-o-the'-kă*). A tooth follicle.

odontotherapy (*o-dont"-o-ther"-ap-ĭ*). Treatment of dental diseases.

odontotomy (*o-dont-ot'-om-ĭ*). The process of cutting into tooth structure.

    prophylactic o. Mechanical modification of the occlusal fissures of teeth in an attempt to prevent dental caries.

odontotripsis (*o-dont-o-trip'-sis*). Wearing away of the teeth.

odontotrypy (*o-dont-ot'-rip-ĭ*). The drilling of a tooth in order to drain the pus from the pulp cavity.

-odynia. Suffix signifying *pain, ache*.

odynolysis (*o-din-ol'-is-is*). The easing or relief of pain.

odynophobia (*o-din-o-fo'-bi-ă*). Morbid fear of pain.

odynphagia (*o''-din-fa'-jĭ-ă*). Deglutition causing pain.

oedema (*e-de'-mă*). An abnormal accumulation of fluid in the body tissues, producing swelling.

oedematous (*e-de'-mat-us*). Relating to or affected by oedema.

oesophagitis (*e-sof-ag-i'-tis*). Inflammation of the oesophagus.

oesophagosalivary reflex. Stimulation of the oesophagus producing salivation; Roger's reflex.

oesophagus (*e-sof'-ag-us*). The gullet; the musculomembranous tube extending between the pharynx and the stomach.

-oid. Suffix signifying *like.*

oil (*oyl*). A liquid which does not mix with, and is generally lighter than, water; oils may be derived from fats, or from chemicals.

ointment (*oynt'-ment*). A fatty, semisolid substance, used as a base for local medicaments for external application.

oleum (*o'-le-um*). Latin for *oil;* used in prescription writing, and abbreviated *ol.*

olfactory (*ol-fak'-tor-ĭ*). Relating to the sense of smell.

olfactory nerve. The first cranial nerve, supplying the olfactory mucosa. *See* Table of Nerves—olfactorius.

oligo-. Prefix signifying *few, deficient.*

oligodontia (*ol-ig-o-don'-shĭ-ă*). The condition of having few teeth; inaccurately called partial anodontia.

oligoptyalism (*ol''-ig-o-ti'-al-izm*). Deficiency of saliva secretion.

oligosialia (*ol''-ig-o-si-al'-i-ă*). Deficiency in salivary secretion, usually pathological.

oliphyodontic gemination. A condition in which a deciduous tooth is fused to a permanent one.

-ology. Suffix signifying *study of, science of.*

-oma. Suffix signifying *tumour.*

omnis. Latin for *every;* used in prescription writing.

omnivorous (*om-niv'-or-us*). Capable of eating anything; as opposed to *herbivorous, carnivorous,* etc.

omohyoid muscle. Depresses hyoid bone and tightens deep cervical fascia in lower part of neck. *See* Table of Muscles—omohyoideus.

onco-, oncho-. Prefix signifying *tumour.*

oncocytoma (*on-ko-si-to'-mă*). A benign circumscribed and encapsulated epithelial adenoma generally affecting only the parotid gland, and occurring in elderly persons.

oncology (*on-kol'-oj-ĭ*). The study of neoplasms.

oncosis (*on-ko'-sis*). Any disease characterized by the development of tumours.

oncotic (*on-kot'-ik*). Relating to oncosis.

Onion's fusible alloy. An alloy containing five parts of bismuth to three parts of lead and two parts of tin.

onlay (*on'-la*). A cast metal cap, which may have an acrylic veneer, an extension of an occlusal rest to cover and fit over the whole of the occlusal surface of a tooth; used as a partial denture support and also to correct closed bite or as a splint to natural teeth.

onychophagia (*on"-ik-o-fa'-ji-ă*). Nail-biting.

opacity (*o-pas'-it-i*). The condition of being impervious to light.

opalescent (*o-pal-es'-ent*). Irridescent, showing various colours.

opalescent dentine, hereditary. Dentinogenesis imperfecta (*q.v.*).

opalgia (*op-al'-ji-ă*). Facial neuralgia; opsialgia.

opaque (*o-pāk'*). Impervious to light; neither transparent nor translucent.

open-bite (*ō'-pen-bīt*). A form of malocclusion in which a group of teeth fail to come into contact when the dental arches are brought into occlusion.

anterior o-b. Open-bite in which the anterior teeth do not come into contact.

posterior o-b. Open-bite in which the posterior teeth

on one side (*unilateral*) or both sides (*bilateral*) do not come into contact.

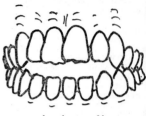

Anterior open-bite

open-cap splint. A form of cap splint in which the occlusal surfaces of the teeth are left exposed.

open-face crown. Half-cap crown (*q.v.*).

operability (*op-er-ab-il'-it-i*). The state allowing of operation with a reasonable expectation of recovery.

operable (*op'-er-abl*). Permitting of an operation; capable of treatment by operation.

operation (*op-er-a'-shun*). 1. Anything performed, especially any procedure by a surgeon, either with instruments or by hand. 2. The mode of action of a drug.
For eponymous operations *see* under the personal name by which the operation is known.

operative (*op'-er-at-iv*). 1. Relating to an operation. 2. Effective.

operculum (*op-er'-kyu-lum*). A cover or lid, in any form.

ophryon (*of'-ri-on*). The midpoint of the transverse supra-orbital line.

ophthalmic artery. Supplies the eyeball, eye muscles, etc. *See* Table of Arteries—ophthalmica.

ophthalmic nerve. *See* Table of Nerves—ophthalmicus.

ophthalmic veins. Veins draining the area supplied by the ophthalmic artery. *See* Table of Veins—ophthalmica.

opisthion (*o-pis'-thi-on*). A craniometric landmark, the midpoint on the lower edge of the foramen magnum.

opisthogenia (*o-pis-tho-je'-ni-ă*). Defective development of the jaws as a result of ankylosis.

opisthognathism (*o-pis-thog'-nath-izm*). Recession of the mandible.

opsialgia (*op-si-al'-ji-ă*). Facial neuralgia.

opsigenes (*op-sij'-en-ēz*). A term meaning late born, applied to third molars.

optic nerve. The second cranial nerve, supplying the retina. *See* Table of Nerves —opticus.

orad (*or'-ad*). In the direction of the mouth.

oral (*or'-al*). Pertaining to the mouth.

oral diaphragm. The partition dividing the submandibular region from the sublingual, and formed by the hyoglossus and the mylohyoid muscles.

oral hygiene. Principles of hygiene as applied to the mouth, to ensure cleanliness of the teeth and promote healthy gingiva.

oral moniliasis. Infection of the mouth with *Candida albicans*; a precancerous condition when chronic.

oral phimosis. Labial phimosis (*q.v.*).

oral plate. Buccopharyngeal membrane (*q.v.*).

oral prophylaxis. Preventive treatment for diseases of the oral cavity.

oral screen. A thin plastic plate constructed so that it is in contact with the tips of protruding maxillary incisors whilst appearing to cover the labial surfaces of all the maxillary teeth; lip pressure tips the incisors lingually. It is also used as an inhibitor of mouth-breathing and thumb-sucking.

oral sepsis. A septic condition in the mouth producing excessive bacterial activity which may affect the general health.

oral vibrator. A prosthetic appliance designed to provide a method of speaking for those patients who, either from operation or paralysis, have no current of air passing through the mouth. It consists of a flexible diaphragm fitted into the palate of an upper denture and vibrated by means of electric batteries, thus creating the necessary current of air.

orale (*o-ra'-lĕ*). The point on the inner surface of the alveolar process marking the end of the incisive suture.

oralogy (*or-al'-oj-ĭ*). The science of the mouth; sometimes used to denote medical and dental co-operation for health.

orbicularis oculi muscle. Closes eyelids. *See* Table of Muscles.

orbicularis oris muscle. Purses lips and puckers up mouth. *See* Table of Muscles.

orbit (*or'-bit*). The bony eye-socket.

orbital (*or'-bit-al*). Relating to the orbit.

orbital aperture. One of the openings in the facial bones which contain the eyeballs.

orbital fissure, *inferior:* A long cleft between the floor and lateral wall of the orbit, opening into the infratemporal fossa. *superior:* An elongated cleft between the great and small wings of the sphenoid bone, giving passage to various blood vessels and nerves.

orbital muscle. Vestigial. *See* Table of Muscles—orbitalis.

orbital nerve. Supplies the orbit. *See* Table of Nerves—orbitalis.

orbital plate. One of the two processes of the frontal bone which form the vaults of the orbits.

orbital process *of the palatine bone.* A bone process from the palate bone, pointing upwards and outwards.

orbital process *of the zygomatic bone.* A process extending backwards from the orbital margin of the zygomatic bone and forming part of the lateral wall and floor of the orbital cavity.

orbitale (*or-bit-a'-lĕ*). The lowest point on the lower border of the orbit.

order (*or'-der*). One of the principle divisions of a class in biological classification.

organ (*or'-gan*). Any separate part of the body having a specific function.
absorbent o. Vascular tissue lying between the roots of a deciduous tooth and its permanent successor, during resorption of the deciduous roots.
enamel o. A proliferation of the dental lamina enclosing the dental papilla; it determines the shape of the tooth crown and forms the dental enamel.

organ, Chievitz's. *See* Chievitz's organ.

organic (*or-gan'-ik*). 1. Relating to, having, or characteristic of an organ or organs. 2. Arising from, or relating to substances arising from, living organisms. 3. In chemistry, relating to carbon compounds.

organism (*or'-gan-izm*). Any individual plant or animal; an organized body of living cells.

orifacial angle. In craniometry, the angle formed by the facial line with the upper occlusal plane.

orifice (*or'-if-is*). An opening; the mouth or entrance of a body cavity.

orificial (*or-if-ish'-al*). Relating to an orifice.

origin (*or'-ij-in*). The beginning of anything.

origin of a muscle. The fixed attachment of a muscle, as opposed to its *insertion*.

oro-. Prefix signifying *mouth, oral.*

orolingual (*or-o-lin'-gwal*). Relating to the mouth and the tongue.

oromaxillary (*or-o-maks-il'-ar-ĭ*). Relating to the mouth and the maxilla.

oronasal (*or-o-na'-zal*). Relating to the mouth and the nose.

oropharyngeal (*or-o-far-in'-jĕ-al*). 1. Relating to the mouth and the pharynx, as one cavity. 2. Relating to the oropharynx.

oropharynx (*or-o-far'-inks*). The continuation of the nasopharynx from below the border of the soft palate to the larynx; the oral portion of the pharynx.

ortho-. Prefix signifying *straight, normal.*

orthocephalic (*or-tho-sef-al'-ik*). Having a vertically straight head, with an index between 70 and 75.

ortho-dentine (*or'-tho-den-tēn*). Straight-tubed dentine, occurring in mammals.

orthodontia (*or-tho-don'-shĭ-ă*). The study of malocclusion and irregularities of the teeth and the methods of treating them.

orthodontics (*or-tho-don'-tics*). The treatment and prevention of malocclusion and irregularities of the teeth.

orthognathia (*or-thog-na'-thĭ-ă*). The study and treatment of conditions causing malposition of the jaws.

orthognathic, orthognath-ous (*or-thog'-nath-ik, or-thog'-nath-us*). Having a straight, unprojecting jaw; having a gnathic index of under 98.

orthopaedics (*or-tho-pe'-diks*).
dental o. Orthodontics (*q.v.*).
dento-facial o. Correction of dental and facial malformations.

orthopnoea (*or-thop'-ne-ă*). Severely laboured breathing except when in an upright position.

orthopnoeic (*or-thop-ne'-ik*). Relating to or characterized by orthopnoea.

oscedo (*os-se'-do*). 1. The act of yawning. 2. Aphthous stomatitis (*q.v.*).

osphresis (*os-fre'-sis*). The sense of smell.

osphretic (*os-fret'-ik*). Relating to the sense of smell.

osseous (*os'-ĕ-us*). Having the characteristics of bone; bony.

ossicle (*os'-ikl*). A small bone.
auditory o's. The stapes,

malleus and incus, in the middle ear.

ossification (os-if-ik-a'-shun). Development of, or conversion into, bone.

ossify (os'-if-i). To develop or become bone or bone-like.

osteal (os'-tĕ-al). Bony.

osteitis (os-tĕ-i'-tis). Inflammation of a bone.
dentoalveolar o. Pyorrhoea alveolaris (q.v.).

osteitis deformans. A chronic disease of bone, characterized by resorption followed by thickening and distortion; Paget's disease of bone.

osteitis interna. Osteomyelitis of the alveolar process caused by infection from a tooth.

osteo-. Prefix signifying bone.

osteoblast (os'-te-o-blast). One of the cells from which bone is developed.

osteocementum (os''-tĕ-o-sement'-um). Secondary cementum and the tissue of which it is formed.

osteochondral (os-te-o-kon'-dral). Relating to bone and cartilage.

osteoclast (os'-te-o-klast). 1. A bone-consuming multinuclear giant cell. 2. A surgical instrument used to break up bone.

osteoclastoma (os''-te-o-klast-o'-mă). A giant-cell tumour affecting the bone.

osteodentine (os''-te-o-den'-tĕn). Bone-like dentine, found in the teeth of certain fish.

osteodentoma (os''-te-o-dent-o'-mă). A tumour composed of both bone tissue and dentine.

osteodystrophy (os''-te-o-dis'-trof-i). Defective bone formation.

osteogenic (os-te-o-jen'-ik). Relating to or derived from the tissue from which bone is developed.

osteoid (os'-te-oyd). Resembling or having the characteristics of bone.

osteology (os-te-ol'-oj-i). The study of bone and bones.

osteolysis (os-te-ol'-is-is). Absorption of bone, especially decalcification.

osteoma (os-te-o'-mă). A hard tumour composed of bone tissue, and developing on bone or on other structures of the body.

osteomalacia (os''-te-o-mal-a'-shi-ă). Softening of the bones, caused by vitamin D deficiency in adult life.

osteomyelitis (os''-te-o-mi-el-i'-tis). Inflammation of the soft tissues of the bone.
alveolar o. Pyorrhoea alveolaris (q.v.).

osteonecrosis (os''-te-o-nek-ro'-sis). Massive bone necrosis.

osteo-odontoma (os''-te-o-o-dont-o'-mă). A tumour arising from the odontoblastic processes.

osteopetrosis (os''-te-o-pet-ro'-sis). A familial bone disease, characterized by osteosclerosis, fibrosis of bone marrow, fragility, and anaemia; Albers-Schönberg disease.

osteoporosis (*os-te-o-por-o'-sis*). Enlargement of the bone marrow and canals, causing fragility and abnormal porosity of bone.

osteopsathyrosis (*os″-te-op-sath-ir-o'-sis*). Fragilitas osseum (*q.v.*).

osteoradionecrosis (*os″-te-o-ra″-di-o-nek-ro'-sis*). Necrosis of bone as a result of irradiation.

osteosarcoma (*os″-te-o-sar-ko'-mă*). A sarcoma composed of osseous tissue.

osteosclerosis (*os″-te-o-skler-o'-sis*). A condition characterized by abnormal hardness or denseness of bone.

osteotomy (*os-te-ot'-om-ĭ*). The surgical operation of cutting through a bone.

otalgia (*o-tal'-ji-ă*). Ear-ache.

otalgia dentalis. Referred pain in the ear caused by dental disease.

otic (*o'-tik*). Relating to the ear.

otitis (*o-ti'-tis*). Inflammation of the ear.

oto-. Prefix signifying *ear*.

oul- Prefix signifying *gingiva*. *See* under ul-.

oula (*u'-lă*). Ula; the gingiva or gum.

overbite (*o'-ver-bīt*). The distance, measured vertically, between the incisal edges of the incisor teeth, with the dental arches in occlusion.
horizontal o. Overjet (*q.v.*).
negative o. Anterior openbite (*q.v.*).

overclosure (*o-ver-klo'-zhur*). A form of malocclusion in an edentulous mouth in which the jaws are in abnormally close relationship.

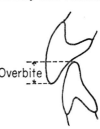

Overbite

overhang (*o'-ver-hang*). 1. To jut out or project over. 2. In dentistry, a filling, especially on a proximal surface, having a projection at the cervical margin of the cavity, causing a shoulder under which food may become lodged.

overjet (*ŏ'-ver-jet*). The distance, measured horizontally, between the labial incisal edges of the incisor teeth, with the dental arches in occlusion.
reverse o. A relationship of the anterior teeth in which, in centric occlusion, the maxillary incisors are lingual to the mandibular incisors (as in Angle's Class III malocclusion).

overlap (*o'-ver-lap*).
horizontal o. Overjet (*q.v.*).
vertical o. Overbite (*q.v.*).

overlay (*o'-ver-la*). Onlay (*q.v.*).

overt (*o-vert'*). In the medical sciences, evident or obvious.

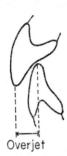

Overjet

Overjet

ovoid (*o'-voyd*). Egg-shaped.

Owen's contour lines (Sir R. Owen, 1804-92. English anatomist). The concentric rings which mark the interglobular spaces in dentine in a transverse section.

oxycephaly (*oks"-ĭ-sef'-al-ĭ*). A condition which is characterized by a pointed and high-domed skull.

oxygen (*oks'-ĭj-en*). A colourless, odourless and tasteless gas, chemical symbol O, which supports combustion and is essential to life in animals and also in many plants. It constitutes one-fifth of the air, and in combination exists in most solids, liquids or gases which are not elements.

oxygeusia (*oks-ĭ-gu'-sĭ-ă*). The condition of having an especially acute sense of taste.

ozena (*o-ze'-nă*). Rhinitis sicca (*q.v.*).

ozostomia (*o-zo-sto'-mĭ-ă*). Foul-smelling breath, of oral origin.

P

P Chemical symbol for phosphorus.

P Abbreviation for *premolar*.

PA Pulpoaxial.

p.ae.; part. aeq. Abbreviation for *partes aequales*—equal parts; used in prescription writing.

Pb Chemical symbol for lead.

PBA Pulpobuccoaxial.

p.c. Abbreviation for *post cibum*—after meals; used in prescription writing.

pH. Abbreviation for hydrogen ion concentration, based on a scale from 0 (pure acidity) to 14 (pure alkalinity), with neutrality at 7.

pil. Abbreviation for *pilula*—a pill; used in prescription writing.

PL Pulpolingual.

PLa Pulpolabial.

PLA Pulpolinguoaxial.

PM Pulpomesial. Also used for *premolar*.

PMA 1. Pulpomesio-axial. 2. An index used to indicate the prevalence and degrees of gingivitis affecting those papillae (P), margins (M) and attached portions of gingiva (A) associated with the incisor teeth.

p.r.n. Abbreviation for *pro re nata*—as required; used in prescription writing.

pulv. Abbreviation for *pulvis*—a powder; used in prescription writing.

P.U.O. Pyrexia of unknown origin.

PVC Polyvinylchloride.

pachy-. Prefix signifying *thick*.

pachycheilia (*pak-ĭ-kī'-lĭ-ă*). The condition of having abnormally thick lips.

pachyglossia (*pak-ĭ-glos'-ĭ-ă*). The condition of having an abnormally thick tongue.

pachygnathous (*pak-ĭ-na'-thus*). Having a thick, abnormally large jaw.

pack (*pak*). A dressing or blanket, either wet or dry, hot or cold, which is laid on or wrapped round a part or the whole body.

periodontal p. A dressing laid on the gums and about the teeth during treatment of periodontal disease or after gingivectomy.

pad (*pad*).
occlusal p. A pad of gingiva covering the occlusal surface of a tooth.

retromolar p. The soft tissue mass at the distal end of the mandibular ridge behind the last molar tooth.

Padgett's operation (E. C. Padgett, 1893-1946. American surgeon). Plastic surgical reconstruction of the lip by tubular grafts from the neck and scalp.

paediatrics (*pe-dĭ-at'-riks*). See pediatrics.

paedo- Prefix signifying *child*. See under pedo-.

Paget's disease of bone (Sir James Paget, 1814-99. British surgeon). Osteitis deformans (*q.v.*).

pain (*pān*). A distressing or unpleasant sensation transmitted by a sensory nerve, usually indicative of injury or of disease.

referred p. Pain felt in a part different from that in which it is caused.

palatal (*pal-a'-tal*). Relating to the palate.

palatal abscess. An apical abscess of the lateral incisors or the palatal roots of the posterior teeth, pointing towards the palate.

palatal arch. The roof of the mouth.

palatal bar. A metal bar extending across the hard palate, connecting and strengthening two parts of an upper partial denture.

palatal index. The ratio of

$$\frac{\text{palatal width} \times 100}{\text{palatal length}}$$

which gives an indication of the size and shape of the palate; *also called* palatine, or palatomaxillary, index.

palatal reflex. Swallowing caused by stimulation of the palate.

palatal root. That root of a multi-rooted maxillary tooth which is situated nearest to the palate.

palatal triangle. Formed by a line across the greatest transverse diameter of the palate, and lines from either end of this base to the alveolar point.

palate (*pal'-at*). The roof of the mouth.

artificial p. An obturator used to close a cleft palate.

bony p. Hard palate (*q.v.*).

cleft p. Congenital fissure of the palate, due to defective development in embryo; it may be associated with harelip. There is a wide range of deformity, from a bifid uvula to complete bilateral cleft of both palate and lip.

gothic p. An abnormally high, pointed palatal arch.

hard p. The bony, front portion of the roof of the mouth.

primary p. The palate in the embryo, corresponding to the premaxillary region.

primitive p. That part of the median nasal process in the embryo from which the middle portion of the upper lip and the primary palate develop.

secondary p. The palate formed by the joining of the palatal processes of the maxilla in the embryo.

soft p. The fleshy rear portion of the roof of the mouth.

palate-hook. An instrument used to retract the uvula.

palatiform (*pal-at'-i-form*). Shaped like a palate.

palatine (*pal'-at-in*). Relating to the palatal processes.

palatine aponeurosis. The fibrous extension of the tensor palati muscles forming the anterior part of the soft palate and to which other palatal muscles are attached.

palatine artery. Supplies the hard and soft palates; four branches: ascending, descending, greater, lesser. *See* Table of Arteries—palatina.

palatine bone. The bone forming the posterior part of the hard palate and the lateral wall of the nose.

palatine canal, *greater (or anterior).* The canal running from the pterygo-palatine fossa to the greater palatine foramen, in the side wall of the nasal cavity, between the maxilla and the palatine bone, through which pass the greater palatine artery and nerve.

lesser (or posterior). One of the branches of the greater palatine canal conveying branches of the greater palatine vessels to the tissues of the soft palate.

palatine crest. A thin transverse ridge of bone across the back of the hard palate.

palatine foramen, anterior. Incisive fossa (*q.v.*, I).

palatine foramen, greater. The opening of the greater palatine canal into the hard palate, between the horizontal portion of the palatine bone and the adjacent maxilla.

palatine foramen, lesser. One of the openings of the

lesser palatine canals, on the anterior surface of the hard palate.

palatine fossa. Incisive fossa (*q.v.,* 1).

palatine nerves. Supplying the palatal mucosa and the uvula; three branches: anterior, middle, and posterior. Anterior *also called* greater palatine n.; middle and posterior, together, *also called* lesser palatine n. *See* Table of Nerves—palatinus.

palatine papilla. Incisive papilla (*q.v.*).

palatine point, Méglin's. *See* Méglin's palatine point.

palatine process *of the maxilla.* The flat plate of bone on the maxilla which forms the front portion of the roof of the mouth and articulates with the palatine bone.

palatine protrusion. Torus palatinus (*q.v.*).

palatine raphe. The narrow mucosal ridge on the midline of the hard palate.

palatine ridges. The median raphe and the lateral mucosal corrugations on the hard palate.

palatine sinus. A variable cavity in the orbital process of the palatine bone, opening into the sphenoidal or a posterior ethmoidal sinus.

palatine tonsil. Tonsil (*q.v.*).

palatine vein, external. The vein draining the palatal region. *See* Table of Veins—palatina externa.

palatitis (*pal-at-i'-tis*). Inflammation of the palate.

palato-. Prefix signifying *palate.*

palatoglossal (*pal"-at-o-glos'-al*). Relating to the palate and the tongue.

palatoglossal arch. The anterior pillar of the fauces.

palatoglossal muscle. Raises tongue and constricts anterior fauces. *Also called* glossopalatine. *See* Table of Muscles—palatoglossus.

palatognathous (*pal-at-og'-nath-us*). Having a congenital cleft palate.

palatograph (*pal'-at-o-graf*). An instrument for recording movements of the palate during speech.

palatolabial (*pal"-at-o-la'-bi-al*). Relating to the palate and the lips.

palatomaxillary (*pal"-at-o-maks-il'-ar-i*). Relating to the palate and the maxilla.

palatomyograph (*pal"-at-o-mi'-o-graf*). An instrument for recording movements of the soft palate.

palatonasal (*pal"-at-o-na'-zal*). Relating to the palate and the nose.

palatopharyngeal (*pal"-at-o-far-in'-jě-al*). Relating to the palate and the pharynx.

palatopharyngeal arch. The posterior pillar of the fauces.

palatopharyngeal muscle. Aids in swallowing. *Also called* pharyngopalatine. *See* Table of Muscles—palatopharyngeus.

palatoplasty (*pal'-at-o-plast-i*). Plastic surgical repair of the palate.

palatoplegia (*pal″-at-o-ple′-ji-ă*). Palatal paralysis.

palatopterygoid (*pal″-at-o-ter′-ig-oyd*). Relating to the palatine bone and the pterygoid processes of the sphenoid bone.

palatorrhaphy (*pal-at-or′-af-ĭ*). Repair of cleft palate by means of sutures; staphylorraphy.

palatosalpingeus (*pal″-at-o-sal-pin′-jĕ-us*). Part of the levator veli palatini muscle. *See* Table of Muscles.

palatoschisis (*pal-at-os′-kis-is*). Cleft palate, palatal fissure.

palirrhoea (*pal-ir-re′-ă*). 1. Regurgitation. 2. Recurrence of a mucous discharge.

pallanaesthesia (*pal-an-es-the′-zi-ă*). Diminution or complete loss of the sense of vibration.

palliation (*pal-ĭ-a′-shun*). The act of alleviating or affording relief, without effecting a cure.

palliative (*pal′-ĭ-at-iv*). 1. Alleviating or relieving without curing. 2. Any medicine which alleviates or relieves.

palm-chin reflex. Palmomental reflex (*q.v.*).

palmomental reflex. Irritation of the thenar eminence on one hand producing contraction of the facial muscles on the same side.

palpation (*pal-pa′-shun*). Examination by touch to determine the position or consistence of an organ or part lying beneath the body surface.

palpebral (*pal′-pe-bral*). Relating to the eyelid.

palpebral artery. Supplies the conjunctiva, eyelid and lacrimal sac; three branches: inferior, middle, and superior. *See* Table of Arteries—palpebralis.

palpebral nerve. Supplies the eyelid. *See* Table of Nerves—palpebralis.

palpebris lateralis artery. Supplies the eyelids and conjunctiva. *See* Table of Arteries.

palsy (*pawl′-zĭ*). Paralysis (*q.v.*).

palsy, Bell's. *See* Bell's palsy.

papilla (*pap-il′-ă*) (*pl.* papillae). Any small nipple-like eminence.

circumvallate p. Vallate papilla (*q.v.*).

fusiform p. Any one of the slender, spindle - shaped papillae on the anterior two-thirds of the dorsum of the tongue.

gingival p. The gingiva in the interproximal space; the interdental papilla.

incisive p. The projection of the palatine mucosa overlying the incisive fossa at the anterior end of the palatine raphe.

interdental p. The gingiva in the space between the mesial surface of one tooth and the distal surface of the one adjacent.

lingual p. Any one of the papillae on the dorsum of the tongue.

palatine p. Incisive papilla (*q.v.*).

vallate p. Any one of the large, flat papillae, having a surrounding rim, found in front of the terminal sulcus of the tongue.

papillitis (*pap-il-i'-tis*). Inflammation of the optic disk.

papilloma (*pap-il-o'-mă*). A benign epithelial tumour.

papillomatosis (*pap-il-o-mat-o'-sis*). The development of multiple papillomas.

papular (*pap'-yu-lar*). Relating to or characterized by papules.

papule (*pap'-yūl*). A circumscribed, nodular elevation of the skin.

para-. Prefix signifying *by the side of;* sometimes used as synonymous with peri-.

paracone (*par'-ă-kōn*). The mesiobuccal cusp of a maxillary molar.

paraconid (*par-ă-ko'-nid*). The mesiolingual cusp of a mandibular molar.

paradental (*par-ă-den'-tal*). Near or next to a tooth; parodontal.

paradental pyorrhoea. Periodontitis with deep pocketing and discharge of pus, even after the removal of local irritants.

paradenitis (*par-ad-en-i'-tis*). Inflammation of the tissues surrounding a gland.

paradentitis (*par-ă-dent-i'-tis*). Periodontitis (q.v.).

paradentosis (*par-ă-dent-o'-sis*). Any disease affecting the tissues round a tooth.

paraesthesia (*par-es-the'-zi-ă*). Perverted sensation;

a burning, prickling or crawling sensation of the skin.

parageusia (*par-ă-gu'-si-ă*). 1. An unpleasant taste in the mouth. 2. Perversion of the sense of taste.

paraglossa (*par-ă-glos'-ă*). Swelling of the tongue.

paraglossia (*par-ă-glos'-i-ă*). Paraglossitis (q.v.).

paraglossitis (*par-ă-glos-i'-tis*). Inflammation of the tissues and muscles below the tongue.

parakeratosis (*par-ă-ker-at-o'-sis*). Any abnormality of the stratum corneum of the epidermis, which may be associated with inflammation of the prickle-cell layer, causing defective formation of keratin. Normally affects the mucous membrane.

paralysis (*par-al'-is-is*). Loss or impairment of muscle function or of sensation due to nerve injury or destruction of neurons.

paralytic (*par-al-it'-ik*). Relating to or affected by paralysis.

paramedian (*par-ă-me'-di-an*). Near to the median line; paramesial.

paramesial (*par-ă-me'-zi-al*). Paramedian (q.v.).

paramolar (*par-ă-mo'-lar*). A small supernumerary tooth which may erupt beside the molar teeth.

paramolar tubercle. An additional cusp occurring on the mesiobuccal aspect of a second or third molar;

it is thought to be a rudimentary paramolar.

paranasal (*par-ă-na'-zal*). Near to or in the region of the nose.

paranasal sinus. One of the air cavities in the skull bones of the face, communicating with the nasal cavity; they are named after the bones in which they occur.

parapharyngeal (*par-ă-far-in'-jĕ-al*). Around, in the area of, the pharynx.

parapharyngeal space. The area contained within the cervical vertebrae, the lateral wall of the pharynx and the internal pterygoid muscle.

pararhizoclasia (*par-ă-ri-zo-kla'-zĭ-ă*). Inflammatory ulcerative destruction of the deep layers of tissue and the alveolar process about the root of a tooth.

parasite (*par'-as-īt*). An organism, plant or animal, living on or within another organism from which it obtains nourishment, to the detriment of the host.

parasitic (*par-ă-sit'-ik*). Relating to parasites.

paratonsillar (*par-ă-ton'-sil-ar*). In the region of a tonsil, around a tonsil.

paratonsillar vein. V. palatina externa. *See* Table of Veins.

parenteral (*par-ent'-er-al*). Descriptive of methods of drug administration other than by the alimentary canal.

paresis (*par-e'-sis*). Slight paralysis.

paraesthesia. *See* paraesthesia.

parietal (*par-i'-et-al*). 1. Relating to the walls of a cavity. 2. Relating to the parietal bone.

parietal abscess. A periodontal abscess occurring at any site away from the apex of a tooth root.

parietal angle. The angle formed at the junction of lines connecting the bregma and the lambda to the highest point on the sagittal curvature above the horizontal plane passing through them.

parietal bone. One of two bones forming the lateral surface of the cranium.

parietal notch. The notch which occurs in the angle between the squamous and mastoid processes of the temporal bone.

parieto-. Prefix signifying *parietal*.

parodontal (*par-o-dont'-al*). Near or next to a tooth; sometimes used as synonymous with *periodontal*.

parodontal abscess. An abscess arising in the periodontal membrane.

parodontid (*par-o-dont'-id*). Any tumour occurring on the gums.

parodontitis (*par-o-dont-i'-tis*). Periodontitis (*q.v.*).

parodontium (*par-o-don'-shi-um*). Periodontium (*q.v.*).

parodontopathy (*par-o-dont-op'-ath-i*). Any periodontal disease.

parodontosis (*par-o-dont-o'-sis*). Periodontosis (*q.v.*).

parotic (*par-o'-tik*). In the region of the ear.

parotid (*par-ot'-id*). In the region of the ear.

parotid artery. Branch of the superficial temporal artery supplying the parotid gland. *See* Table of Arteries—parotidea.

parotid gland. One of a pair of salivary glands lying below the ear, between the ascending ramus of the mandible and the mastoid process.

parotid notch. An indentation between the mastoid process of the temporal bone and the ascending ramus of the mandible.

parrot jaw. The facies associated with severe protrusion of the maxilla and the consequent abnormal relation of the anterior teeth.

parrot tongue. A horny, dry tongue, seen in typhus and low fever, which cannot be protruded.

pars alveolaris. The alveolar process, either mandibular or maxillary.

partes aequales. Latin for *equal parts*; used in prescription writing, and abbreviated *p. ae.*, or *part. aeq.*

partial (*par'-shi-al*). In part, incomplete.

partial denture. A denture which replaces some of the natural teeth in one jaw.

particle (*par'-tikl*). A small piece of a substance.

parulis (*par'-u-lis*). A subperiosteal abscess; a gumboil.

Parvobacteriaceae (*par"-vo-bak-te-ri-a'-se-e*). A family of bacteria of the order Eubacteriales.

Passavant's bar (P. G. Passavant, 1815-93. German surgeon). A bulge

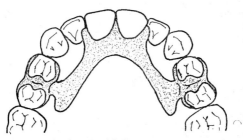

Partial denture

which appears on the posterior wall of the pharynx, caused by the contraction of the superior and middle constrictor pharyngis muscles during speech; occurs generally in a person having a cleft palate. *Also called P's cushion.*

passive (*pas'-iv*). Not produced by active efforts, not active or spontaneous.

patent (*pa'-tent*). In the medical sciences, open (not closed).

patho-. Prefix signifying *disease.*

pathodontia (*path-o-don'-shi-ă*). The study of diseases of the teeth; dental pathology.

pathogen (*path'-o-jen*). Any agent which produces or is able to produce disease.

pathogenesis (*path-o-jen'-es-is*). The development of disease from its inception to the appearance of characteristic symptoms or lesions.

pathognomonic (*path-og-no-mon'-ik*). Characteristic of one specific disease or pathological condition as distinct from any others.

pathologic, pathological (*path-ol-oj'-ik*). Relating to pathology.

pathologic reflex. Any reflex which is the result of a pathologic condition, and not normal; a diagnostic sign.

pathology (*path-ol'-oj-ĭ*). That branch of medicine which is concerned with the structural

and functional changes caused by disease.

patho-occlusion (*path"-o-ok-lu'-zhun*). Malocclusion (*q.v.*).

pathosis (*path-o'-sis*). A disease condition.

-pathy. Suffix signifying *disease.*

pearl, enamel. Enameloma (*q.v.*).

pearls, epithelial, Bohn's. Epstein's pearls (*q.v.*).

pearls, Epstein's. *See* Epstein's pearls.

pectinate (*pek'-tin-āt*). Comb-like.

pediadontology (*ped-ĭ-ă-dont-ol'-oj-ĭ*). Pedodontics (*q.v.*).

pediatrics (*pe-dĭ-at'-riks*). That branch of medicine which deals with the growth and development, diseases and treatment of children.

pediodontia (*ped-ĭ-o-don'-shi-ă*). Pedodontics (*q.v.*).

pedodontics (*ped-o-dont'-iks*). The care and treatment of teeth and oral conditions in children.

peduncle (*ped-unkl*). A stem or stalk-like process supporting a part or tumour.

pedunculated (*ped-un'-kyula-ted*). Having a peduncle.

pelican (*pel'-ik-an*). An old form of forceps used in extracting teeth; so called because of its 'beaked' jaws.

pellicle (*pel'-ikl*). 1. A thin membrane or skin. 2. A scum or film on the surface of a liquid.
acquired p. An acellular layer of organic material

deposited on the tooth surface after eruption.

brown p. Acquired pellicle (*q.v.*).

pellicular, pelliculous (*pel-ik'-yu-lar; pel-ik'-yu-lus*). Relating to a pellicle.

pellucid (*pel-lu'-sid*). Translucent; not opaque.

pemphigoid (*pem'-fig-oyd*). Relating to or affected by pemphigus.

pemphigus (*pem'-fig-us*). A skin disease characterized by the formation of irregularly distributed bullae which leave pigmented spots, and accompanied by inflammation and itching.

pendulous (*pen'-dyu-lus*). Hanging loosely.

penetration (*pen-et-ra'-shun*). 1. The act of piercing or entering beyond the surface. 2. The focal depth of a lens.

penta-. Prefix signifying *five*.

per-. Prefix signifying 1. *through*; 2. *very*.

perforate (*per'-for-āt*). To pierce with a hole or holes.

perforation (*per-for-a'-shun*). 1. The process of boring a hole through a part. 2. The hole thus pierced.

peri-. Prefix signifying *around, surrounding*.

periadenitis mucosa necrotica recurrens. A disease characterized by chronic recurrent ulceration of the buccal and pharyngeal mucosa, extending also to the tongue and the genitals.

periapical (*per-i-a'-pik-al*). In the region of the tooth apex.

periapical abscess. An abscess erupting around the apex of a tooth root.

pericemental (*per-i-se-ment'-al*). Relating to the periodontal membrane (*q.v.*).

pericemental abscess. A parodontal abscess (*q.v.*) not arising from a diseased pulp or as an extension of a periodontal pocket.

pericementitis (*per-i-se-ment-i'-tis*). Periodontitis (*q.v.*).

alveolar p. Pyorrhoea alveolaris (*q.v.*).

pericementoclasia (*per-i-se-ment-o-kla'-zi-ă*). Periodontitis (*q.v.*) with chronic pocket formation.

pericementum (*per-i-sement'-um*). The periodontal membrane.

periclasia (*per-i-kla'-zi-ă*). Periodontoclasia (*q.v.*).

pericoronal (*per-i-kor-o'-nal*). Around, in the region of, a tooth crown.

pericoronal abscess. An abscess arising about the crown of an unerupted tooth.

pericoronitis (*per-i-kor-on-i'-tis*). Inflammation of the gingiva surrounding a partially erupted tooth crown.

peridens (*per'-i-denz*). A supernumerary tooth found in any position in the mouth other than in the midline.

peridental (*per-i-den'-tal*). Periodontal.

peridentine (*per-i-den'-tēn*). Cementum (*q.v.*).

peridentitis (*per-i-dent-i'-tis*). Periodontitis (*q.v.*).

peridentoclasia (*per-ĭ-dent-o-klā'-zĭ-ă*). Pyorrhoea alveolaris (*q.v.*).

peridontoclasia (*per-ĭ-dont-o-klā'-zĭ-ă*). Periodontoclasia (*q.v.*).

periglossitis (*per-ĭ-glos-i'-tis*). Inflammation of the tissues surrounding the tongue.

periglottic (*per-ĭ-glot'-ik*). Situated near or around the tongue.

periglottis (*per-ĭ-glot'-is*). The mucous membrane of the tongue.

perignathic (*per-ĭ-na'-thik*). Situated near or around the jaw.

perikymata (*per-ĭ-ki'-mat-ă*). The shallow grooves on the surface of the tooth enamel which mark the ends of the striae of Retzius.

perilymph (*per'-ĭ-limf*). The liquid within the space between the bony and membranous labyrinth of the ear.

perimeter (*per-im'-et-er*).
dental p. An instrument to measure the circumference of a tooth.

periodontal (*per-ĭ-o-dont'-al*). Pertaining to the gums and the supporting tissues of the teeth.

periodontal abscess. A parodontal abscess formed as a result of periodontal disease.

periodontal hoe. An instrument used for removing dental calculus and other deposits from the tooth surface.

periodontal membrane. The layer of fibrous tissue surrounding the root of the tooth, attached to the cementum, the alveolar bone and the free gingiva and supporting the tooth in the socket.

periodontal pack. A dressing laid on the gums and about the teeth during treatment of periodontal disease or after gingivectomy.

periodontal pocket. An abnormally deep gingival sulcus associated with periodontal disease.
false p.p. A periodontal pocket due to the enlargement of the free gingivae in ginvigitis.
true p. p. A periodontal pocket due to the apical migration of the gingival attachment, associated with periodontitis.

periodontal traumatism. Degenerative changes occurring in the periodontium as a result of excessive stress transmitted through the teeth over a prolonged period of time.

periodontia, periodontics (*per-ĭ-o-don'-shĭ-ă*). Periodontology (*q.v.*).

periodontitis (*per-ĭ-o-dont-i'-tis*). Inflammation of the periodontal tissues resulting in destruction of the periodontal membrane and the supporting alveolar bone.
acute. p An acute inflammation of the periodontium of (usually) a single tooth, arising as a result of acute trauma to the tooth, or, when localized to the periapical area,

as a result of irritation from bacterial toxins, drugs or instruments following pulpal infection and subsequent root canal therapy.

chronic p. A form of periodontitis in which the progress of the condition is slow and usually generalised.

periodontitis complex. A clinical condition thought to be due to chronic periodontitis (*q.v.*) and periodontosis (*q.v.*) co-existing in the same mouth.

periodontitis simplex. Chronic periodontitis (*q.v.*).

periodontium (*per-ĭ-o-don'-shĭ-um*). The tissues which support and surround the teeth: the cementum, the periodontal membrane, the alveolar bone and the gingiva.

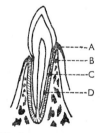

A Gingiva.
B Alveolar bone.
C Periodonta membrane.
D Cementum.

Periodontium

periodontoclasia (*per-ĭ-o-dont-o-kla'-zĭ-ă*). Any destructive or degenerative disease of the periodontium.

periodontology (*per-ĭ-o-dont-ol'-oj-ĭ*). The study of diseases of the supporting tissues of the teeth and of the gingivae.

periodontopathy (*per-ĭ-o-dont-op'-ath-ĭ*). Any non-inflammatory disease of the periodontium.

periodontosis (*per-ĭ-o-dont-o'-sis*). Non-inflammatory degenerative destruction of the periodontal membrane and the associated alveolar bone.

perioral (*per-ĭ-or'-al*). Around, in the region of, the mouth.

periosteal (*per-ĭ-os'-tĕ-al*). Relating to the periosteum.

periosteitis (*per-ĭ-os-tĕ-ī'-tis*). Inflammation of the periosteum.

periosteoma (*per-ĭ-os-tĕ-o'-mă*). A morbid osseous growth around bone tissue.

periosteum (*per-ĭ-os'-tĕ-um*). The fibrous membrane covering any bone surface except articulating surfaces.

periosteum alveolaris. The periodontal membrane.

periostitis (*per-ĭ-os-ti'-tis*). Inflammation of the periosteum.

alveolar p. Pyorrhoea alveolaris (*q.v.*).

peripheral (*per-if'-er-al*). Relating to the periphery.

peripheral nerve. Any nerve whose distribution is to the skin, loosely used of any branch of the central nervous system.

periphery (*per-if'-er-ĭ*). The outer edge, farthest from the centre.

peripyema (*per-ĭ-pi-e'-mă*). Suppuration around an organ or part, such as a tooth; rarely used.

periradicular (*per-ĭ-rad-ik'-yu-lar*). Around a root, especially the root of a tooth.

perirhizoclasia (*per-ĭ-ri-zo-kla'-zĭ-ă*). Inflammatory destruction of the periradicular tissues.

peristomal, peristomatous (*per-ĭ-sto'-mal*). Around, in the region of, the mouth.

perithelioma (*per-ĭ-the-lĭ-o'-mă*). Telangiectatic sarcoma.

peritonsillar (*per-ĭ-ton'-sil-ar*). Situated about or near a tonsil.

peritonsillar abscess. Quinsy (*q.v.*).

perlèche (*per-lesh'*). Cheilosis (*q.v.*).

perlingual (*per-lin'-gwal*). Through the tongue; used of drugs administered by resorption through the tongue's surface.

permeable (*per'-me-abl*). Affording passage through; not impassable.

permeability (*per-me-ab-il'-it-ĭ*). The condition of being permeable; in physiology used of the property in membranes which permits the transit of molecules and ions in solution through fine pores.

permeation (*per-me-a'-shun*). The spreading or extension through tissues or organs, used especially of malignant tumours extending by continuous growth through the lymphatics.

pernicious (*per-nish'-us*). Destructive, generally fatal.

peroral (*per-or'-al*). Through the mouth; administered by mouth.

pestle (*pes'-tl*). An instrument used for rubbing or pounding substances in a mortar.

petechia (*pe-te'-kĭ-ă*) (*pl.* petechiae). A small spot or mark beneath the epidermis, caused by an effusion of blood.

petrosa (*pet-ro'-să*). The petrous part of the temporal bone.

petrosal artery. Branch of the middle meningeal artery, supplying the tympanic cavity. *See* Table of Arteries—petrosa.

petrosal nerves. Supply the palatal mucosa and glands. *See* Table of Nerves—petrosus.
lesser deep p.n. N. caroticotympanicus.

petrosal process. A small pointed process at the lower end of the sphenoid bone, articulating with the apex of the petrous portion of the temporal bone.

petrosal sinuses. *See* Table of Veins—sinus petrosus.

petrosquamous fissure. The narrow cleft between the petrous and squamous portions of the temporal bone.

petrotympanic fissure. The narrow opening posterior to the glenoid fossa, through which passes the chorda tympani nerve.

petrous (*pet'-rŭs*). Rock-like.

petrous bone. The petrous part of the temporal bone.

phagadenic gingivitis. Acute ulcerative gingivitis (*q.v.*).

phagodynamometer(*fag''-o-di-nam-om'-et-er*). An instrument used to measure the force applied during mastication.

phantom odontalgia. Toothache felt in the socket from which a tooth has been extracted.

pharmacal (*far'-mak-al*). Relating to pharmacy.

pharmaceutic, pharmaceutical (*far-mas-yu'-tik*). Relating to pharmacy.

pharmaceutical chemistry. The chemistry of drugs.

pharmaceutics (*far-mas-yu'tiks*). 1. The art of pharmacy (*q.v.*, 1). 2. Pharmaceutical chemistry.

pharmacist (*far'-mas-ist*). A specialist in pharmacy.

pharmaco-. Prefix signifying *drug*.

pharmacochemistry (*far''-mak-o-kem'-ist-ri*). Pharmaceutical chemistry.

pharmacodiagnosis (*far''-mak-o-di-ag-no'-sis*). The use of drugs as an aid to diagnosis.

pharmacodynamics (*far''-mak-o-di-nam'-iks*). The study of drug-action.

pharmacognosist (*far-mak-og'-nos-ist*). A specialist in pharmacognosy.

pharmacognosy (*far-mak-og'-nos-i*). That branch of pharmacology which is concerned with crude drugs.

pharmacologist (*farm-ak-ol'-oj-ist*). One who studies the composition and action of drugs.

pharmacology (*far-mak-ol'-oj-i*). The study of drugs, and of drug-actions in particular.

pharmacomania (*far''-mak-o-ma'-ni-ă*). Morbid craving to take or administer drugs.

pharmacophobia (*far''-mak-o-fo'-bi-ă*). Morbid fear of drugs.

pharmacopoeia, pharmacopeia (*far-mak-o-pe'-ă*). A collection of formulae and methods of preparation of drugs; particularly an authoritative book containing recognised standard formulae and methods.

pharmacotherapy (*far''-mak-o-ther'-ap-i*). The treatment of disease with drugs.

pharmacy (*far'-mas-i*). 1. The preparation of medicines from prescription. 2. The shop where medicines are made up and sold.

pharyngeal (*far-in'-jĕ-al*). Relating to the pharynx.

pharyngeal artery. Supplies pharynx, and also membranes of brain, neck muscles and nerves, etc.; two branches: pharyngeal, and ascending pharyngeal. *See*

Table of Arteries—pharyngea.

pharyngeal nerve, Bock's. See Bock's pharyngeal nerve.

pharyngeal nerves. Supply the pharyngeal mucosa and the pharyngeal muscles. See Table of Nerves—pharyngeus.

pharyngeal plexus. The plexus from which arise the pharyngeal veins. See Table of Veins—plexus pharyngeus.

pharyngeal reflex. Contraction of the constrictor pharyngis muscles produced by stimulation of the posterior pharyngeal wall.

pharyngitis (far-in-ji'-tis). Inflammation of the pharynx.

pharyngo-. Prefix signifying *pharynx.*

pharyngoglossal (far″-in-go-glos'-al). Relating to both the pharynx and the tongue.

pharyngoglossus (far″-in-go-glos'-us). Muscle fibres extending from the superior constrictor pharyngis to the tongue.

pharyngomaxillary (far″-in-go-maks-il'-ar-ĭ). Relating to the pharynx and the maxilla.

pharyngomaxillary space. Parapharyngeal space (*q.v.*).

pharyngo-oral (far″-in-go-or'-al). Relating to the pharynx and the mouth.

pharyngopalatine (far″-in-go-pal'-at-ĭn). Relating to both the pharynx and the palate.

pharyngopalatine muscle. M. palatopharyngeus. See Table of Muscles.

pharyngoplasty (far-in'-go-plast-ĭ). A plastic surgery operation performed on the pharynx.

pharyngotympanic (far-in″-go-tim-pan'-ik). Relating to the pharynx and the ear drum.

pharyngotympanic tube. A canal connecting the upper pharynx with the middle ear; *also called* Eustachian tube.

pharynx (far'-inks). The musculo-membranous canal forming the upper end of the digestive tract, between the mouth and nostrils and the oesophagus.

phatne (fat'-nĕ). Alveolus (*q.v.*); an obsolete term.

phatnoma (fat-no'-mă). Alveolus (*q.v.*); an obsolete term.

phatnorrhagia (fat-nor-a'-jĕ-ă). Bleeding from a tooth socket.

philtrum (fil'-trum). The groove occurring at the median line of the upper lip.

phimosis (fim-o'-sis). *labial p.* Imperforation of the mouth. *oral p.* Labial phimosis (*q.v.*).

phlebo-. Prefix signifying *vein.*

phlegm (flem). Mucus, especially that secreted by the mucosa of the nose and throat.

phlegmon (fleg'-mon). Acute inflammation of the subcutaneous connective tissue.

phlegmon of the tongue. Acute diffuse glossitis.

phosphonecrosis (*fos-fo-nek'-ro'-sis*). Jaw necrosis caused by phosphorus poisoning; *also called* phossy jaw.

phosphorous (*fos'-for-us*). Relating to phosphorus.

phosphorus (*fos'-for-us*). A non-metallic element, chemical symbol P, occurring in two forms: white, or yellow, phosphorus, a semi-transparent solid, which is poisonous and highly inflammable; and red, or amorphous phosphorus, which is a non-poisonous and non-inflammable red-brown powder.

phossy jaw. Jaw necrosis caused by phosphorus poisoning.

photo-. Prefix signifying *light*.

photomicrograph (*fo"-to-mi'-kro-graf*). A photograph of a minute object made with the aid of a microscope, so that the result is visible to the naked eye.

phyma (*fi'-mă*) (*pl.* phymata). 1. A tumour or neoplasm composed of skin or subcutaneous tissue. 2. A circumscribed swelling on the skin caused by exudation, and larger than a tubercle.

physical (*fiz'-ik-al*). 1. Relating to nature. 2. Relating to material substance, or to the body. 3. Relating to physics.

physiologic, physiological (*fiz-i-ol-oj'-ik-al*). Relating to physiology.

physiological root. Clinical root (*q.v.*).

physiology (*fiz-i-ol'-oj-ĭ*). The study of the body functions.

physocephaly (*fi-so-sef'-al-ĭ*). Emphysematous swelling of the head.

phytosis (*fi-to'-sis*). Any disease produced by bacteria.

pick (*pik*). Toothpick (*q.v.*).

Pickerill's lines. Horizontal imbrication lines on the surface of tooth enamel.

picrogeusia (*pik-ro-gu'-sĭ-ă*). Pathologic bitterness of taste.

pier (*pe'-er*). An abutment (*q.v.*).

pier-band. Any band constructed to fit an abutment tooth.

pigment (*pig'-ment*). 1. Any colouring matter of the body, normal or abnormal. 2. A dye or other colouring agent.

pigmentation (*pig-ment-a'-shun*). 1. The deposit of pigment. 2. The condition resulting from such deposit.

pigmented (*pig-ment'-ed*). Marked by a deposit of pigment.

pilation (*pil-a'-shun*). A hair-like fracture.

pill (*pil*). A small solid mass, either oval or globular, for the internal administration of a medicine.

pillars of fauces. Curved muscular folds on either side of the pharyngeal opening, running from the palate to the base of the tongue and the pharynx; they enclose the tonsils. The *anterior* pillars are also known as the palatoglossal arch, and the *posterior* as the palatopharyngeal arch.

pilula (*pil'-yu-lă*). Latin for *a pill*; used in prescription writing, and abbreviated *pil.*, or *p*.

pin (*pin*). 1. A thin metal rod used to secure the ends of bones in treatment of fracture. 2. A short peg or post (*q.v.*), used in dentistry to attach an artificial crown to a tooth root.

piniform (*pin'-ĭ-form*). Conical.

pinlay (*pin'-la*). 1. A gold inlay which is retained by pins, where the tooth surface is too much abraded to permit of a cavity being cut. 2. Pinledge (*q.v.*).

pinledge (*pin'-ledj*). The anchorage for a bridge, held in position by pins extending into the root of the abutment tooth.

pinna (*pin'-nă*). The external ear.

pipe jaw. A painful condition of the jaw caused by constant carrying of a tobacco pipe in the mouth.

piriform (*pir'-ĭ-form*). Pear-shaped.

piriform aperture. The pear-shaped nasal opening in the skull.

Pirogoff's triangle (N. I. Pirogoff, 1810-81. Russian surgeon and anatomist). The triangular space bounded by the posterior border of the mylohyoid, the intermediate tendon of the digastric, and the hypoglossal nerve.

pit (*pit*). *In dentistry:* A sharp, pointed depression in the enamel of a tooth.
basilar p. A pit in the crown of a maxillary incisor above the cervix.

pityriasis linguae (*pit-ĭ-ri'-as-is*). Geographic tongue (*q.v.*).

pivot (*piv'-ot*). A metal post or dowel inserted in the root canal of a natural tooth as a means of attachment for an artificial crown.

pivot crown. An artificial crown attached by means of a metal post into the root canal of a natural tooth.

placebo (*plas-e'-bo*). A medicine having no pharmacological value given to humour or quieten a patient; it is used also in certain forms of drug trial.

placode (*plak'-ōd*). A thickened epithelial plate, found in the embryo and forming the anlage of some organ or part.

plane (*plān*). A flat smooth surface, or any imaginary surface tangent to the body or dividing it.
auriculo-infraorbital p. Frankfort plane (*q.v.*).
auriculo-nasal p. Camper's plane (*q.v.*).
auriculo-orbital p. Frankfort plane (*q.v.*).
axiobuccolingual p. A plane through the buccal and lingual surfaces of a tooth parallel to its axis.

axiolabiolingual p. A plane through the labial and lingual surfaces of a tooth parallel to its axis.

axiomesiodistal p. A plane through the mesial and distal surfaces of a tooth parallel to the axis.

base p. An imaginary horizontal plane used in the setting up of artificial dentures.

bite p. 1. Occlusal plane (*q.v.*). 2. Bite plate (*q.v.*, 2).

buccolingual p. Any plane passing through both the buccal and lingual surfaces of a tooth.

condylar p. The plane passing through the most posterior points on the condylar head and on the ascending ramus in the region of the angle of the mandible, and perpendicular to the sagittal plane.

facial p. The plane passing through the nasion and the pogonion and perpendicular to the sagittal plane.

labiolingual p. Axiolabiolingual plane (*q.v.*).

mandibular p. The plane passing through the lowest point of the lower border of the mandible in the region of the angle and through the menton, and perpendicular to the sagittal plane.

maxillary p. In cephalometrics, the plane, perpendicular to the sagittal plane, passing through the anterior and posterior nasal spines as seen on a lateral skull radiograph.

mesiodistal p. Axiomesoidistal plane (*q.v.*).

occlusal p. The imaginary plane between the maxillary and mandibular teeth in occlusion; it is used in the construction of artificial dentures.

S-N p. In cephalometrics, that plane which passes through the centre of the shadow of the sella turcica and the nasion and which is perpendicular to the sagittal plane.

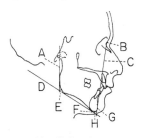

Mandibular plane

A Condylar plane.
B Nasion.
C Facial plane.
D Mandibular plane.
E Gonion.
F Menton.
G Pogonion.
H Gnathion.

plane, Bolton. *See* Bolton plane, Bolton-Broadbent plane.

plane, Bolton-Broadbent. *See* Bolton plane, Bolton-Broadbent plane.

plane, Frankfort. *See* Frankfort plane.

planoconcave (*pla″-no-kon-kāv'*). Level on one side and concave on the other.

planoconvex (*pla″-no-kon'-veks*). Level on one side and convex on the other.

plaque (*plak*). Dental plaque, (*q.v.*, 1).
  bacterial p. Dental plaque, (*q.v.*, 1).
  dental p. 1. A soft, concentrated mass, consisting of a large variety of bacteria, together with a certain amount of cellular debris, found adhering to the surfaces of the teeth when oral hygiene is neglected; it cannot be removed by rinsing 2. Acquired pellicle (*q.v.*).
  mucin p. Acquired pellicle (*q.v.*).

plasma (*plaz'-mă*). The fluid part of blood or lymph, in which cells or corpuscles are suspended.

plasmocytoma (*plaz″-mo-si-to'-mă*). A tumour composed of plasma cells.

plaster of Paris. Calcined gypsum, $CaSO_4.H_2O$, which will set hard on drying after being mixed with water. It is used to make dental impressions and casts.

plastic (*plas'-tik*). 1. Able to be moulded. 2. Material which can be moulded in processing by pressure or heat. 3. Relating to those processes by which tissue is restored or replaced, and defects rectified, as in *plastic* surgery.

plastics (*plas'-tiks*). *In dentistry*: Those materials used for fillings or prostheses which are soft enough to be moulded whilst being inserted.

plate (*plāt*). 1. Any flat structure, especially a flattened bone process. 2. In dentistry, a thin sheet of metal, rubber, or plastic, either forming part of an orthodontic appliance or holding teeth in an artificial denture.
  base p. The plate of an artificial denture, to which the teeth are attached.
  bite p. A temporary base plate of rigid material carrying a rim of wax or plastic (bite rim) on which the bite is recorded. 2. An orthodontic appliance designed to correct an abnormal bite by interposing a ledge of metal, vulcanite or acrylic behind the maxillary incisors, on which the mandibular incisors strike. Where this ledge is sloped and not flat this appliance is known as a *bite plane*.
  cortical p. The superficial outer layer of bone in the alveolar process.
  dental p. A plate of metal, acrylic or other material, shaped to fit the roof of the mouth, to which artificial teeth are attached.
  die p. A sheet of metal containing dies for forming cusps on a shell crown.

oral p. Buccopharyngeal membrane (*q.v.*).

orbital p. One of the two processes of the frontal bone which form the vaults of the orbits.

retention p. 1. The foundation for an obturator. 2. Any orthodontic retaining appliance.

simple p. A plate base without teeth attached; generally used for radium or similar therapy.

spring p. A dental plate which is retained by the elasticity of its material pressing against the abutment teeth.

stomodeal p. Buccopharyngeal membrane (*q.v.*).

suction p. A dental plate which is retained in the mouth by suction or atmospheric pressure.

trial p. A temporary dental plate of soft material or wax, used to hold the artificial teeth for fitting in the mouth.

X p. An orthodontic screw-adjusted appliance used to retract protrusive incisors and prevent excessive overbite.

plate, Coffin. *See* Coffin split plate.

plate culture. A bacterial culture grown on a glass plate, or in a Petri dish.

platelet (*plāt'-let*). One of the minute circular or oval discs found in the blood of all mammals and concerned in its coagulation mechanism.

platy-. Prefix signifying *flat, broad.*

platycephalic (*plat-i-sef-al'-ik*). Having a broad, flattened skull.

platyglossal (*plat-i-glos'-al*). Having a flat and broad tongue.

platysma muscle. Raises skin from underlying structures, and, with M. risorius, retracts angle of mouth. *See* Table of Muscles.

platystaphyline (*plat-i-staf'-il-īn*). Having a broad and flat palate.

Plaut's angina (H. K. Plaut, 1858-1928. German physician). Acute ulcerative tonsillitis (*q.v.*).

Plaut-Vincent gingivitis (H. K. Plaut, 1858- 1928. German physician. J. H. Vincent, 1862-1950. French physician and bacteriologist). Acute ulcerative gingivitis (*q.v.*).

pledget (*plej'-et*). A small compress of cotton-wool, lint, or gauze.

pleomorphic (*ple-o-mor'-fik*). Occurring in several distinct shapes.

pleomorphic fibroadenoma. Adenofibroma (*q.v.*).

pleurodont (*plu'-ro-dont*). Having teeth attached to the side of a bony socket or to the side of the jaw.

plexus (*pleks'-us*). A network of nerves or blood vessels. *dental p.* A network of nerve fibres about the roots of the teeth; those of the maxilla are branches of the maxillary nerve, and those of the mandible are branches of the inferior dental nerve.

lingual p. A nerve plexus about the lingual artery.

maxillary p. One of the nerve plexuses about the facial and maxillary arteries.

nasopalatine p. A nerve plexus of the nasopalatine nerves in the incisive foramen.

pterygoid p. A venous plexus accompanying the maxillary artery through the pterygoid muscles.

venous p. For venous plexuses, see Table of Veins —plexus.

plexus of Raschow. See Raschow's plexus.

plica (*pli'-kă*). A pleat or fold.

plici-dentine (*pli-si-den-tēn*). A form of dentine made up of complex folds, found in the teeth of reptiles and of some fish.

pliers (*pli'-ers*). Small pincers, with variously shaped jaws, depending on the purpose for which they are designed, used to hold small objects or bend or cut metal strips or wire.

plugger (*plug'-er*). An instrument used to pack or to condense filling material into a tooth cavity.

amalgam p. An instrument used to condense amalgam in a tooth cavity.

Plummer-Vinson syndrome (H. S. Plummer, 1874-1936, American physician; P. P. Vinson, b. 1890.

American physician). Dysphagia associated with splenomegaly and hypochromic anaemia, glossitis, and atrophy of the mucous membranes of the mouth, pharynx and upper end of the oesophagus.

plumper (*plump'-er*). The labial flange on a denture or obturator built up to hold the cheek and lip in their normal positions.

Pneumococcus (*nyu-mo-kok'-us*). Diplococcus pneumoniae (*q.v.*).

pocket (*pok'-et*). 1. A pouch, small bag, or cavity, into which something may be put. 2. In dentistry, an abnormal space developing between the tooth root and the gum.

complex p. A periodontal pocket involving more than one tooth surface but having an outlet on only one surface.

compound p. A periodontal pocket involving more than one tooth surface.

gingival p. Periodontal pocket (*q.v.*).

infra-bony p. A form of true periodontal pocket (*q.v.*) in which the base of the pocket lies below the level of the alveolar bone.

intra-oral p. In oral plastic surgery, a pocket created within the mouth, lined with a skin graft, which is used to support a prosthesis in restoration of the facial contours caused by the loss or absence of a large portion of the mandible.

periodontal p. An abnormally deep gingival sulcus associated with periodontal disease. A *false* periodontal pocket is one due to the enlargement of the free gingivae in gingivitis; a *true* periodontal pocket is one due to the apical migration of the gingival attachment, associated with periodontitis.

supra-bony p. A form of true periodontal pocket (*q.v.*) in which the base of the pocket lies above the level of the alveolar bone.

pocket measuring probe. A periodontal probe for determining the size of a periodontal pocket.

pocket probe. Pocket measuring probe (*q.v.*).

pogonion (*po-go'-ni-on*). The extreme anterior point on the midline of the mandible; a subsurface landmark.

poikilodentosis (*poy"-kil-o-dent-o'-sis*). Mottled tooth enamel.

point (*poynt*). 1. The sharp end of an object, or a small spot. 2. To approach the surface at one place, as of the pus in an abscess.

'A' p. Subspinale (*q.v.*).

alveolar p. The midpoint between the central incisors, on the maxillary alveolar arch.

'B' p. Supramentale (*q.v.*).

contact p's. The areas of contact on the surfaces of proximal teeth.

craniometric p. Any one of the landmarks on the skull used in craniometry.

irritation p. In the testing of vital tooth pulp with an electric current, the average reading at which, on application of the current, a tingling sensation is felt, but before pain is produced.

jugal p. The craniometric point at the angle of the maxillary and masseteric edges of the zygoma.

mental p. Gnathion (*q.v.*, 1).

nasal p. Nasion (*q.v.*).

'S' p. Sella turcica (*q.v.*, 2).

silver p. A fine cone of silver used to fill a root canal after the removal of the pulp.

point, Bolton. *See* Bolton point.

point, palatine, Méglin's. *See* Méglin's palatine point.

point angle. An angle formed at the junction of three tooth surfaces or of three cavity walls. The cavity point angles are named after the walls which form them; e.g. distobuccopulpal, gingivolinguoaxial.

Poirier's line (P. J. Poirier, 1853-1907. French anatomist). The line joining the lambda to the nasion.

poison (*poy'-zon*). Any substance which, when absorbed into the system of a living body, is liable to cause injury and endanger life.

poly-. Prefix signifying *many*; in medicine it signifies *too many*, or *affecting many parts*.

polycystic (*pol-i-sist'-ik*). Composed of or containing many cysts.

polydontia (*pol-ĭ-don'-shĭ-ă*). Polyodontia (*q.v.*).

polylophodont (*pol-ĭ-lof'-o-dont*). Having teeth with multi-ridged crowns.

polymer (*pol'-ĭ-mer*). The product resulting from the combination of two or more molecules of the same substance, the molecular weight being a whole multiple of the molecular weight of the original substance.

polymerization (*pol-ĭ-mer-ĭ-za'-shun*). The process whereby two or more molecules of the same substance combine to form a polymer (*q.v.*).

polyodontia (*pol-ĭ-o-don'-shĭ-ă*). The condition of having supernumerary teeth.

polyostotic (*pol-ĭ-os-tot'-ĭk*). Affecting several bones.

polyp (*pol'-ip*). See polypus.

polyphyodont (*pol-ĭ-fi'-o-dont*). Having several successive sets of natural teeth.

polypoid (*pol'-ip-oyd*). Resembling a polypus.

polyposis (*pol-ip-o'-sis*). A condition characterized by the presence of multiple polypi.

polypous (*pol'-ip-us*). Having the characteristics of a polypus.

polyprotodont (*pol-ĭ-pro'-to-dont*). Having numerous incisors.

polypus (*pol'-ip-us*) (*pl.* polypi). A pedunculated growth or tumour arising from mucous membrane.

polysialia (*pol-ĭ-si-al'-ĭ-ă*). Ptyalism (*q.v.*).

polystomatous (*pol-ĭ-sto'-mat-us*). Having many mouths, or many openings.

pontic (*pon'-tik*). A suspended member on a bridge or partial denture, replacing a natural crown.

pontine artery. Branch of basilar artery supplying the pons. *See* Table of Arteries —pontina.

porcelain (*por'-sel-ān*). A ceramic product of the fusion of kaolin, feldspar and quartz, with other minerals, used in the making of artificial teeth, inlays, etc.

porcelain cusp crown. A crown having porcelain and not metal on the occlusal surface.

porcelain veneer crown. A metal crown covered by a thin veneer of porcelain.

pore (*pawr*). A minute opening on a free surface, especially one of the sweat gland ducts.

porion (*paw'-rĭ-on*) (*pl.* poria). The median point on the upper margin of the opening of the external auditory canal.

porosity (*por-os'-it-ĭ*). The quality of being porous.

porous (*pawr'-us*). Having pores.

Porte polisher (*port pol'-ish-er*). A handpiece or carrier used to hold dental polishing instruments.

porus (*por'-us*). A pore or meatus.

p. acusticus externus: The opening of the external

auditory canal in the tympanic portion of the temporal bone.

p. acusticus internus: The opening of the internal auditory canal into the cranial cavity.

posed (*pōzd*). In position, placed; in dentistry it is applied to tooth position.

post (*pōst*). A peg or pin of metal used to attach an artificial crown to the root of a natural tooth; *also called* a dowel.

post cibum. Latin for *after meals;* used in prescription writing, and abbreviated *p.c.*

post crown. Any artificial crown attached to the tooth root by means of a post or dowel; *also called* a pivot crown.

post-. Prefix signifying *after,* or *behind.*

postbuccal (*pōst-buk'-al*). Behind the buccal region in the mouth.

postcondylar (*pōst-kon'-di-lar*). Behind the condyle.

postcondylar notch. An indentation on the lower surface of the occipital bone, occurring between the condyle and the foramen magnum.

post-dam (*pōst'-dam*). A groove along the palatal edge on a model for a denture, which produces a ridge on the finished denture serving as a perfect seal for retention purposes and to prevent food debris from collecting under the plate.

posterior (*post-e'-rĭ-or*). Behind, in the rear.

posterior facial vein. V. retromandibularis. *See* Table of Veins.

posterior occlusion. The occlusion resulting when the mandibular teeth occlude posterior to their normal position in relation to the maxillary teeth.

posterior open-bite. Openbite (*q.v.*) in which the posterior teeth on one side (*unilateral*) or on both sides (*bilateral*) do not come into contact.

posterior teeth. The premolars and molars, collectively.

posteroclusion (*post-er-ok-lu'-zhun*). Posterior occlusion (*q.v.*).

post-eruption cuticle. Acquired pellicle (*q.v.*).

postoperative (*pōst-op'-er-at-iv*). After a surgical operation is completed.

post-oral (*pōst-or'-al*). Behind the mouth.

post-palatine (*pōst-pal'-at-īn*). Behind the palate, or behind the fauces of the throat.

postpermanent (*pōst-per'-man-ent*). Relating to those teeth which occasionally erupt after the second permanent dentition.

pouch, Rathke's. *See* Rathke's pouch.

pre-. Prefix signifying *before.*

precancerous (*pre-kan'-ser-us*). Relating to any abnormal growth which is likely to develop into cancer.

precarious (*pre″-ka′-ri-us*). Occurring before or early in the development of caries.

precision attachment. A prefabricated form of attachment for the retention of a bridge or partial denture; it consists of a male and a female portion, one being incorporated in the prosthesis and the other in the retainer cemented to the supporting tooth or root.

predentine (*pre″-den′-tēn*). The inner, uncalcified layer of dentine.

pregnancy epulis. A form of epulis developing during or as a result of pregnancy.

pregnancy gingivitis. Gingivitis thought to be caused by endocrine changes occurring during pregnancy.

premaxilla (*pre-maks-il′-ă*). The frontal bone between the maxillae in the foetus; the intermaxillary bone.

premaxillary (*pre-maks-il′-ar-ĭ*). 1. Relating to the premaxilla. 2. In front of the maxilla.

premolar tooth (*pre-mo′-lar*). A bicuspid, found in front of the molar teeth; there are two in each quadrant in the permanent dentition in man.

prenatal (*pre-na′-tal*). Present before birth.

preoperative (*pre-op′-er-at-iv*). Before a surgical operation is commenced.

pre-oral (*pre-or′-al*). In front of the mouth.

prepalatal (*pre-pal-a′-tal*). In front of the palate.

prescribe (*prĕ-scrīb′*). To write instructions for the preparation, composition and administration of a medicine.

Premolar tooth

prescription (*prĕ-skrip′-shun*). A written instruction on the preparation, composition and administration of a medicine.

presenile (*pre-se′-nīl*). Relating to premature old age.

presenility (*pre-sen-il′-it-ĭ*). Premature old age.

prevalence (*prev′-al-ens*). The number of cases of a disease at any given time in any given place.

preventive (*pre-vent′-iv*). Designed to avert the onset of something.

prickle cell. One having delicate fibrous processes connecting it to neighbouring cells.

prickle-cell layer. The stratum germinativum of the epidermis, excluding the basal cells.

Priestley's mass (J. Priestley, 1733-1804. English scientist). A green or brown stain on the anterior teeth of the young or where reduced enamel epithelium remains over the enamel.

primary enamel cuticle.
An acellular layer of organic material attached to the surface of enamel; it is thought to be the final product of ameloblasts.

primary palate. The palate in the embryo, corresponding to the premaxillary region.

primer (*pri'-mer*). Liner (*q.v.*).

cavity p. Cavity liner (*q.v.*).

primitive (*prim'-it-iv*). Original; in its first, simplest form.

primitive palate. That part of the median nasal process in the embryo from which develops the middle portion of the upper lip and the primary palate.

primordium (*pri-mor'-di-um*). The first discernible signs of any organ or part.

prism (*prizm*). A solid figure whose sides are parallelograms and which has a triangular or polygonal cross-section.

enamel p. One of the prismatic rods of which tooth enamel is made up.

prismatic (*pris-mat'-ik*). Relating to a prism.

prismos (*priz'-mos*). Tooth-grinding; bruxism.

pro re nata. Latin for *as required*; used in prescription writing, and abbreviated *p.r.n.*

pro-. Prefix signifying *before*, *in front of*.

probe (*prōb*). A slender, flexible instrument used to explore a cavity or wound.

pocket p. Pocket measuring probe (*q.v.*).

pocket measuring p. A periodontal probe for determining the size of a periodontal pocket.

probes, Brackett's. See Brackett's probes.

procelous (*pro-se'-lus*). Concave at the front.

procerus muscle. Wrinkles skin over nose. See Table of Muscles.

process (*pro'-ses*). *In anatomy*: A slender projection of bone, or a tissue protuberance.

alveolar p. A bony ridge on the border of the maxilla or the mandible containing the tooth sockets.

ameloblastic p. A projection of cytoplasm from an enamel cell, about which calcification occurs.

condyloid p. One of the two mandibular condyles.

coronoid p. A thin and flattened projection of bone from the anterior upper border of the ramus of the mandible, into which the temporal muscle is inserted.

ethmoid p. A projection from the upper border of the inferior nasal concha.

frontal p. A projection of the maxilla articulating with the frontal bone and forming part of the side of the nasal cavity and of the margin of the orbit.

frontonasal p. The front portion of bone in the head of an embryo which develops

into the forehead and the
bridge of the nose.

frontosphenoidal p. A thick
ascending serrated process of
the zygomatic bone articulating with the frontal bone
and the great wing of the
sphenoid.

globular p. One of the
bulbous expansions at either
angle of the nose in the
embryo, later fusing to form
the philtrum.

hamular p. A hook-like
descending process of the
medial pterygoid plate.

infraorbital p. A sharp
pointed projection on the
anterior surface of the zygomatic bone, articulating with
the mandible.

mandibular p. That part of
the mandibular arch in the
embryo from which the
mandible will develop.

maxillary p. in the embryo. A
protuberance from the mandibular arch in the embryo
from which the maxilla, the
zygomatic bone, and the
upper cheek and lip region
will develop.

*maxillary p. of the palatine
bone.* A thin plate pro-
jecting forward from the
anterior border of the palatine bone, closing the lower
posterior end of the opening
of the maxillary sinus.

*maxillary p. of the zygomatic
bone.* A blunt descending
process of the zygomatic
bone, articulating with the
maxilla.

nasal p. of the maxilla.
Frontal process (*q.v.*).

odontoblastic p's. The branching processes of the odontoblasts which occur in the
dentinal canals.

orbital p. of the palatine bone.
A bone process from the
palatine bone, pointing upwards and outwards.

*orbital p. of the zygomatic
bone.* A process extending
backwards from the orbital
margin of the zygomatic
bone and forming part of
the lateral wall and floor of
the orbital cavity.

palatine p. of the maxilla.
The flat plate of bone on
the maxilla which forms the
front portion of the roof of
the mouth and articulates
with the palatine bone.

petrosal p. A small pointed
process at the lower end of
the sphenoid bone, articulating with the apex of the
petrous portion of the
temporal bone.

pterygoid p. One of two
descending processes from
the junction of the body of
the sphenoid bone with the
greater wings.

retromandibular p. The
narrow part of the parotid
gland found in the fossa
behind the mandible.

*sphenoidal p. of the palatine
bone.* A thin bony plate
running upwards and in-
wards from the palatine
bone and articulating with
the sphenoid bone and the
vomer.

*styloid p. of the temporal
bone.* A sharp spine pro-
jecting downwards from the

lower surface of the petrous portion of the temporal bone.

temporal p. The posterior angle of the zygomatic bone which articulates with the zygomatic process of the temporal bone.

zygomatic p. of the frontal bone. A thick strong lateral projection of the frontal bone which articulates with the zygomatic bone.

zygomatic p. of the maxilla. A rough triangular eminence articulating with the maxillary process of the zygomatic bone.

zygomatic p. of the temporal bone. A long process from the lower squamous portion of the temporal bone, articulating with the zygomatic bone.

processes, Tomes'. Ameloblastic processes (*q.v.*).

procheilia (*pro-ki'-li-ă*). The condition in which one lip is forward of its normal position.

procheilon (*pro-ki'-lon*). The central prominence on the upper border of the upper lip.

procynodontos (*pro-si-no-dont'-os*). A canine tooth, especially one which is protruded.

profunda linguae artery. Supplies the lower surface of the tongue. *Also called* ranine artery. *See* Table of Arteries.

proglossis (*pro-glos'-is*). The tip of the tongue.

prognathic (*prog-na'-thik*). Having a projecting jaw.

prognathism (*prog'-nath-izm*). Protrusion of the jaw.

prognathometer (*prog"-nath-om'-et-er*). An instrument for measuring the degree of prognathism.

prognathous (*prog'-nath-us*). Having a gnathic index of over 103; having a protruding jaw.

prognosis (*prog-no'-sis*). A forecast, from the symptoms, of the probable course of an attack of a disease and the prospects for recovery.

prolabium (*pro-la'-bi-um*). The red outer part of the lip.

proliferation (*pro-lif-er-a'-shun*). Reproduction or multiplication.

prominent (*prom'-in-ent*). Projecting, standing out.

prong (*prong*). A tooth root; obsolete term.

prop (*prop*).
jaw p. An appliance for holding the jaws open during an operation performed under general anaesthesia.

prophylactic (*pro-fil-ak'-tik*). Relating to prophylaxis; a preventive remedy.

prophylactic odontotomy. Mechanical modification of the occlusal fissures of teeth in an attempt to prevent dental caries.

prophylactodontia, prophylactodontics (*pro-fil-akt-o-don'-shi-ă*). Prevention and preventive treatment for diseases of the mouth and teeth, and for malformation.

pro 248 pro

prophylactodontist (*pro-fil-akt-o-dont'-ist*). One who specializes in preventive dentistry.

prophylaxis (*pro-fil-aks'-is*). The prevention of disease.
dental p. Preventive treatment for diseases of the teeth.
oral p. Preventive treatment for diseases of the oral cavity.

propriodentium (*prop"-ri-o-den'-shi-un*). The tooth tissues.

prosencephalon (*pros-en-sef'-al-on*). The anterior brain vesicle in the embryo, from which develop the cerebral hemispheres, the olfactory lobes and corpora striata; the forebrain.

prosopalgia (*pro-sop-al'-ji-ă*). Facial pain; facial neuralgia.

prosopanoschisis (*pros-o-pan-os'-kis-is*). A congenital oblique facial cleft.

prosopo-. Prefix signifying *face.*

prosopodiplegia (*pros-o-po-di-ple'-ji-ă*). Paralysis of both sides of the face.

prosopodynia (*pros-o-po-din'-i-ă*). Facial neuralgia.

prosoponeuralgia (*pros-o-po-nyu-ral'-ji-ă*). Facial neuralgia.

prosopoplegia (*pros-o-po-ple'-ji-ă*). Facial paralysis.

prosoposchisis (*pros-o-pos'-kis-is*). Congenital facial cleft or fissure.

prosopospasm (*pros'-o-po-spazm*). Spasm of the facial muscles; risus sardonicus.

prosopus varus. Congenital hemiatrophy of the cranium and the facial bones, resulting in an oblique facies.

prosthesis (*pros-the'-sis*). A manufactured appliance to take the place of a natural part or to correct a congenital abnormality.
dental p. Partial or full dentures, crown, or bridge, or any appliance to correct cleft palate.
maxillofacial p. An artificial substitute for some facial structure which has been too severely damaged to be repaired by surgery.

prosthetic (*pros-thet'-ik*). Relating to a prosthesis.

prosthetics (*pros-thet'-iks*). The design, construction and fitting of prostheses.

prosthion (*pros'-thi-on*). The alveolar point (*q.v.*).

prosthodontia, prosthodontics (*pros-tho-don'-shi-ă*). Prosthetic dentistry; the design and construction of artificial dentures, and crown- and bridge-work.

prosthodontist (*pros-tho-dont'-ist*). One who practises prosthetic dentistry.

proteolysis (*pro-te-ol'-is-is*). The process of digestion of protein and its conversion by enzymes into peptones, proteoses, etc.

proteolytic (*pro-te-o-lit'-ik*). 1. Relating to or effecting proteolysis. 2. Any agent effecting proteolysis.

Proteus (*pro'-te-us*). A genus of Enterobacteriaceae family of bacteria, Gram-negative, rod-shaped organisms, capable of rapid decomposition of carbohydrates and of proteins.

proto-. Prefix signifying *first.*

protocone (*pro'-to-kōn*). The mesiolingual cusp on a maxillary molar.

protoconid (*pro-to-kon'-id*). The mesiobuccal cusp on a mandibular molar.

protomere (*pro'-to-mēr*). *In dentistry:* The buccal half of the enamel organ of a tooth.

protraction (*pro-trak'-shun*) *of the jaws.* The condition in which the jaw is forward of its normal position in relation to the orbital plane.

protrusion (*pro-tru'-zhun*). A forward thrust; in dentistry, the forward thrust of teeth, usually the incisors.
palatine p. Torus palatinus (*q.v.*).

protrusion *of the jaws.* Protraction (*q.v.*).

protrusive occlusion. The occlusion produced by a protruding mandible.

protuberance (*pro-tyu'-ber-ans*). A swelling, eminence or knob of tissue.
maxillary p. One of the eminences marking the embryonic rudiments of the jaws.
mental p. The prominence at the angle of the mandible in the midline of the face.

proximal (*proks'-im-al*). Next to, adjacent.

proximal cavity. A cavity affecting either a mesial or a distal surface; a class III cavity.

proximal surfaces of the teeth. Those surfaces which adjoin each other in the same dental arch.

proximobuccal (*proks"-im-o-buk'-al*). Relating to the proximal and buccal surfaces of a posterior tooth.

proximo-incisal (*proks"-im-o-in-si'-zal*). Relating to the proximal surface and the incisal edge of an anterior tooth.

proximo-incisal cavity. A cavity affecting either a mesial or distal surface and also the incisal surface of an incisor or canine; a class IV cavity.

proximolabial (*proks"-im-o-la'-bi-al*). Relating to the proximal and labial surfaces of an anterior tooth.

proximolingual (*proks"-im-o-lin'-gwal*). Relating to the proximal and lingual surfaces of a tooth.

proximo-occlusal (*proks"-im-o-ok-lu'-zal*). Relating to both the proximal and occlusal surfaces of a posterior tooth.

proximo-occlusal cavity. A cavity in the occlusal and distal or the occlusal and mesial surfaces of a tooth; a class II cavity.

pseudoalveolar (*su"-do-al-ve'-o-lar*). Simulating an alveolus, or alveolar tissue.

pseudo-anodontia (*su"-do-an-o-don'-shi-ă*). A condition in which the teeth, although developed, are all unerupted.

pseudocolloid *(su-do-kol'-oyd) of the lips.* Fordyce's spots *(q.v.)*.

pseudoexposure *(su"-do-eks-po'-zhur).* A dental condition in which the caries has progressed through the dentine but has not quite exposed the pulp.

pseudomembrane *(su"-do-mem'-brān).* A false membrane; a skin-like layer formed by a fibrinous exudate containing leukocytes and bacteria.

Pseudomonadaceae *(su"-do-mon-ad-a'-se-e).* A family of micro-organisms of the order Eubacteriales.

Pseudomonas *(su-do-mo'-nas).* A genus of the Pseudomonadaceae family of bacteria, Gram-negative, aerobic and motile.

psilosis *(si-lo'-sis).* Sprue *(q.v., 1)*.

psoriasis buccalis. Leukoplakia buccalis *(q.v.)*.

psoriasis linguae. Leukoplakia of the tongue.

psychosomatic *(si"-ko-so-mat'-ik).* Relating to the mind and the body; in medicine particularly relating to the interdependence of mental processes and bodily function.

pterion *(ter'-e-on).* The point of articulation of the great wing of the sphenoid bone, at the junction of the frontal, parietal and temporal bones.

pterygoid *(ter'-ig-oyd).* In the shape of a wing.

pterygoid artery. Branch of the maxillary artery to the pterygoid muscles. *See* Table of Arteries—pterygoidea.

pterygoid canal, artery of. *See* Table of Arteries—canalis pterygoidea.

pterygoid canal, nerve of. Supplies lacrimal gland and glands of nose and palate. *See* Table of Nerves—canalis pterygoidea.

pterygoid fissure. The angular cleft between the pterygoid processes of the sphenoid bone.

pterygoid fossa. A groove between the medial and lateral plates of the pterygoid process of the sphenoid bone.

pterygoid muscles. *See* Table of Muscles—pterygoideus.

pterygoid nerves. Supply pterygoid muscles. *See* Table of Nerves—pterygoideus.

pterygoid plexus. *See* pterygoid venous plexus.

pterygoid process. One of two descending processes from the junction of the body of the sphenoid bone with its greater wings.

pterygoid venous plexus. A plexus of veins lying in the infra-temporal fossa, between the pterygoid muscles. *See* Table of Veins—plexus venosus pterygoidus.

pterygomandibular *(ter"-ig-o-man-dib'-yu-lar).* Relating to the pterygoid process and the mandible.

pterygomandibular raphe. A sinewy ligament dividing

the buccinator muscle from the constrictor pharyngis superior.

pterygomaxillary (*ter-ig-o-maks-il'-ar-ĭ*). Relating to the pterygoid process and the maxilla.

pterygomaxillary fissure. A narrow cleft between the lateral pterygoid plate and the maxilla, through which passes the maxillary artery.

pterygomaxillary notch. The notch at the junction of the maxilla with the pterygoid process of the sphenoid bone.

pterygopalatine (*ter"-ig-o-pal'-at-ĭn*). Relating to the pterygoid process and the palatine bone.

pterygopalatine canal. The lesser, or posterior, palatine canal (*q.v.*).

pterygopalatine fossa. A small cleft between the pterygoid process of the sphenoid bone and the palatine bone and the maxilla.

pterygopalatine ganglion. Meckel's ganglion (*q.v.*).

pterygopalatine groove. 1. A groove on the ventral aspect of the pterygoid process of the sphenoid bone. 2. A groove on the vertical portion of the palatine bone.

pterygopalatine nerve. Supplies the mucosa of the hard palate and the nose. *See* Table of Nerves—pterygopalatinus.

pterygopharyngeal muscle.

Part of constrictor pharyngis superior. *See* Table of Muscles — pterygopharyngeus.

ptyalism (*ti'-al-izm*). Excessive secretion of saliva; salivation.

ptyalith (*ti'-al-ith*). Ptyalolith (*q.v.*).

ptyalo-. Prefix signifying *saliva*.

ptyalocele (*ti-al'-o-sēl*). A cyst or cystic tumour containing saliva.
sublingual p. Ranula (*q.v.*).

ptyalogogue (*ti-al'-o-gog*). Sialogogue (*q.v.*).

ptyalolith (*ti-al'-o-lith*). A salivary calculus (*q.v.*, 1).

ptyalolithiasis (*ti-al-o-lith-i'-as-is*). The condition of having multiple salivary calculi.

ptyalorrhoea (*ti-al-or-e'-ă*). Abnormal flow of saliva.

ptyalosis (*ti-al-o'-sis*). Salivation (*q.v.*).

ptychodont (*ti'-ko-dont*). An animal in which the crowns of the molar teeth are formed in folds.

ptysma (*tiz'-mă*). Saliva.

Puente's disease. Cheilitis glandularis (*q.v.*).

pulmonary artery. The artery which conveys de-oxygenated blood from the heart to the lungs.

pulmonary vein. One of the short thick blood vessels conveying oxygenated blood from the lungs to the heart.

pulp (*pulp*). Any soft and juicy tissue.
dental p. The vascular and connective tissue, highly

innervated, found at the core of a tooth.

enamel p. The stellate reticulum (*q.v.*).

pulp amputation. Pulpotomy (*q.v.*).

pulp canal. Root canal (*q.v.*).

pulp cavity. The cavity at the core of a tooth, comprising the pulp chamber and the root canal.

pulp chamber. The cavity at the core of a tooth crown, surrounded by dentine and containing dental pulp.

pulp horn. Horn-like projections of the pulp chamber into the crown of a tooth.

pulp protection. The act of inserting intermediate linings in a cavity to prevent conduction of heat or cold to the pulp from the filling material.

pulpal (*pulp'-al*). Relating to the dental pulp.

pulpal wall. The wall which overlies the pulp in an occlusal or incisal cavity; it runs horizontally to the axial surface.

pulpalgia (*pulp-al'-ji-ă*). Pain affecting the dental pulp.

pulpectomy (*pulp-ekt'-om-i*). Removal of the pulp of a tooth.

pulpitis (*pulp-i'-tis*). Inflammation of the tooth pulp.

pulpless (*pulp'-les*). Having no pulp.

pulpoaxial (*pulp"-o-aks'-i-al*). Relating to the pulpal and axial walls in the step portion of a proximo-incisal cavity.

p. angle. The angle formed at the junction of these walls; a *line* angle.

pulpobuccoaxial (*pulp"-o-buk"-o-aks'-i-al*). Relating to the pulpal, buccal and axial walls in the step portion of a proximo-occlusal cavity in a molar or premolar.

p. angle. The angle formed at the junction of these three walls; a *point* angle.

pulpodistal (*pulp"-o-dis'-tal*). Relating to the pulpal and distal walls in the step portion of a proximo-incisal cavity.

p. angle. The angle formed at the junction of these walls; a *line* angle.

pulpodontics (*pulp-o-don'-tiks*). That branch of endodontics concerned with the pulp of the tooth.

pulpolabial (*pulp"-o-la'-bi-al*). Relating to the pulpal and labial walls in the step portion of a proximo-incisal cavity.

p. angle. The angle formed at the junction of these walls; a *line* angle.

pulpolingual (*pulp"-o-lin'-gwal*). Relating to the pulpal and lingual walls in the step portion of a proximo-occlusal cavity.

p. angle. The angle formed at the junction of these walls; a *line* angle.

pulpolinguoaxial (*pulp"-o-lin"-gwo-aks'-i-al*). Relating to the pulpal, lingual and axial walls in the step portion of a proximo-occlusal cavity in a molar or premolar.

p. angle. The angle formed at the junction of these walls; a *point* angle.

pulpomesial (*pulp″-o-me′zi-al*). Relating to the pulpal and mesial walls of a cavity.

p. angle. The angle formed at the junction of these walls; a *line* angle.

pulpotomy (*pulp-ot′-om-ĭ*). Surgical removal of a portion of the tooth pulp.

pulpstone (*pulp′-stōn*). A deposit of calcareous matter within the tooth pulp, associated with degenerative changes; *also called* a denticle.

pulsation (*pul-sa′-shun*). A rhythmic throb or beating, as that of the heart.

pulse (*puls*). The expansion and contraction of an artery due to increased tension of its walls following contraction of the heart and subsequent relaxation. It is usually felt at the wrist, but may be felt over any palpable artery.

pulvis (*pul′-vis*). Latin for *a powder*; used in prescription writing, and abbreviated *pulv*.

pumice (*pum′-is*). A hard, abrasive substance of volcanic origin, used in dentistry as a polishing agent.

punch (*punsh*). 1. Any instrument used to pierce or indent. 2. An instrument used to extract a tooth root.

puromucous (*pyu-ro-myu′-kus*). Mucopurulent; containing both pus and mucus.

purpura (*pur′-pur-ă*). A disease characterized by the presence on the skin and mucous membranes of purple patches, caused by subcutaneous haemorrhage.

purpuric (*pur′-pur-ik*). Relating to or affected with purpura.

purulence (*pyu′-ru-lens*). The condition of containing pus.

purulent (*pyu′-ru-lent*). Relating to or forming pus.

pus (*pus*). A fluid consisting of liquefied cells and liquor puris, produced as a result of inflammation.

pustular (*pus′-tyu-lar*). Relating to or characterized by pustules.

pustule (*pus′-tyūl*). A small circumscribed elevation of the skin containing pus or lymph.

putrefaction (*pyu-tre-fak′-shun*). The decomposition of organic matter through the action of micro-organisms, resulting in the production of various solid and liquid compounds and gases, giving off a foul odour.

putrescent (*pyu-tres′-ent*). In the process of rotting; undergoing putrefaction.

putrid (*pyū-trid*). Rotten, in a state of putrefaction.

pyaemia (*pi-e′-mi-ă*). Generalized septicaemia caused by pyogenic micro-organisms in the blood stream, and marked by the formation of multiple abscesses.

pyemia. *See* pyaemia.

pyic (*pi'-ik*). Relating to pus.

pyo-. Prefix signifying *pus*.

pyogenic (*pi-o-jen'-ik*). Pus-producing.

pyorrhea. *See* pyorrhoea.

pyorrhoea (*pi-or e'-ă*). 1. A discharge of pus. 2. In dentistry, used by the layman to denote any form of periodontal disease.
paradental p. Periodontitis with deep pocketing and discharge of pus, even after the removal of local irritants.
Schmutz p. A form of paradental pyorrhoea caused by persistently poor dental hygiene.

pyorrhoea alveolaris. Usually applied to advanced forms of chronic periodontitis where pus can be expressed from the associated periodontal pockets.

pyosis (*pi-o'-sis*). Suppuration.

pyostomatitis (*pi''-o-sto-mat-i'-tis*). Inflammation and suppuration in the mouth.

pyramidal fracture. Le Fort fracture, class II (*q.v.*).

pyrexia (*pi-reks'-i-ă*). Fever.

pyrexial (*pi-reks'-i-al*). Relating to or affected with pyrexia.

pyro-. Prefix signifying *burning, fire.*

pyroglossia (*pi-ro-glos'-i-ă*). A burning sensation affecting the tongue.

Q

q.d. Abbreviation for *quater in die*—four times a day; used in prescription writing.

q.h., qq.h. Abbreviation for *quaque hora*—every hour; used in prescription writing.
q.2h. *Quaque secunda hora*—every two hours.
q.3h. *Quaque tertia hora*—every three hours.

q.i.d. Abbreviation for *quater in die*—four times a day; used in prescription writing.

q.l. Abbreviation for *quantum libet*—as much as desired; used in prescription writing.

quadrangle (*kwad'-ran-gl*). *Of an instrument:* Having four angles in the shank.

quadrant (*kwad'-rant*). *In dentistry:* One half of each dental arch, the dividing line being the mid-point of the arch; the quadrants are then designated 'upper right', 'upper left', 'lower right', 'lower left'.

quadratus labii inferioris muscle. M. depressor labii inferioris. *See* Table of Muscles.

quadratus labii superioris muscle. M. levator labii superioris. *See* Table of Muscles.

quadratus menti. M. depressor labii inferioris. *See* Table of Muscles.

quadri-. Prefix signifying *four.*

quadriscuspid (*kwad-ri-kus'-pid*). Having four cusps.

quadritubercular (*kwad''-ri-tu-ber'-kyu-lar*). Having four tubercles.

quantum libet. Latin for *as much as desired*; used in prescription writing, and abbreviated *q.l.*

quaque hora. Latin for *every hour*; used in prescription writing, and abbreviated *q.h.* or *qq.h.*

quater in die. Latin for *four times a day*; used in prescription writing, and abbreviated *q.i.d.*, or *q.d.*

quaternary amalgam. An amalgam containing mercury and three other metals.

Quatrefages' angle (J. L. A. Quatrefages de Bréau, 1810-92. French anthropologist). Parietal angle (*q.v.*).

queen's metal. An alloy composed of tin and antimony.

Queyrat's erythroplasia (A. Queyrat, b. 1872. French dermatologist). A precancerous condition of the epithelial mucosa, characterized by circumscribed red velvety lesions, tending to malignancy.

quicksilver (*kwik'-sil-ver*). Mercury (*q.v.*).

quinary amalgam. An amalgam containing mercury and four other metals.

quinquecuspid (*kwin-kwĕ-kus'-pid*). Having five cusps.

quinquetubercular (*kwin"-kwĕ-tu-ber'-kyu-lar*). Having five tubercles.

quinsy (*kwin'-zi*). Acute suppurative tonsillitis.

quotidian (*kwot-id'-i-an*). Recurring daily.

R

R Abbreviation for *recipe*—take; used in prescription writing.

rep. Abbreviation for *repetatur*—let it be repeated; used in prescription writing.

radectomy (*rad-ek'-tom-i*). Radiectomy (*q.v.*).

radiability (*ra-di-ab-il'-it-i*). The condition of being easily penetrated by x rays.

radiciform (*rad-is'-i-form*). In the shape of a root, especially a tooth root.

radicular (*rad-ik'-yu-lar*). Relating to a root.

radicular cyst. A cyst occurring about the root of a tooth, arising from a granuloma in that area.

radiectomy (*rad-i-ek'-tom-i*). Excision of all or part of a tooth root.

radiodontia, radiodontics (*ra"-di-o-don'-shi-ă*). The radiography and interpretation of x-ray films of the teeth and surrounding structures.

radiography (*ra-di-og'-raf-i*). Photography by means of x rays.

radiology (*ra-di-ol'-oj-i*). The science of radiant energy; more particularly the application of radiant energy to medical diagnosis and treatment.

radiolucent (*ra-di-o-lu'-sent*). Offering little resistance to x rays in radiography; almost transparent.

radionecrosis (*ra"-di-o-nek-ro'-sis*). Tissue destruction or ulceration caused by radiation.

radio-opaque (*ra"-di-o-op-āk'*). Resistant to the passage of x rays in photography and appearing opaque on a radiograph.

radula (*rad'-yu-lă*). Any scraping instrument such as a scaler, used to remove dental calculus from the teeth.

rake teeth. Descriptive of widely separated teeth.

rampart (*ram'-part*). A broad encircling ridge.

maxillary r. A ridge of epithelial cells found in the embryo in that part of the jaw which will develop into the alveolar border.

ramus (*ra'-mus*). 1. A branch or process projecting from a bone, as the *ramus* of the mandible. 2. A branch, especially of a blood-vessel or nerve.

ranine (*ra'-nīn*). 1. Relating to a ranula. 2. Relating to the under surface of the tongue.

ranine artery. A. profunda linguae. *See* Table of Arteries.

Ranke's angle (J. Ranke, 1836-1916. German anthropologist). The angle made by a line through the centre of the nasofrontal suture and the centre of the maxillary alveolar process with the horizontal plane of the skull.

ranula (*ran'-yul-ă*). A retention cyst of the sublingual or submandibular glands, occurring under the tongue.

ranular (*ran'-yu-lar*). Relating to a ranula.

raphe (*rāf*, or *rah'-fĕ*). A suture, ridge or crease marking the line of union between two symmetrical halves.

buccal r. The line marking the union of those parts of the cheek derived from the maxillary process with those derived from the mandibular process.

lingual r. The furrow along the midline of the dorsal surface of the tongue, corresponding to the fibrous septum which divides the tongue in two.

palatine r. The narrow mucosal ridge on the midline of the hard palate.

pterygo-mandibular r. A sinewy ligament dividing the buccinator muscle from the constrictor pharyngis superior.

rarefaction (*rar-ĕ-fak'-shun*). The lessening in density but not in volume of any substance.

Raschow's plexus. A fine nerve plexus below the odontoblasts in the dental papilla, found during the formation of dentine.

rash (*rash*). A temporary cutaneous eruption.

gum r. Strophulus (*q.v.*).

tooth r. Strophulus (*q.v.*).

wandering r. Geographic tongue (*q.v.*).

Rathke's pouch (M. H. Rathke, 1793-1860. German anatomist). A dorsal diverticulum from the embryonic buccal cavity which develops into the anterior lobe of the pituitary body.

ratio (*ra'-she-o*). A quantative or numerical relationship between two substances or between groups, expressed in its lowest terms.

re-. Prefix signifying *again, back*.

reaction (*re-ak'-shun*). Response to a stimulus.

reamer (*re'-mer*). A thin corkscrew-like instrument, used either by hand or with a dental engine, for enlarging root canals.

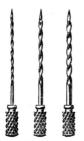

Reamers

reattachment (*re-at-atch'-ment*). 1. The process of replacing a loosened artificial tooth crown or a bridge. 2. The process whereby a loosened or a replanted tooth becomes attached again to the alveolus.

rebase (*re-bās'*). The process of fitting a new denture base without altering the

occlusal relations of the teeth.

recession (*re-sesh'-un*). The drawing or falling away. In dentistry the gradual shrinking back of the gums leaving the tooth cervix, and part of the root, exposed.

recipe. Latin for *take*; used in prescription writing, and abbreviated R.

recrudescence (*rek-ru-des'-ens*). The return of symptoms or the recurrence of disease after a temporary remission.

rectus muscles. *See* Table of Muscles.

recurrence (*re-kur'-ens*). The return of symptoms or of a disease, after a period of remission, or of a malignant tumour after surgical removal.

recurrent (*re-kur'-ent*). 1. Returning at intervals. 2. Turning back on itself or on its course.

recurrent nerve. N. laryngeus recurrens. *See* Table of Nerves.

reduced dental epithelium. Reduced enamel epithelium (*q.v.*).

reduced enamel epithelium. A cellular layer, the remnants of the enamel organ, attached to the enamel surface of a tooth on eruption.

reflect (*re-flekt'*). Turn back on itself; transmit, as with light rays, back in the direction from which something came.

reflection (*re-flek'-shun*). A turning or bending back upon itself.

reflex (*re'-fleks*). 1. Reflected. 2. An involuntary invariable reaction to certain stimuli.

chin r. Jaw jerk reflex (*q.v.*).

conditioned r. A reflex which is not normal and instinctive, but which is developed as a result of repeated association.

faucial r. Vomiting or gagging caused by irritation of the fauces.

gag r. Pharyngeal reflex (*q.v.*).

jaw clonus r. Jaw jerk reflex (*q.v.*).

jaw jerk r. Clonic contraction of the muscles of mastication and upward jerking of the mandible, produced by a downward blow on the relaxed and open jaw. Observed in sclerosis of the lateral columns of the spinal cord.

laryngeal r. Coughing caused by irritation of the larynx and fauces.

mandibular r. Jaw jerk reflex (*q.v.*).

nasal r. Bekhterev's reflex (*q.v.*).

nasomental r. Contraction of the mentalis muscle causing elevation of the lower lip, as a result of a tap on the side of the nose with a percussion hammer.

nociceptive r. Any reflex produced by a painful stimulus.

oesophagosalivary r. Stimulation of the oesophagus producing salivation; Roger's reflex.

palatal r. Swallowing caused by stimulation of the palate.

palm-chin r. Palmomental reflex (*q.v.*).

palmomental r. Irritation of the thenar eminence on one hand producing contraction of the facial muscles on the same side.

pathologic r. Any reflex which is the result of a pathologic condition and not normal; a diagnostic sign.

pharyngeal r. Contraction of the constrictor pharyngis muscles produced by stimulation of the posterior pharyngeal wall.

zygomatic r. Lateral movement of the mandible to the percussed side in response to a tap over the zygoma with a percussion hammer.

reflex, Bekhterev's. See Bekhterev's reflex.

reflex, Roger's. Oesophagosalivary reflex (*q.v.*).

regional anaesthesia. Anaesthetic block (*q.v.*, 1).

registration (*rej-is-tra'-shun*). The record of jaw relations in certain desired positions.

regression (*re-gresh'-un*). 1. A going or turning back; a return to an earlier state. 2. Subsidence of fever or symptoms of a disease.

regressive (*re-gres'-iv*). Relating to or characterized by regression.

regurgitation (*re-gur-jit-a'-shun*). The return of

undigested or partially digested food from the stomach or oesophagus to the mouth, or of fluid or semifluid to the nose.

Reid's base line (R. W. Reid, 1851-1939. Scottish anatomist). An imaginary line from the infra-orbital ridge through the external auditory meatus to the midline of the skull.

reimplantation (*re-im-plant-a'-shun*). Replacement of a tooth into the socket from which it has been removed.

relation (*rĕ-la'-shun*).
centric r. The relation of the jaws which obtains when the condyles are in the most retruded unstrained position in the glenoid fossa from which lateral excursions of the jaw can be made. In an edentulous mouth it is applied to the position of the alveolar processes with the jaws at rest.

relief (*re-lĕf'*). 1. The easing of pain or anxiety. 2. The outline of ridges and hollows within the mouth which are reproduced in a denture.

relief chamber. A recess in the surface of a denture base to reduce pressure on a specific area of the mouth.

reline (*re-lin'*). To resurface or rebase a denture for a more accurate fit.

remedy (*rem'-ed-ĭ*). Any cure or preventive measure.

remission (*re-mish'-un*). 1. The abatement of disease symptoms. 2. The period of such an abatement.

removable appliance. Any orthodontic or prosthetic appliance which can be easily removed by the wearer.

removable bridge. A dental bridge which can be removed by the wearer for cleaning or other purposes.

repetatur. Latin for *let it be repeated*; used in prescription writing, and abbreviated *rep*.

replantation (*re-plant-a'-shun*). Reimplantation (*q.v.*).

resection (*re-sek'-shun*). The cutting away of part of an organ, used especially of the ends of bones which form a joint.

residual (*rez-id'-yu-al*). Left behind; relating to a residue.

residue (*rez'-id-yu*). That which is left after some part has been removed; a remainder.

resin (*rez'-in*). An amorphous, inflammable vegetable substance, exuded from plants and trees; it is transparent or translucent, insoluble in water but readily soluble in ether, alcohol or volatile oils, and readily fusible.
acrylic r. A synthetic form of resin used in the manufacture of dentures, etc.

resinous (*rez'-in-us*). Relating to resin.

resistance form (*rez-ist'-ans*) *of a cavity.* The shape of a cavity designed to withstand the stress to which the restoration is subjected during mastication.

resorption (*re-zorp'-shun*). Physiological reabsorption of tissues or secreted matter. In dentistry applied to absorption of the roots of deciduous teeth, and of the alveolar process after extraction.

rest (*rest*). 1. Repose after activity. 2. The remnants of embryonic epithelial tissue retained within a fully developed organism. 3. In dentistry, an extension on a partial denture or orthodontic appliance to assist in its support or stabilization.

incisal r. An extension or projection on a partial denture which rests on or engages with the incisal edge of an anterior tooth.

lingual r. An extension or projection on a partial denture which rests on or engages with the lingual surface of an anterior tooth.

occlusal r. A cast metal projection on a partial denture, extending over and resting upon the occlusal or other prepared surface of a natural tooth, and acting as an indirect retainer.

r's of Malassez. The remains of Hertwig's epithelial sheath found in the periodontal membrane, and contributing to the formation of dental cysts.

restbite (*rest'-bīt*). The relationship of the dental arches with the jaws at rest.

restoration (*res-tor-a'-shun*). Replacement of missing or removed substance or tissue, as in the filling of teeth, or in prosthetic work in the mouth.

retainer, retaining appliance (*re-ta'-ner*). 1. In prosthetic dentistry, any form of attachment by which a restoration is fastened to an abutment tooth. 2. In orthodontics, any appliance which holds in position teeth which have been moved.

continuous bar r. A metal bar along the lingual surfaces of the teeth, used in prosthetic dentistry to stabilize them and to act as an indirect retainer (*q.v.*).

direct r. An attachment or clasp on a partial denture which connects with the abutment tooth.

indirect r. Part of a partial denture which acts indirectly on the opposite side of the fulcrum line to the direct retainers, to prevent displacement in free-end dentures.

retainer, Hawley. See Hawley retainer.

retardation (*re-tard-a'-shun*). Delay or slowness of development, or hindrance of function.

retention (*re-ten'-shun*). 1. Keeping in place permanently, as of dentures in the mouth. 2. Keeping within the body matter normally excreted, as of urine in the bladder.

retention cyst. A cyst caused by the retention of glandular secretion.

retention form. The shape of a cavity, designed to prevent displacement of the restoration by lifting or tipping stress.

retention plate. 1. The foundation for an obturator. 2. Any orthodontic retaining appliance.

reticular (*ret-ik'-yu-lar*). Relating to a net or net-like structure.

reticulo-endothelial system. The system of specialised reticular and endothelial cells concentrated in the bone marrow, liver, spleen and lymph glands; they are concerned in the formation and destruction of blood cells, and in iron metabolism, and are part of the defensive mechanisms in inflammation and immunity.

reticulo-endothelium (*ret-ik"-yu-lo-en-do-the'-li-um*). The tissue which forms the reticulo-endothelial system.

reticulum (*ret-ik'-yu-lum*). Fibrous net-like tissue. *stellate r.* The second layer of tissue laid down by the enamel organ before the formation of enamel.

retina, central artery. See Table of Arteries—centralis retinae.

retraction (*re-trak'-shun*) *of the jaws.* The condition in which the jaw is drawn back from its normal position in relation to the orbital plane.

retractor (*re-trakt'-or*). A surgical instrument for drawing back the edges of a wound to allow access to deeper structures.

retractor, chin, Angle's. See Angle's chin retractor.

retractor, Moorehead's. See Moorehead's retractor.

retro-. Prefix signifying *behind, backward.*

retrobuccal (*ret-ro-buk'-al*). Relating to the region of the mouth behind the cheeks.

retrocheilia (*ret-ro-ki'-li-ă*). The condition in which one lip is farther back than normal.

retrognathia (*ret-ro-na'-thi-ă*). Retrognathism (q.v.).

retrognathism (*ret-rog'-nath-izm*). The condition of having a retruded lower jaw.

retrolingual (*ret-ro-lin'-gwal*). Behind the tongue.

retromandibular (*ret-ro-man-dib'-yu-lar*). Relating to the region of the mouth behind the mandible.

retromandibular process. The narrow part of the parotid gland found in the fossa behind the mandible.

retromandibular vein. Joins common facial vein and drains into the external jugular. See Table of Veins —retromandibularis.

retromaxillary (*ret-ro-maks-il'-ar-i*). Behind the maxilla, relating to that region of the mouth situated behind the maxilla.

retromolar (*ret-ro-mo'-lar*). Situated behind the molar teeth.

retromolar pad. The soft tissue mass at the distal

end of the mandibular ridge behind the last molar tooth.

retronasal (ret-ro-na′-zal). Behind the nose.

retropharyngeal (ret-ro-far-in′-jē-al). Behind the pharynx.

retropharyngeal space. The space, containing areolar tissue, behind the pharynx.

retroposed (ret′-ro-pōzd). Displaced backward.

retrusion (re-tru′-zhun) of the jaws. Retraction (q.v.).

retrusion of the teeth. Malposition of teeth behind the line of the normal arch.

retrusive occlusion. The occlusion produced by a receding mandible.

Retzius' lines (M. G. Retzius, 1842-1919. Swedish anatomist). Lines visible under a microscope which mark the successive layers of calcification in tooth enamel; striae of Retzius.

reverse overjet. A relationship of the anterior teeth in which, in centric occlusion, the maxillary incisors are lingual to the mandibular incisors (as in Angle's Class III malocclusion).

reverse pin facing. A porcelain facing in which the pins attaching it to the metal crown are fixed into the tooth.

rhabdomyoma (rab″-do-mi-o′-mă). A myoma made up of striated muscular fibres.

rhabdomyosarcoma (rab″-do-mi″-o-sar-ko′-mă). A mixed tumour containing

elements of both a rhabdomyoma and of a sarcoma.

rhagades (rag-ad′-ēz). Chaps or excoriations of the skin; often syphilitic lesions, appearing on the lips and round the mouth.

rhinion (ri′-ni-on). The lower end of the internasal suture.

rhinitis sicca (ri-ni′-tis sik′-ă). Inflammation and wasting of the mucous membranes of the nose, with no secretion. Part of the syndrome complex known as *Sjögren's syndrome*.

rhino-. Prefix signifying *nose*.

rhinocheiloplasty (ri″-no-ki′-lo-plast-ĭ). Plastic surgery of both the nose and the upper lip.

rhinolalia (ri-no-lal′-ĭ-ă). A nasal intonation, caused by defect or disease in the nasal passages.

rhinolith (ri′-no-lith). A calculus or concretion occurring in the nose.

rhinopharyngitis mutilans. Gangosa (q.v.).

rhinorrhagia (ri-nor-a′-jĭ-ă). Nosebleed; epistaxis.

rhinoschisis (ri-nos′-kis-is). Congenital nasal cleft.

rhinoscopy (ri-nos′-kop-ĭ). Examination of the nasal passages by means of a speculum.

rhizagra (ri-zag′-ră). An old instrument used to extract the roots of teeth.

rhizo-. Prefix signifying *root*.

rhizodontropy (*ri-zo-dont'-rop-i*). The attachment of an artificial crown to the tooth root by means of a pivot.

rhizodontrypy (*ri-zo-dont'-rip-i.*) Surgical perforation of a tooth root to allow for the discharge of fluid.

rhizotomy (*ri-zot'-om-i*). Surgical division of either a tooth root or a nerve root.

ribbon arch. An orthodontic appliance of flattened wire conforming to the dental arch, used for anchorage in the movement of teeth; a type of expansion arch.

riboflavin (*ri-bo-fla'-vin*). Vitamin B2, occurring in milk, liver, cheese, eggs, and malt, and in other foods; used therapeutically in deficiency states.

Richmond crown (C. M. Richmond, 1835-1902. American dentist). A porcelain-veneer faced gold-crown attached by means of a dowel to the tooth root.

rictal (*rik'-tal*). Relating to a rictus or fissure.

rictus (*rik'-tus*). 1. A fissure or cleft. 2. Any gaping condition.

rictus lupinus. Cleft palate (*q.v.*).

ridge (*ridj*). A projecting or raised edge.
   alveolar r. The crest remaining in an edentulous mouth after the resorption of the alveolar process.
   basal r. Cingulum (*q.v.*).
   buccocervical r. A ridge on the buccal surface of a deciduous molar near to the cervix of the tooth.
   buccogingival r. (*q.v.*). Bucco-cervical ridge (*q.v.*).
   dental r. Any elevation on a tooth, forming a cusp or a tooth margin.
   linguocervical r. A ridge on the lingual surface of an anterior tooth near to the cervix.
   linguogingival r. Linguo-cervical ridge (*q.v.*).
   marginal r. Any one of the ridges forming the outer margins on the occlusal surface of a molar or premolar, or on the lingual surface of an incisor or canine.
   mylohyoid r. The ridge on the internal surface of the mandible to which the mylohyoid muscle is attached.
   oblique r. A ridge running obliquely across the occlusal surface of a maxillary molar.
   palatine r's. The median raphe, and the lateral corrugations on the hard palate.
   supplemental r. Any abnormal or extra ridge on a tooth surface.

Riga's aphthae (A. Riga, 1832-1919). Italian physician). Cachetic aphthae of the tongue, mucous membranes of the mouth and gastrointestinal tract.

Riga's disease (A Riga, 1832-1919. Italian physician). 1. Fede's disease (*q.v.*); *also called* Riga-Fede's disease. 2. Riga's aphthae (*q.v.*).

Riggs' disease (J. M. Riggs, 1810-85. American dentist). Pyorrhoea alveolaris (q.v.).

rim (rim). A narrow edging or well-defined edge.
bite r. Occlusal rim (q.v.)
occlusal r. A rim of wax mounted on a denture base; it is used in the recording of the relationships of the jaws.

rima glottidis. The glottis (q.v.).

rima oris. The mouth opening.

ring (ring).
infancy r. A line marking the arrested calcification of tooth enamel, formed at about 12 months.
neonatal r. Neonatal line (q.v.).

ring, Bickel's. See Bickel's ring.

Ringer's solution (S. Ringer, 1835-1910. English physiologist). A solution of sodium chloride, calcium chloride and potassium chloride used, in dentistry, as a vehicle in anaesthetic injection.

risorius muscle. Draws angle of mouth sideways. See Table of Muscles.

risus sardonicus. A grinning distortion of the face produced by spasm of the facial muscles; seen in tetanus.

Rivinus' gland (A. Q. Rivinus, 1652-1723. German anatomist). The sublingual gland (q.v.).

Roach's attachment. A form of attachment for removable partial dentures, consisting of a ball and socket joint, the socket being

in a prepared crown or inlay.

rod (rod).
enamel r. Enamel prism (q.v.).

rodent ulcer. A basal-cell carcinoma of superficial origin, arising in the epidermis, and occurring generally on the face or neck.

roentgenogram (rent'-gen-o-gram). A photograph taken using roentgen or x rays.

roentgenology (rent-gen-ol'-oj-i) (W. K. von Roentgen, 1845-1923. German physician). The science of the diagnostic and therapeutic uses of roentgen rays or x rays.

Roger's reflex (G. H. Roger, 1860-1946. French physiologist). Oesophagosalivary reflex (q.v.).

roll (rōl).
cotton wool r. A small and tightly -packed roll of cotton wool used in the mouth to absorb saliva and assist in keeping the operative field dry.

rongeurs (ron-zhur'). Bone-cutting forceps.

root (rūt). *In dentistry:* The part of the tooth in the gums, covered by cementum.
anatomical r. That portion of a tooth which is covered by cementum.
clinical r. That portion of a tooth which is embedded in the gums, from the gingival sulcus.
palatal r. That root of a multi-rooted maxillary tooth which is situated nearest to the palate.

physiological r.   Clinical root (*q.v.*).

root *of the tongue.*   The pharyngeal, fixed portion of the tongue.

root abscess.   An apical granuloma (*q.v.*).

root amputation. 1. Surgical excision of a tooth root. 2. Apicectomy (*q.v.*).

root canal.   The canal, containing dental pulp, leading from the root of the tooth to the pulp chamber.

root sheath.   An epithelial covering surrounding the root of a developing tooth.

Root trunk

root trunk.   That portion of a multi-rooted tooth between the cervical line and the branching of the roots.

rostral (*ros'-tral*). 1. Relating to a rostrum or beak. 2. Relating to the front end of a body, as opposed to *caudal.*

rostrum (*ros'-trum*).   A beak or beak-like appendage.

rotation (*ro-ta'-shun*).   *In dentistry:* The turning of a tooth about its central axis, either correcting a malposed tooth, or the gradual twisting of a normal one to malposition.

-rraphy.   Suffix signifying *suturing.*

-rrhagia.   Suffix signifying *excessive discharge.*

rubber dam.   A thin sheet of rubber, pierced to fit over the mouth leaving certain teeth exposed, used to exclude moisture from the field of operation during cavity preparation and other dental procedures.

rubber-dam clamp.   A form of spring clip which holds the rubber dam round the neck of an exposed tooth.

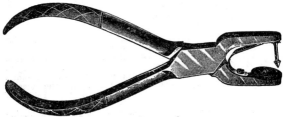

Rubber-dam punch

rubber-dam clamp forceps.
Specially designed forceps
for placing rubber-dam
clamps on the teeth.

rubber-dam holder. A
strap device for holding a
rubber dam in position over
the mouth, and for keeping
the edges back clear of the
field of operation.

rubber-dam punch. An
instrument used to punch
holes of various sizes in a
rubber dam.

rudiment (*ru'-dĭ-ment*). An
organ or part either im-
perfectly developed or at
an early stage in its development.

rudimentary (*ru-dĭ-ment'-
ar-ĭ*). Only partially, or
imperfectly, developed.

ruga (*ru'-gă*) (*pl.* rugae). A
ridge, fold, or wrinkle.

ruga palatinae. One of the
ridges on the hard palate.

S

sig. Abbreviation for *signatur*
—let it be labelled; used
in prescription writing.

sing. Abbreviation for *sing-
ulorem*—of each; used in
prescription writing.

Sn Chemical symbol for tin.

'S' point. Stella turcica
(*q.v.*, 2).

S N A. In cephalometrics,
the angle between the S-N
plane and the line joining the
nasion to the subspinale
(point 'A').

S N B. In cephalometrics,
the angle between the S-N

plane and the line joining
the nasion to the supra-
mentale (point 'B').

S-N plane. In cephalometrics, that plane which
passes through the centre
of the shadow of the sella
turcica and the nasion and
which is perpendicular to
the sagittal plane.

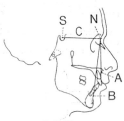

S-N Plane

S Sella turcica.
N Nasion.
A 'A' point.
B 'B' point.
C S-N plane.

saburra (*să-bur'-ă*). A foul
condition of the mouth and
teeth or of the stomach
due to food debris.

sac (*sak*). A pouch or bag-like
covering.
dental s. The vascular tissue
enclosing the enamel organ.

saccular nerve. Supplies
filaments for the macula
sacculi. *See* Table of
Nerves—saccularis.

sacro-. Prefix signifying
flesh.

saddle (*sad'-l*). In prosthetic dentistry, that part of a partial denture which is supported by and in contact with the underlying alveolar tissue.

sagittal (*saj'-it-al*). 1. Shaped like an arrow. 2. In anatomy, running antero-posteriorly.

sagittal sinus, *inferior:* A venous sinus joining the great cerebral vein to form the straight sinus. *See* Table of Veins—sinus sagittalis inferior. *superior:* A venous sinus draining into the transverse sinus. *See* Table of Veins—sinus sagittalis superior.

Saint Apollonia's disease. Toothache.

saline (*sa'-lin*). Salty; relating to a salt.

saline solution. A solution of sodium chloride.

saliva (*sal-i'-vă*). Clear, slightly alkaline fluid secreted by the salivary glands, assisting in the mastication and digestion of food.

saliva ejector. An apparatus whereby saliva is sucked from the mouth during operative dentistry, thus keeping the field of operation free from moisture.

salivant (*sal'-iv-ant*). Producing a flow of saliva.

salivary (*sal-i'-var-i*). Relating to saliva.

salivary calculus. 1. An abnormal concretion occurring in a salivary gland or duct. 2. Supragingival calculus (*q.v.*).

salivary gland. Any one of three pairs of saliva-secreting glands in the mouth, i.e. the parotid, sublingual, and submandibular glands.

salivation (*sal-iv-a'-shun*). 1. Production and secretion of saliva. 2. Excessive secretion of saliva.

salivatory (*sal-iv-a'-tor-i*). Causing or promoting salivation.

salivolithiasis (*sal"-iv-o-lith-i'-as-is*). The condition of having a salivary calculus (*q.v.*, 1).

Salmonella (*sal-mon-el'-ă*) (D. E. Salmon, 1850-1914. American pathologist). A genus of Enterobacteriaceae; non-spore forming, motile rods, Gram negative, found primarily as intestinal parasites, pathogenic to man.

salpingopalatal (*sal-ping-o-pal-a'-tal*). Relating to the pharyngotympanic tube and the palate.

salpingopalatine (*sal-ping-o-pal'-at-in*). Salpingopalatal (*q.v.*).

salpingopharyngeal muscle. Part of M. palatopharyngeus. *See* Table of Muscles—salpingopharyngeus.

Salter's lines (Sir Samuel J. A. Salter, 1825-97. English dentist). Owen's lines (*q.v.*).

sandarac varnish (*san'-dar-ak*). A solution of transparent resin in alcohol, used as a separating fluid and protective coating for plaster casts in dentistry.

Sandwith's bald tongue (F. M. Sandwith, 1853-1918. British physician). The smooth tongue surface seen in the later stages of pellagra.

sanguine (*san'-gwin*). 1. Bloody. 2. Hopeful, optimistic.

sanguineous (*san-gwin'-e-us*). Relating to blood; bloody.

sapid (*sap'-id*). Of agreeable flavour.

sapro-. Prefix signifying *rotten, decaying.*

saprodontia (*sap-ro-don'-shi-ă*). Dental caries (*q.v.*).

saprophyte (*sap'-ro-fīt*). A plant living on decaying or putrefying matter.

Sarcina (*sar'-sin-ă*). A genus of Micrococcaceae family of bacteria, in which cell division occurs in three planes.

sarcoma (*sar-ko'-mă*). A malignant tumour arising from any non-epithelial embryonic tissue.

sarcomatous (*sar-ko'-mat-us*). Relating to a sarcoma.

saucerize (*saw'-ser-īz*). To shape a wound or bone cavity, as in osteomyelitis, to a wide and shallow depression.

sausarism (*saw'-sar-izm*). 1. Lingual paralysis. 2. A dry condition of the tongue.

saw (*saw*). An instrument having a thin blade with a sharp serrated edge, used for cutting bone or other hard tissue.

scaler (*ska'-ler*). A hand instrument used for the removal of calculus and other deposits from the tooth surface.

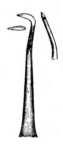

Scaler

scaling (*ska'-ling*). The removal of calculus and other accretions from the surfaces of the teeth with instruments.

scalpel (*skal'-pel*). A small, straight surgical knife.

scalpriform (*skal'-pri-form*). In the shape of a chisel.

scalpriform teeth. The chisel-like incisors of a rodent, used for cutting or gnawing.

scaphocephalic (*skaf-o-sef-al'-ik*). Having a ridged, keel-shaped skull.

scaphocephalous (*skaf-o-sef'-al-us*). Scaphocephalic (*q.v.*).

scaphoid fossa. A depression in the lower surface of the median pterygoid plate of the sphenoid bone, from which arises the tensor veli palatini muscle.

scar (*skar*). The mark left in tissue after the healing of a wound or sore.

Scarpa's foramen (A. Scarpa, 1747-1832. Italian anatomist and surgeon). A foramen occasionally present in the midline fossa in the hard palate.

Scarpa's nerve (A. Scarpa, 1747-1832. Italian anatomist and surgeon). The nasopalatine nerve (*q.v.*).

-schisis. Suffix signifying *fissure* or *cleft*.

schisto-. Prefix signifying *fissure* or *cleft*.

schistoglossia (*skis″-to-glos′-i-ă*). A tongue fissure.

schistoprosopia (*skis-to-pros-o′-pĭ-ă*). Congenital facial cleft.

schizodontia (*skit-so-don′-shĭ-ă*). The development of two separate teeth from one follicle; it usually occurs in the permanent upper anterior teeth.

schizognathism (*skit-zo-na′-thizm*). Jaw cleft.

Schizomycetes (*skit″-zo-mi-se′-tēz*). A class of bacterial fungi.

schizoprosopia (*skit-so-pro-so′-pĭ-ă*). Any congenital fissure of the face.

Schmutz pyorrhoea. A form of paradental pyorrhoea (*q.v.*) caused by persistently poor dental hygiene.

Schreger's lines (C. H. T. Schreger, 1768-1833. German anatomist). *In dentine:* Concentric rings which appear in transverse section

parallel to the amelo-dentinal junction and mark the coincidence of the primary curvatures of dentinal tubules. *In enamel:* A series of lines or bands in the enamel, visible, in a longitudinal section of a human tooth, by reflected light.

scion tooth. A tooth used for transplantation, to replace one extracted.

scirrhous (*skir′-us*). Hard; especially relating to a hard carcinoma or schirrus.

scirrhus (*skir′-us*). A hard carcinoma containing dense connective tissue.

scleroderma (*skler-o-der′-ma*). A systemic disease affecting the fibrous connective tissue and characterized by progressive hardening and thickening of patches of the skin and mucous membranes; it may also involve the periodontal membrane.

scleroid (*skler′-oyd*). Hard; of a hard texture.

sclerosis (*skler-o′-sis*). Hardening of a vessel or part; applied particularly to arteries, and to proliferation of connective tissue in the nervous system as a result of degeneration.
dentinal s. Calcification of the dentinal tubules producing translucent areas and tissue changes in the tooth.

sclerotic (*skler-ot′-ik*). Relating to or affected by sclerosis.

scobinate (*sko′-bin-āt*). Having a rough or roughened surface.

scoliodontic (*sko-li-o-don'-tik*). Having a tooth which has twisted in its socket.

scorbutic (*skor-byu'-tik*). Relating to or affected with scurvy.

screen (*skrēn*).
oral s. A thin plastic plate constructed so that it is in contact with the tips of protruding maxillary incisors, whilst appearing to cover the labial surface of all the maxillary teeth; lip pressure tips the incisors lingually. It is also used as an inhibitor of mouth-breathing and thumb-sucking.

screw (*skru*). A threaded pin, post, or peg, used for attachment.
traction s. A screw used in orthodontics to produce a pulling force sufficient to move malposed teeth.

screw elevator. An instrument which can be screwed into a retained root in order to draw it out.

scrotal tongue (*skro'-tal*). A tongue having a surface much furrowed and with deep depressions, resembling the skin on the scrotum.

scurvy (*skur'-vi*). A disease produced by vitamin C deficiency and characterized by general weakness and anaemia, swollen gums and mucocutaneous haemorrhage; it used to be common amongst sailors, but is now chiefly seen amongst the elderly.

seamless band. A band stamped out from a metal tube, having no joins.

seamless crown. A shell crown contoured from a metal cap, without soldering.

seat (*sēt*). *Of a cavity:* In simple cavities, the floor of the cavity; in proximo-occlusal or proximo-incisal cavities, the gingival wall.
basal s. The tissue area on which a denture base rests.

sebaceous (*se-ba'-shus*). Relating to sebum.

sebaceous cyst. A cyst caused by the blocking of the duct of a sebaceous gland and the retention of its secretion.

sebaceous gland. One of the glands which secrete sebum.

Sebileau's hollow (P. Sebileau, 1860-1953. French surgeon). The depression beneath the tongue between the sublingual glands.

sebum (*se'-bum*). A semi-fluid substance containing fat, keratin and epithelial debris secreted by the sebaceous glands.

secodont (*sek'-o-dont*). Having cutting edges on the tubercles of the molar teeth.

secondary dentine. A new deposit of dentine laid down in the pulp chamber as a protection against caries or tooth damage.

secondary palate. The palate formed by the joining of the palatal processes of the maxilla in the embryo.

secretion (*se-kre'-shun*). 1. The production and ejection of a specific fluid material by a gland. 2. Any substance thus produced and ejected.

secretory nerve. Any efferent nerve whose stimulation increases activity in the gland to which it is distributed.

sectorial (*sek-tor'-i-al*). Cutting.

sectorial teeth. The cutting teeth of Carnivora.

sedation (*sed-a'-shun*). 1. A condition of decreased functional activity. 2. The production of calm, or lessened excitement.

sedative (*sed'-at-iv*). 1. Relating to sedation. 2. Any agent which produces sedation.

selenodont (*se-le'-no-dont*). Having teeth with longitudinal crescentic ridges, as, for example, the molar teeth in man.

sella turcica (*sel'-ă turs'-ik-ă*). 1. The depression on the inner part of the upper surface of the sphenoid bone, forming the pituitary fossa. 2. A cephalometric landmark, 'S', in the centre of the shadow of the sella turcica on a lateral skull radiograph.

semi-. Prefix signifying *half.*

semicohesive (*sem-i-ko-he'-ziv*). Only partially cohesive.

semispinalis capitis muscle. Extends head. *Also called* complexus muscle. *See* Table of Muscles.

semispinalis cervicis muscle. Extends vertebral column and rotates it. *Also called* semispinalis colli muscle. *See* Table of Muscles.

semispinalis colli muscle. M. semispinalis cervicis. *See* Table of Muscles.

senescence (*sen-es'-ens*). Ageing.
dental s. The changes occurring in the mouth and in the teeth as a result of ageing.

senile (*se'-nīl*). Relating to old age.

senility (*sen-il'-it-i*). Old age.

sensory nerve. An afferent nerve, transmitting sensations of pain, touch, etc., to the central nervous system from the periphery.

separating strip. A strip of metal, having one side coated with a coarse abrasive, used to increase the space between adjacent teeth.

separating varnish. Any varnish used to coat a plaster mould and prevent adhesion of fresh plaster poured in to produce a model.

separator (*sep'-ar-a-tor*). Anything used to effect a separation. In dentistry, a device for forcing apart adjoining teeth.

sepsis (*sep'-sis*). Poisoning as a result of the absorption of putrefactive products.
focal s. A local source of infection which may spread to cause systemic disease.
oral s. A septic condition in the mouth producing

excessive bacterial activity which may affect the general health.

septal (*sep'-tal*). Relating to a septum.

septal abscess. An abscess forming on the proximal surface of a tooth root.

septal artery. Supplies the nasal mucous membrane. *See* Table of Arteries—septi.

septal cartilage. The cartilage lying within the nasal septum, dividing the right and left nasal cavities.

septic (*sep'-tik*). Relating to or caused by sepsis.

septicaemia (*sep-tĭ-se'-mĭ-ă*). A systemic condition due to the presence of bacteria and their poisons in the blood.

septicaemic (*sep-tĭ-se'-mik*). Relating to or affected with septicaemia.

septicemia. *See* septicaemia.

septum (*sep'-tum*). A thin partition between two masses of soft tissue or two cavities.
  alveolar s. Interalveolar septum (*q.v.*).
  gingival s. Gingival papillae (*q.v.*).
  interalveolar s. The bony wall dividing two tooth sockets.
  interdental s. That portion of the alveolar process between adjoining tooth sockets.
  interradicular s. The bony partition in a tooth socket between the roots of a multi-rooted tooth.

intra-alveolar s. A bony partition within the tooth socket.
lingual s. The median, vertical, fibrous partition of the tongue.

sequela (*se-kwel'-ă*) (*pl.* sequelae). Any condition following on a disease, of which it is the direct or indirect result.

sequential (*se-kwen'-shal*). 1. In sequence. 2. Relating to sequelae.

sequestrectomy (*se-kwes-trek'-tom-i*). The removal of a bone sequestrum by surgery.

sequestrum (*se-kwes'-trum*). A piece of necrotized bone which has become detached from the sound bone.

sero-. Prefix signifying *serum*.

serous (*se'-rus*). 1. Relating to a serum. 2. Serum-producing.

serpiginous (*ser-pij'-in-us*). Creeping.

serpiginous ulcer. An ulcer which is constantly spreading in one direction whilst healing in another.

serrated (*ser-a'-ted*). Having a toothed edge, like a saw.

serration (*ser-a'-shun*). 1. A structure having a toothed, saw-like edge. 2. A notch, as between two teeth on a saw edge.

Serres' glands (A. E. R. A. Serres, 1786-1868. French physiologist). Pearly masses of epithelial cells found on the gums of infants.

serum (*se'-rum*) (*pl.* sera). 1. The clear, amber-coloured

fluid obtained by the separating out of the solid elements in blood by clotting.
2. Blood serum obtained from immune animals or humans and used in the prevention and treatment of disease.

serumal, seruminal calculus. Subgingival calculus (*q.v.*).

sesqui-. Prefix signifying *one-and-one-half; in the ratio of two to three.*

sesquihora (*ses-kwĭ-or'-ă*). An hour and a half.

sessile (*ses'-ĭl*). Having a broad base; as opposed to *pedunculated.*

setiform (*set'-ĭ-form*). Bristle-shaped.

setiform teeth. Ciliiform teeth (*q.v.*).

shaft (*shaft*) *of an instrument.* The handle.

shank (*shank*) *of an instrument.* The slender portion joining the handle to the blade or nib.

Sharpey's fibres (W. Sharpey, 1802-80. English anatomist). 1. The collagenic fibres of connective tissue between bone and periosteum. 2. In dentistry, those parts of the collagenic fibres of the periodontal membrane which are embedded in the alveolar bone or in the cementum of the tooth.

sheath (*shēth*). A covering or sac; applied to the outer envelope of nerves and arteries.

carotid s. The envelope containing the common carotid artery, the internal jugular vein and the vagus nerve.

dentinal s. Neumann's sheath (*q.v.*).

root s. An epithelial covering surrounding the root of a developing tooth.

sheath of Hertwig. *See* Hertwig's sheath.

sheath of Neumann. *See* Neumann's sheath.

shell crown. A crown consisting of a metal shell, contoured to fit over the crown of an existing natural tooth; *also called* a cap crown.

shingles (*shin'-gels*). Herpes zoster (*q.v.*).

shock (*shok*). Acute circulatory failure, marked by a fall in blood pressure, rapid and feeble pulse, pallor and clamminess of the skin, shallow respiration, and similar symptoms.

shoulder crown. A crown which has been shaped at the base to sit on the prepared root without a metal collar.

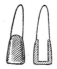

Shoulder crown

siagonagra (*si-ag-on-ag'-ră*). Pain of the jaw-bone.

siagonantritis (*si-ag-on-an-tri'-tis*). Inflammation of the maxillary antrum.

sialadenitis (*si-al-ad-en-i'-tis*). Sialoadenitis (*q.v.*).

sialadenoncus (*si''-al-ad-en-on'-kus*). Any salivary gland tumour.

sialagogue (*si-al'-ag-og*). Sialogogue (*q.v.*).

sialaporia (*si-al-ă-por-e'-ă*). Deficiency in the amount of saliva secreted.

sialic (*si-al'-ik*). Relating to or characteristic of saliva.

sialitis (*si-al-i'-tis*). Sialoadenitis (*q.v.*).

sialo-. Prefix signifying *saliva*.

sialoadenitis (*si''-al-o-ad-en-i'-tis*). Inflammation of a salivary gland.

sialo-angiectasis (*si''-al-o-an-jĕ-ek'-tas-is*). Distension of the salivary ducts.

sialocele (*si-al'-o-sēl*). A tumour or cyst of the salivary glands.

sialodochitis (*si-al-o-dok-i'-tis*). Sialoductitis (*q.v.*).

sialoductitis (*si-al-o-dukt-i'-tis*). Inflammation of the salivary ducts.

sialogenous (*si-al-oj'-en-us*). Saliva-producing.

sialogogue (*si-al'-og-og*). 1. Saliva-producing. 2. An agent which promotes a flow of saliva.

sialography (*si-al-og'-raf-ĭ*). Radiography of the salivary glands and ducts.

sialoid (*si'-al-oyd*). 1. Relating to saliva. 2. Saliva-like.

sialolith (*si-al'-o-lith*). A salivary calculus (*q.v.*, 1).

sialolithiasis (*si''-al-o-lith-i'-as-is*). The process of formation of salivary calculi (*q.v.*, 1).

sialoma (*si-al-o'-mă*). A salivary tumour.

sialoncus (*si-al-on'-kus*). A tumour of the sublingual gland caused by obstruction of the duct.

sialorrhoea (*si-al-or-e'-ă*). Salivation (*q.v.*, 2).

sialoschesis (*si-al-os'-kes-is*). Suppression of the secretion of the salivary glands.

sialosemeiology (*si''-al-o-se-mī-ol'-oj-i*). Diagnosis by chemical examination and analysis of saliva.

sialosis (*si-al-o'-sis*). Salivation (*q.v.*, 2).

sialotic (*si-al-ot'-ik*). Relating to or characterized by saliva.

sialozemia (*si-al-o-ze'-mi-ă*). Uncontrolled flow of saliva, often with dribbling.

sigmoid notch (*sig'-moyd*). The crescent-shaped border of the ramus, between the coronoid process and the condyle of the mandible; *also called* the mandibular notch.

sigmoid sinus. A venous sinus, continuous with the transverse sinus and draining into the internal jugular vein. *See* Table of Veins—sinus sigmoideus.

signatur (*sig-na'-tur*). Latin for *let it be labelled*; used in prescription writing, and abbreviated *sig*.

signature (*sig'-nat-yur*). That part of a prescription, written on the label of the medicine, which gives the directions for administration.

silicone (*sil'-ik-on*). A plastic material based on silicon. In dentistry it is used as a impression compound.

silver (*sil'-ver*). A soft, white, malleable and ductile metal, chemical symbol Ag; soluble in dilute nitric acid, hot concentrated sulphuric acid, and solutions of alkali cyanides.

silver cone. Silver point (*q.v.*).

silver point. A fine cone of silver used to fill a root canal after the removal of the pulp.

sinciput (*sin'-sip-ut*). The top of the head.

singulorum (*sin-gyu-lor'-um*). Latin for *of each*; used in prescription writing, and abbreviated *sing*.

sino-, sinu-. Prefix signifying *sinus*.

sinus (*si'-nus*). 1. A hollow or cavity. 2. A channel for venous blood, especially in the cranium. 3. An air cavity, especially one communicating with the nose. 4. A tract lined with granulations and leading from a suppurating cavity to the body surface.
air s. Sinus (*q.v.*, 3).
ethmoidal s. One of the many small intercommunicating cavities forming the labyrinth of the ethmoid bone, opening into the nasal cavity.

frontal s. One of two cavities in the frontal bone, varying in size in different skulls, and found above the root of the nose.
maxillary s. A large air sinus in the maxilla communicating with the middle meatus of the nose; *also called* the antrum of Highmore.
palatine s. A variable cavity in the orbital process of the palatine bone, opening into the sphenoidal or a posterior ethmoidal sinus.
paranasal s. One of the air cavities in the skull bones of the face, communicating with the nasal cavity; they are named after the bones in which they occur.
sphenoidal s. A cavity, of variable size, in the body of the sphenoid bone, above the nasopharynx and the nasal cavity; it is divided by a bone septum into a right and left sinus.
venous s. For venous sinuses, *see* Table of Veins —sinus.

sinusal (*si'-nus-al*). Relating to a sinus.

sinusitis (*si-nus-i'-tis*). Inflammation of the maxillary sinus.

skeletal (*skel-e'-tal*). Relating to a skeleton.

skeletal classification of malocclusion. *See* under malocclusion.

skeletal fixation, external. *In surgery:* A method of immobilizing the ends of a fractured bone by external metal pins or screw appliances, used especially for an edentulous mouth.

skeleton (*skel'-et-on*). The bony framework of an animal body.

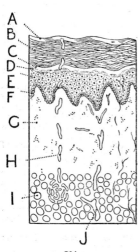

Skin

A Skin surface.
B Stratum corneum.
C Stratum lucidum.
D Stratum granulosum.
E Stratum spinosum.
F Stratum germinativum.
G Dermis.
H Duct of sweat gland.
I Subcutaneous tissue.
J Blood vessel.

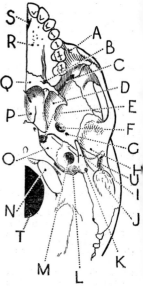

Skull (inferior aspect)

A Infraorbital foramen.
B Greater palatine foramen.
C Inferior orbital fissure.
D Lateral pterygoid plate.
E Foramen lacerum.
F Foramen ovale.
G Foramen spinosum.
H Articular fossa.
I Styloid process.
J Mastoid process.
K Stylomastoid foramen.
L Jugular foramen.
M Carotid canal.

N Occipital condyle.
O Petrous portion of temporal bone.
P Vomer.
Q Horizontal plate of palatine bone.
R Palatine process of maxilla.
S Incisive fossa.
T Foramen magnum.
U External auditory meatus.

skeleton denture. A form of partial denture which is mainly tooth-borne, and which has connectors of the smallest size consistent with adequate strength, leaving the mucous membrane and gingival margins exposed.

skiagram (*ski'-ă-gram*). A radiograph or roentgeno-gram.

skin (*skin*). The outer covering of the body, consisting of the epidermis and the dermis.

skull (*skul*). The bony framework of the head.

slant culture. One grown on a slanting surface, to obtain a greater area for growth.

slough (*sluf*). The necrotizing tissue which scales or peels off in ulcerative conditions.

smoker's tongue. Leuko-plakia (*q.v.*).

smooth muscle. Muscle consisting of spindle-shaped, unstriped fibres; involuntary muscle is usually of this type.

socket (*sok'-et*). The cavity or depression into which a corresponding part fits.

dry s. An acute inflammatory condition of the walls of

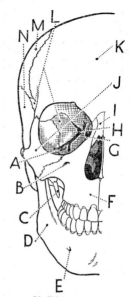

Skull (front view)

A Inferior orbital fissure.
B Infraorbital foramen.
C Styloid process.
D Mandible.
E Mental foramen.
F Maxilla.
G Lacrimal bone.
H Superior orbital fissure.
I Nasal bone.
J Zygomatic bone.
K Frontal bone.
L Sphenoid bone.
M Parietal bone.
N Temporal bone.

a tooth socket following the extraction of the tooth; alveolalgia.

tooth s. An alveolus (*q.v.*).

sodium (*so'-di-um*). A silver-white alkaline metallic element which oxidizes rapidly on exposure to air; chemical symbol Na.

sodium fluoride. NaF, a white powder form of fluoride used to adjust the concentration of fluoride ion in a water supply to an optimum level of 1 p.p.m. in water fluoridation (*q.v.*), in tablet form for administration where the water supply is not so adjusted and in solution as a topical application for the prevention of dental caries.

soft palate. The fleshy, rear portion of the roof of the mouth.

sol (*sol*). A colloidal solution, in which the colloid disperse phase is dispersed in some medium, either gas, liquid, or solid.

solder (*sol'-der*). 1. A fusible alloy used to join two metal surfaces or edges. 2. The process of joining a metal in this way.

solubility (*sol-yu-bil'-it-ĭ*). The degree to which any substance is soluble.

soluble (*sol'-yu-bl*). Capable of dissolving in a liquid to make a solution.

solution, disclosing. *See* disclosing solution.

solution, Hartman's. *See* Hartman's solution.

solution, Ringer's. *See* Ringer's solution.

somatic nerve. One of the nerves supplying voluntary muscles, tendons, joints, skin, and parietal serous membranes.

sophronistae dentes. Old term for wisdom teeth.

soporific (*sop-or-if'-ik*). Sleep-producing.

sorbifacient (*zor-bĭ-fa'-shunt*). 1. Causing or promoting absorption. 2. Any agent which causes or promotes absorption.

sordes (*sor'-dēz*). 1. Dirt; particularly the dark brown crust which forms on the teeth and lips in continued low fever. 2. In dentistry, food debris (*q.v.*).

sore (*sawr*). 1. Painful. 2. Any lesion of the skin or mucous membrane.

cold s. Herpes labialis (*q.v.*).

hard s. Chancre (*q.v.*).

space (*spās*).

apical s. The area between the bony wall of the tooth socket and the apex of the tooth root; the site of an apical abscess.

freeway s. The slight gap between the upper and lower teeth when the mandible is at rest.

interdental s. The space below the contact point between two adjacent teeth.

interglobular s's. Large spaces found in dentine, close to the amelo-dentinal junction, caused by incomplete calcification.

interproximal s. Interdental space (q.v.).

Nance's leeway s. The difference between the space occupied by the deciduous canine and two molars and that occupied by the permanent canine and premolars in each side of the dental arch.

parapharyngeal s. The area contained within the cervical vertebrae, the lateral wall of the pharynx and the internal pterygoid muscle.

pharyngomaxillary s. Parapharyngeal space (q.v.).

retropharyngeal s. The space, containing areolar tissue, behind the pharynx.

subgingival s. The space between the tooth enamel and the adjacent gingiva.

submandibular s. The space formed by the division of the deep cervical fascia about the submandibular salivary gland.

submasseteric s. The space between the masseter muscle and the ascending ramus of the mandible.

space-maintainer. An orthodontic appliance used to prevent overcrowding of teeth or closure of a space into which a tooth is expected to erupt.

span bridge. Fixed bridge (q.v.).

spasm (*spazm*). A sudden, involuntary and violent muscular contraction.

spasmodic (*spaz-mod'-ik*). Relating to or characterized by spasm.

spatula (*spat'-yu-lă*). A flexible blunt knife-shaped instrument used for mixing or spreading plaster or ointment.

spatulator (*spat'-yu-la-tor*). A mechanical apparatus for mixing cements or amalgams.

species (*spe'-shēz*). A group of organisms having certain characteristics which distinguish them from similar organisms within the same genus.

specific (*spes-if'-ik*). 1. Relating to a species. 2. Produced by one type of microorganism. 3. A medicine indicated for use in the treatment of a particular disease.

Spee, curve of (F. Graf von Spee, 1855-1937. German embryologist). *See* curve of Spee.

spheno-. Prefix signifying *sphenoid bone*.

sphenoid (*sfe'-noyd*). Shaped like a wedge.

sphenoid bone. The wedge-shaped bone at the base of the skull.

sphenoid fissure. Superior orbital fissure (q.v.).

sphenoidal process *of the palatine bone.* A thin bony plate running upwards and inwards from the palatine bone and articulating with the sphenoid bone and the vomer.

sphenoidal sinus. A cavity, of variable size, in the body of the sphenoid bone, above the nasopharynx and the nasal cavity; it is divided by a bony septum into a right and left sinus.

sphenomandibular (*sfe"-no-man-dib'-yu-lar*). Relating to the sphenoid bone and mandible.

sphenomaxillary (*sfe"-no-maks-il'-ar-ĭ*). Relating to both the sphenoid bone and the maxilla.

sphenomaxillary fissure. Pterygomaxillary fissure (*q.v.*).

sphenomaxillary fossa. Pterygopalatine fossa (*q.v.*).

sphenopalatine (*sfe"-no-pal'-at-ĭn*). Relating to the sphenoid bone and the palate.

sphenopalatine artery. Supplies the lateral nasal wall and septum. *Also called* nasopalatine. *See* Table of Arteries—sphenopalatina.

sphenopalatine foramen. The space between the orbital and sphenoid processes of the palatine bone, opening into the nasal cavity.

sphenopalatine ganglion. Meckel's ganglion (*q.v.*).

sphenopalatine nerve. N. pterygopalatinus. *See* Table of Nerves.
long s.n. N. nasopalatinus.
short s.n. N. nasalis posterior superior lateralis.

sphenopalatine notch. A deep depression which divides the sphenoid and the orbital processes of the palatine bone.

sphenoparietal sinus. A venous sinus draining the dura mater and terminating

in the cavernous sinus. *See* Table of Veins—sinus spheno-parietalis.

spheroid (*sfe'-royd*). In the shape of a sphere.

spheroiding (*sfe'-royd-ing*). The tendency of amalgam to become round, as a result of the presence of mercury in the mass, when mixed too soft.

sphincter muscle (*sfink'-ter*). A muscle which surrounds and closes a natural opening.

spinal (*spi'-nal*). Relating to a spine.

spinalis capitis muscle. Extends head; inconstant. *See* Table of Muscles.

spinalis cervicis muscle. Extends vertebral column; inconstant. *Also called* spinalis colli muscle. *See* Table of Muscles.

spinalis colli muscle. M. spinalis cervicis. *See* Table of Muscles.

spine (*spīn*). 1. A thorn-like, slender bone process. 2. The vertebral column of the body.
anterior nasal s. A median spine of bone projecting from the maxillae and supporting the septal cartilage of the nose.
mental s. Mental tubercle (*q.v.*).
posterior nasal s. The spine at the lower, posterior end of the nasal crest of the palatine bone.

spine, Spix's. *See* Spix's spine.

spinous (*spi'-nus*). Relating to a spine.

Spirilleae (*spir-il'-e-e*). A tribe of the Pseudomonadaceae family of bacteria.

Spirillum (*spir-il'-um*) (*pl.* Spirilla). A genus of microorganisms of the Pseudomonadaceae family, seen as spiral rods.
S. buccale. A species found in dental calculus.

Spirochaetaceae (*spi"-ro-keta'-se-e*). A family of slender spiral micro-organisms of the order Spirochaetales.

Spirochaetales (*spi-ro-keta'-lēz*). An order of spiral micro-organisms.

Spix's spine (J. B. Spix, 1781-1826. German anatomist). The bony spine on the median border of the inferior dental foramen, to which is attached the spheno-mandibular ligament.

splanchnology (*splank-nol'-oj-i*). The study of the viscera of the body.

splenius capitis muscle. Extends head. *See* Table of Muscles.

splenius cervicis muscle. Extends spinal column. *Also called* splenius colli muscle. *See* Table of Muscles.

splenius colli muscle. M. splenius cervicis. *See* Table of Muscles.

splint (*splint*). 1. An appliance, which may be rigid or flexible, used to immobilize the ends of fractured bones or to restrict the movement of joints. 2. To immobilize by the use of such an appliance. In dentistry, to immobilize either loose teeth with a fixed appliance or to immobilize fractured jaws.
acrylic s. A plastic splint or stent used in dental surgery to immobilize fractures of the mandible or the maxilla, or to support bone grafts of the jaw.
anchor s. A splint used in fracture of the jaw, which has metal loops fitting over the teeth.
cap s. A cast metal dental splint fitting accurately over the crowns and occlusal surfaces of the teeth and cemented in place; used to assist in immobilizing jaw fractures.
dental s. Any form of appliance or device used to fasten and immobilize the teeth.
flange s. A metal splint used in fracture of the mandible; it is cemented to several of the posterior mandibular teeth, and has a high flange which rests on the buccal surfaces of the opposing maxillary teeth.
interdental s. A type of splint used in fracture of the jaw, held in place by wires passed round the teeth.
open-cap s. A form of cap splint in which the occlusal surfaces of the teeth are left exposed.

splint, Gilmer. *See* Gilmer splint.

splint, Gunning. *See* Gunning splint.

splint, Kingsley's. *See* Kingsley's splint.

splinter (*splin'-ter*). 1. A small, sharp-pointed fragment. 2. To break up into small fragments.

splinting (*splint'-ing*). The process of applying a splint or splints.

split-dowel crown. A removable crown attached to the tooth by means of a split-pin, which is fitted into a gold-lined root canal.

sponge gold. Cohesive gold in the form of spongy crystals.

spongiosa (*spon-jĭ-o'-să*). Substantia spongiosa (*q.v.*).

spoon denture. A form of upper partial denture for the restoration of one or more anterior teeth, the teeth being attached to a plastic base plate which extends over the whole of the hard palate, but does not cover the gingival margins of the natural teeth.

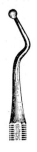

Spoon excavator

spoon excavator. A type of excavator having a spoon-shaped head.

spot grinding. The correction of occlusion by grinding down high areas on the teeth, fillings, or prosthetic appliances, disclosed by articulating paper.

spots, Filatov's. Koplik's spots (*q.v.*).

spots, Fordyce's. See Fordyce's spots.

spots, Koplik's. See Koplik's spots.

sprew (*spru*). See sprue.

spring (*spring*). A coil of fine wire, which possesses the property of elasticity.

spring plate. A dental plate which is retained by the elasticity of its material pressing against the abutment teeth.

sprue (*spru*). 1. A chronic disease affecting the intestines, characterized by diarrhoea, blood changes, wasting, and a raw mouth and tongue. 2. In dentistry, the hole through which molten metal is poured into a closed mould; also the small sprig of waste metal which is left in this hole, or on the casting.

sprue former. A small pin used to remove a wax pattern from a cavity.

spur (*spur*). *In dentistry:* A small metal projection on an appliance or partial denture.

sputum (*spyu'-tum*). Matter expelled from the mouth by spitting; it may be saliva alone, or mixed with mucous secretions from the respiratory tract.

squama (*skwa'-mă*). A scale, or scale-like matter.

squamomandibular (*skwa''-mo-man-dib'-yu-lar*). Relating to the squamous portion of the temporal bone, or of the occipital bone, and the mandible.

squamous (*skwa'-mus*). Scale-like; scaly.

squamous-cell carcinoma. Carcinoma developing from the squamous epithelium; a type of epidermoid carcinoma.

squash bite. A bite taken to register the relationship of the cusps of the upper and lower teeth, but not to give any clear reproduction of the teeth.

stab culture. A culture made by inoculating the medium by means of a needle thrust deeply into it.

stagnation (*stag-na'-shun*). 1. The cessation of flow of any circulating fluid in the body. 2. In dentistry, the accumulation of debris on a tooth.

stain (*stān*). 1. Any mark discolouring a surface. 2. Any colouring agent used to colour tissues for microscopical examination.

stainless steel. A form of steel containing some nickel or chromium, or both; it does not easily tarnish.

stannous fluoride. SnF_2; a form of fluoride used in toothpaste and for topical application for the prevention of dental caries.

stapedius muscle. Retracts stapes. *See* Table of Muscles.

stapedyle (*staf'-il-ă*). The uvula (*q.v.*).

staphyline (*staf'-il-īn*). Relating to the uvula; also used to refer to the palate as a whole.

staphylion (*staf-il'-i-on*). The point in the midline on the posterior edge of the hard palate, a craniometric landmark.

staphylococcal (*staf''-il-o-kok'-al*). Relating to or caused by staphylococci.

Staphylococcus (*staf''-il-o-kok'-us*). A genus of the Micrococcaceae family of bacteria, seen as irregular clusters of cells, or as short chains; species of this genus of bacteria are found in suppurative lesions, boils, inflammatory conditions, etc.

staphylorraphy (*staf-il-or'-af-i*). Surgical repair of a soft palate cleft.

staphyloschisis (*staf-il-os'-kis-is*). Cleft uvula, or cleft of the uvula and the soft palate.

stato-acusticus nerve. N. vestibulocochlearis. *See* Table of Nerves.

staurion (*staw'-ri-on*). The point at which the transverse palatine suture intersects the median suture; a craniometric point.

steel (*stēl*). A metal formed by the combination of iron and a small quantity of carbon; it is tough and elastic.

stainless s. A form of steel containing some nickel or chromium, or both; it does not easily tarnish.

stelengis (*stel-en'-jis*). Grinding of the teeth.

stellate (*stel'-āt*). Star-shaped.

stellate reticulum. The second layer of tissue laid down by the enamel organ before the formation of enamel.

stenion (*sten'-ĭ-on*). One of two craniometric points on the sphenosquamosal suture, located nearest to the midline on each side, being at each end of the smallest transverse diameter of the temporal region.

stenocephalic (*sten-o-sef-al'-ik*). Having an abnormally narrow skull.

stenocompressor (*sten"-o-kom-pres'-or*). An instrument used in oral and dental surgery to close Stensen's duct.

stenodont (*sten'-o-dont*). Having abnormally narrow teeth.

stenosis (*sten-o'-sis*). Constriction or narrowing of an aperture, canal, or duct.

stenostenosis (*sten-o-sten-o'-sis*). Constriction of Stensen's (parotid) duct.

stenostomia (*sten-o-sto'-mĭ-ă*). Constricture of the mouth.

Stensen's duct (N. Stensen, 1638-86. Danish anatomist). The duct through which saliva secreted by the parotid gland flows into the mouth;

its opening lies opposite to the maxillary molars on the buccal surface.

stent (*stent*). A mould of plastic compound used to immobilize certain forms of skin graft.

acrylic s. A plastic splint or stent used in dental surgery to immobilize fractures of the mandible or the maxilla, or to support bone grafts of the jaws.

Stent's composition or mass (C. Stent, 19th century English dentist). A resinous, thermo-plastic material, which sets very hard, used in dentistry as an impression compound and in plastic surgery for moulds to immoblize skin grafts.

step (*step*). *Of a cavity*: The auxiliary part of a compound mortise form, in complex cavities, consisting of the pulpal and axial walls.

stephanial (*stef-a'-nĭ-al*). Relating to the stephanion.

stephanion (*stef-a'-ni-on*). The junction of the coronal suture and the temporal line of the frontal bone.

stereo-. Prefix signifying *three-dimensional*.

sterile (*ster'-īl*). 1. Aseptic, germ-free. 2. Infertile.

sterile abscess. An abscess containing no microorganisms.

sterilization (*ster-il-i-za'-shun*). 1. The process of rendering germ-free or aseptic. 2. The process of rendering incapable of reproduction.

sterilizer (*ster'-il-i-zer*.) An apparatus used for sterilization.

sternocleidomastoid artery. Two branches, from the occipital and the superior thyroid arteries, supplying the sternocleidomastoid muscle. *See* Table of Arteries—sternocleidomastoidea.

sternocleidomastoid muscle. Flexes head and turns it to the opposite side. *Also called* sternomastoid muscle. *See* Table of Muscles—sternocleidomastoideus.

sternohyoid muscle. Depresses hyoid bone. *See* Table of Muscles—sternohyoideus.

sternomastoid muscle. M. sternocleidomastoideus. *See* Table of Muscles.

sternothyroid muscle. Depresses thyroid cartilage and larynx. *See* Table of Muscles—sternothyroideus.

Stevens-Johnson syndrome. Erythema multiforme with involvement of the conjunctiva and the oral tissues; dermatostomatitis.

Stillman's cleft. A fissure in the gum margin, seen in periodontal disease.

Stillman's cleft

stimulus (*stim'-yu-lus*). Any agent or impulse which excites or promotes a functional reaction.

stippled (*stip'-eld*). Having a mottled or spotted appearance with light and dark patches.

stoma (*sto'-mă*) (*pl.* stomata). A mouth, orifice, or opening.

stomacace (*stom-ak'-as-ē*). Ulcerative stomatitis (*q.v.*).

stomadeum (*sto-ma'-dĕ-um*). Stomodeum (*q.v.*).

stomatal (*sto'-mat-al*). Relating to a stoma.

stomatalgia (*sto-mat-al'-ji-ă*). Pain in the mouth.

stomatic (*sto-mat'-ik*). Relating to the mouth; oral.

stomatitis (*sto-mat-i'-tis*). Inflammation of the mouth. *acute ulcerative s.* A severe form of stomatitis, characterized by painful shallow ulcers on the tongue, lips and buccal mucosa and necrosis of the oral tissues. *aphthous s.* A form of stomatitis, often recurring, characterized by painful aphthae affecting the oral mucous membranes. *gangrenous s.* Noma, cancrum oris (*q.v.*). *herpetic s.* An oral form of herpes simplex (*q.v.*). *mycotic s.* Thrush (*q.v.*). *ulceromembranous s.* Acute ulcerative stomatitis (*q.v.*).

stomato-. Prefix signifying mouth.

stomatocace (*sto-mat-ok'-as-ē*). Acute ulcerative stomatitis (*q.v.*).

stomatodeum (*sto-mat-o'-dĕ-um*). Stomodeum (*q.v.*).

stomatodynia (*sto-mat-o-din'-ĭ-ă*). Pain in the mouth; stomatalgia.

stomatodysodia (*sto-mat-o-dis-o'-dĭ-ă*). Halitosis (*q.v.*).

stomatogastric (*sto-mat-o-gas'-trik*). Relating to the mouth and the stomach.

stomatognathic (*sto-mat-o-na'-thik*). Relating to the mouth and the jaws.

stomatolalia (*sto-mat-o-lal'-ĭ-ă*). Speaking through the mouth with the nostrils obstructed.

stomatologic, stomatological (*sto-mat-ol-oj'-ik*). Relating to stomatology.

stomatologist (*sto-mat-ol'-oj-ist*). A dentist, especially one concerned principally with oral diseases.

stomatology (*sto-mat-ol'-oj-ĭ*). The medical specialty concerned with the mouth and its diseases; sometimes used as synonymous with dentistry.

stomatomalacia (*sto"-mat-o-mal-a'-shĭ-ă*). Pathological softening of the mouth structures.

stomatomenia (*sto"-mat-o-me'-nĭ-ă*). Vicarious menstruation occurring in the mouth.

stomatomycosis (*sto"-mat-o-mi-ko'-sis*). Any fungous disease of the mouth.

stomatonecrosis (*sto"-mat-o-nek-ro'-sis*). Gangrene of the mouth, noma.

stomatonoma (*sto-mat-o-no'-mă*). Noma (*q.v.*).

stomatopanus (*sto-mat-o-pan'-us*). Inflammation of the oral lymph glands.

stomatopathy (*sto-mat-op'-ath-ĭ*). Any disease or disorder of the mouth.

stomatophylaxis (*sto"-mat-o-fil-aks'-is*). Prevention of diseases of the mouth and teeth; oral prophylaxis.

stomatophyma (*sto-mat-o-fi'-mă*). Any circumscribed swelling.

stomatoplasty (*sto-mat'-o-plast-ĭ*). Plastic surgery of the mouth.

stomatorrhagia (*sto-mat-or-a'-ji-ă*). Oral haemorrhage.

stomatoschisis (*sto-mat-os'-kis-is*). Hare lip (*q.v.*).

stomatosis (*sto-mat-o-'sis*). Stomatopathy.

stomenorrhagia (*sto-men-or-ra'-ji-ă*). Vicarious menstruation occurring in the mouth.

stomodeal plate. Buccopharyngeal membrane (*q.v.*).

stomodeum (*sto-mo-de'-um*). The primitive oral cavity in the embryo; an invagination of the embryonic ectoderm which later develops into the mouth and the upper pharynx.

stomoschisis (*sto-mos'-kis-is*). Mouth fissure.

stone (*stōn*). 1. A hard mineral concretion. 2. In prosthetic dentistry, a hard form of plaster of Paris, which sets like cement, and is used to make casts. 3. In conservative dentistry, a rotary abrasive head, mounted for use in a handpiece and used for grinding and smoothing.

straight enamel. Enamel in which the prismatic rods run straight.

straight sinus. A venous sinus formed by the union of the inferior sagittal sinus and the great cerebral vein. *See* Table of Veins—sinus rectus.

straight-pin teeth. Porcelain tooth facings having vertical pin attachments.

strawberry tongue. A tongue having prominent red fungiform papillae, seen in scarlet fever.

Streptococcus (*strep-to-kok'-us*). A genus of the Lactobacteriaceae family of bacteria, Gram-positive, seen as spherical cells forming chains.

Streptothrix (*strep'-to-thriks*). A genus of microorganisms of the Chlamydobacteriaceae, not clearly differentiated from *Actinomyces*.

stress (*stres*). 1. Force exerted by some mechanical means; pressure. 2. In dentistry, the pressure or force exerted by the mandibular teeth on the maxillary teeth during mastication.

striae of Retzius (M. G. Retzius, 1842-1919. Swedish anatomist). Retzius' lines (*q.v.*).

striate, striated (*stri'-āt*). Striped or streaked.

striated muscle. Muscle in which the fibres have

cross striations; voluntary muscle is usually of this type.

striation (*stri-a'-shun*). 1. A stripe or streak, or a series of stripes or streaks. 2. The condition of being striped.

stricture (*strik'-tyur*). Abnormal contraction of any aperture or vessel.

stridor (*stri'-dor*). A harsh whistling sound produced by the respiratory system.

stridor decutum. The noise made by the grinding of teeth.

stridor dentium. Grinding the teeth.

strip (*strip*). 1. A thin and narrow piece of material. 2. To peel off, in layers, so revealing the surface below. *separating s.* A strip of metal, having one side coated with a coarse abrasive, used to increase the space between adjacent teeth.

striped muscle. Striated muscle (*q.v.*).

stroma (*stro'-mă*). The tissue forming the matrix or the framework of an organ.

strophulus (*strof'-yu-lus*). A popular eruption sometimes seen on the gums of infants who are cutting teeth.

struma (*stru'-mă*). 1. Goitre (*q.v.*). 2. Scrofula (*q.v.*).

struma of the tongue. A thyroid tumour developing on the dorsum of the tongue.

stump *of a tooth.* That part of the tooth which remains after the destruction or removal of the crown.

styloglossal (*sti-lo-glos'-al*). Relating to the styloid process of the temporal bone and the tongue.

styloglossal muscle. Raises tongue. *See* Table of Muscles—styloglossus.

stylohyoid muscle. Raises tongue and hyoid bone, and draws them back. *See* Table of Muscles—stylohyoideus.

styloid (*sti'-loyd*). Long and pointed; like a stylus.

styloid process *of the temporal bone.* A sharp spine projecting downwards from the lower surface of the petrous portion of the temporal bone.

stylomandibular (*sti"-lo-man-dib'-yu-lar*). Relating to both the styloid process and the mandible.

stylomastoid (*sti"-lo-mas'-toyd*). Relating to both the styloid process and the mastoid process.

stylomastoid artery. Supplies the middle ear. *See* Table of Arteries—stylomastoidea.

stylomastoid foramen. An opening between the styloid and the mastoid processes, through which pass the stylomastoid artery and the facial nerve.

stylomaxillary (*sti"-lo-maks-il'-ar-i*). Relating to both the styloid process and the maxilla.

stylomyloid (*sti"-lo-mi'-loyd*). Relating to the styloid process and the molar teeth.

stylopharyngeal muscle. Raises and opens pharynx. *See* Table of Muscles—stylopharyngeus.

stylostaphyline (*sti-lo-staf'-il-in*). Relating to the styloid process of the temporal bone and the soft palate.

styptic (*stip'-tik*). An astringent haemostatic agent.

sub-. Prefix signifying *below, underneath.*

subacute (*sub-ak-ūt'*). Less severe than acute; the stage between chronic and acute illness.

subapical (*sub-a'-pik-al*). Below the apex.

subclavian artery. Two arteries, *right* from the brachiocephalic trunk, and *left* from the aortic arch, supplying the upper limb, spinal cord, brain, etc. *See* Table of Arteries—subclavia.

subclinical (*sub-klin'-ik-al*). Relating to a mild form of infection, with no clinical symptoms or manifestations.

subcranial (*sub-kra'-ni-al*). Below the cranium.

subcutaneous (*sub-ku-ta'-ně-us*). Beneath the skin.

subdental (*sub-den'-tal*). Below a tooth or teeth.

subgingival (*sub-jin'-jiv-al*). Below or beneath the gums.

subgingival calculus. Dental calculus attached to the tooth within with gingival pocket.

subgingival space. The space between the tooth enamel and the adjacent gingiva.

sub 289 **sub**

subglossal (*sub-glos'-al*). Below the tongue.

subglossitis (*sub-glos-i'-tis*). Inflammation of the sublingual tissues, or of the under side of the tongue.

subjugal (*sub-ju'-gal*). Beneath the malar bone.

sublingual (*sub-lin'-gwal*). Under the tongue.

sublingual artery. Supplies the lower jaw muscles, sublingual glands, etc. See Table of Arteries—sublingualis.

sublingual caruncle. Caruncula sublingualis (*q.v.*).

sublingual cyst. A ranula (*q.v.*).

sublingual duct. One of the ducts of the sublingual gland; Bartholin's duct.

sublingual fossa. A depression on the inner surface of the mandible, by the sublingual gland.

sublingual gland. One of a pair of salivary glands forming a ridge on either side of the floor of the mouth, below the tongue.

sublingual ptyalocele. Ranula (*q.v.*).

sublinguitis (*sub-lin-gwi'-tis*). Inflammation of the sublingual salivary glands.

subluxation (*sub-luks-a'-shun*). A partial dislocation or sprain.

submandibular (*sub-man-dib'-yu-lar*). Below the mandible.

submandibular gland. One of a pair of salivary glands lying on the inner edge of the mandible, in the region of the angle.

submandibular space. The space formed by the division of the deep cervical fascia about the submandibular salivary gland.

submarine alloy. One which can be used in those cavities which cannot be kept free from moisture.

submasseteric (*sub-mas-et-er'-ik*). Beneath the masseter muscle.

submasseteric space. The space between the masseter muscle and the ascending ramus of the mandible.

submaxilla (*sub-maks-il'-ă*). Mandible (*q.v.*).

submaxillaritis (*sub-maks-il-ar-i'-tis*). Adenitis occurring in one of the submandibular (submaxillary) glands.

submaxillary (*sub-maks-il'-ar-i*). Below the mandible or lower maxilla; submandibular.

submaxillary fossa. A depression on the inner surface of the mandible, by the submandibular, or submaxillary, glands.

submaxillary ganglion. A small ganglion on the hyoglossus muscle from which arises the nerve supply for the submandibular and sublingual glands.

submaxillary gland. Submandibular gland (*q.v.*).

submental (*sub-men'-tal*). Beneath the chin.

submental artery. Branch of facial artery, supplying the tissues below the jaw. See

Table of Arteries—submentalis.

subumcosa (*sub-myu-ko'-să*). The layer of tissue beneath the mucous membrane.

subnasale (*sub-na-za'-lĕ*). The point at which the nasal septum forms an angle with the philtrum; a cephalometric soft tissue landmark.

subnasion (*sub-na'-zĭ-on*). The lowest point on the midsagittal plane of the lower anterior margin of the nasal aperture.

suboccipital plexus. *See* suboccipital venous plexus.

suboccipital venous plexus. A plexus of veins found in the posterior portion of the scalp, draining into the vertebral vein. *See* Table of Veins—plexus venosus suboccipitalis.

suborbital (*sub-or'-bit-al*). Below the orbit.

suborbital fossa. Canine fossa (*q.v.*).

subperiosteal (*sub-per-ĭ-os'-tĕ-al*). Below or beneath the periosteum.

subperiosteal amputation. Amputation in which the stump of bone is covered by a periosteal flap.

subpulpal (*sub-pul'-pal*). Beneath the tooth pulp.

subpulpal wall. The base of the pulp-chamber in a cavity where the pulp has been removed and the pulp wall, therefore, does not exist.

subscription (*sub-skrip'-shun*). That part of a prescription containing directions for the preparation and compounding of the ingredients of a medicine.

subspinale (*sub-spin-a'-lĕ*). The deepest point on the midline of the premaxilla, between the anterior nasal spine and the lower border of the alveolus; a subsurface landmark.

substantia adamantina. Tooth enamel.

substantia spongiosa. Cancellous bone.

substructure (*sub'-struk-tyur*). *In dentistry*: That part of an implant denture which is covered by the tissues.

succedaneous (*suk-sed-a'-nĕ-us*). Succeeding and replacing.

succedaneous teeth. Those teeth in the permanent dentition which replace deciduous teeth.

suction chamber. Air chamber (*q.v.*).

suction disc. A flexible disc attached to the fitting surface of an upper denture in an attempt to improve its retention. This method is no longer used.

suction plate. A dental plate which is retained in the mouth by suction or atmospheric pressure.

sulcular (*sul'-kyu-lar*). Relating to a sulcus.

sulcus (*sul'-kus*). 1. A long groove or depression. 2. In dentistry, a long groove or depression in a tooth surface, the sides meeting at an angle.

alveolabial s. The sulcus between the lips and the alveolar process.

alveolingual s. The sulcus between the tongue and the alveolar process and the teeth.

gingival s. Gingival crevice (*q.v.*).

labiodental s. Vestibular lamina (*q.v.*).

lingual s., medial: A narrow and shallow groove on the dorsum of the tongue in the midline. *terminal:* A shallow groove on the posterior portion of the dorsum of the tongue, dividing it from the root of the tongue.

sulfonamide. *See* sulphonamide.

sulphonamide (*sul-fon'-am-īd*). Any one of the compounds derived from sulphanilamide, and used in the treatment of bacterial infections.

super-. Prefix signifying *above,* or *excessive.*

superciliary arch. The slight bulge over the medial part of the supra-orbital margin of the frontal bone.

superficial (*su-per-fish'-ĭ-al*). Immediately below the surface; as opposed to *deep.*

superior (*su-pe'-rĭ-or*). Above; higher of two parts.

superior sagittal sinus. A venous sinus draining into the transverse sinus. *See* Table of Veins—sinus sagittalis superior.

supermaxilla (*su-per-maks-il'-ă*). Maxilla (*q.v.*).

supernumerary (*su"-per-nu'-mer-ar-ĭ*). More than the usual number.

supernumerary tooth. An extra tooth, above the normal number occurring in the mouth.

superscription (*su-per-skrip'-shun*). The symbol R— *recipe*—at the beginning of a prescription.

supplemental cusp. Any abnormal or extra cusp on a tooth surface.

supplemental ridge. Any abnormal or extra ridge on a tooth surface.

supplemental tooth. A supernumerary tooth which is identical in form to the normal teeth in that area of the mouth in which it occurs.

suppuration (*sup-yur-a'-shun*). The formation and discharge of pus.

suppurative (*sup'-yur-at-iv*). Relating to or characterized by suppuration; pus-producing.

supra-. Prefix signifying *over, above, upon.*

supra-bony pocket. A form of true periodontal pocket (*q.v.*) in which the base of the pocket lies above the level of the alveolar bone.

suprabuccal (*su-pra-buk'-al*). Above, or in the upper part of, the cheek region.

suprabulge (*su-prǎ-bulj'*). That part of the tooth crown which converges on the occlusal surface.

supraclusion (*su-pră-klu'-zhun*). Supra-occlusion (*q.v.*).

supracondylism (*su"-pră-kon'-dil-izm*). Deviation of the mandibular condyles in an upward direction.

supragingival (*su-pră-jin'-jiv-al*). Above the gingival margin.

supragingival calculus. Dental calculus attached to the tooth above the gingival margin.

suprahyoid artery. Supplies muscles above the hyoid bone. *See* Table of Arteries—suprahyoidea.

supralabial (*su-pră-la'-bĭ-al*). Above the area of the lips.

supramandibular (*su-pră-man-dib'-yu-lar*). Above the mandible.

supramaxilla (*su-pră-maks-il'-ă*). Maxilla (*q.v.*).

supramaxillary (*su-pră-maks-il'-ar-ĭ*). 1. Relating to the maxilla. 2. Above the maxilla.

supramental (*su-pră-men'-tal*). Above the chin.

supramentale (*su"-pră-ment-a'-lĕ*). The deepest point on the midline of the mandible between the pogonion and the upper border of the alveolus; a subsurface landmark.

supra-occlusion (*su"-pră-ok-lu'-zhun*). The condition of having the teeth extruded from their sockets more that is normal, so that the occluding surfaces are above the normal occlusal plane.

supra-orbital (*su-pră-or'-bit-al*). Above the orbit.

supra-orbital artery. Supplies the supra-orbital muscles. *See* Table of Arteries—supraorbitalis.

supra-orbital nerve. Supplies skin of forehead and upper eyelid. *See* Table of Nerves—supraorbitalis.

supratrochlear artery. Supplies the antero-medial part of the forehead. *See* Table of Arteries—supratrochlearis.

supratrochlear nerve. Supplies skin of forehead, bridge of nose and upper eyelid. *See* Table of Nerves—supratrochlearis.

supraversion (*su-pră-ver'-shun*). Close-bite (*q.v.*).

surface anaesthesia. Local anaesthesia produced by the application of an agent externally before injection or some other operation liable to cause pain.

surface analgesia. Surface anaesthesia (*q.v.*).

surgery (*sur'-jer-ĭ*). That branch of medical science which is concerned with the manual or operative treatment of disease or injury.

surgical (*sur'-jik-al*). Relating to surgery.

sutural (*su'-tyur-al*). Relating to a suture.

suture (*su'-tyur*). 1. The line of junction between bones of the skull. 2. A surgical stitch.

intermandibular s. Symphysis menti (*q.v.*).

metopic s. The suture joining

the two halves of the frontal bone; the frontal suture. The sutures between facial bones are named after the bones which they join.

suture shears. A pair of scissors having short blades, the upper one straight and the lower one with a half-moon notch at the end, used for cutting ligatures or sutures.

Suzanne's gland (J. G. Suzanne, b. 1859. French physician). An oral mucous gland found in the alveolingual sulcus near the midline.

swage (*swāj*). 1. The contouring of metal using dies and counterdies. 2. A tool used in this work.

symbiosis (*sim-bi-o'-sis*). 1. An intimate association of two organisms of different species; it includes parasitism and commensalism. 2. More specifically it is used of an association which is to the mutual advantage of both partners.

symbiotic (*sim-bi-ot'-ik*). Relating to symbiosis.

symmetrical (*sim-et'-rik-al*). Relating to symmetry.

symmetry (*sim'-et-ri*). The correspondence or balance of parts about a common axis, or their regular distribution and relationship within a plane.

sympathetic abscess. A secondary abscess arising at some distance from the orginal focus of infection.

sympathetic nerve. Any one of the nerves of the sympathetic nervous system.

symphysion (*sim-fiz'-i-on*). The midpoint of the anterior border of the mandibular alveolar process; a craniometric point.

symphysis (*sim'-fis-is*). The line of junction or union of two bones.

symphysis mandibulae. Symphysis menti (*q.v.*).

symphysis menti. The central line of the chin, where the two halves of the mandible fused at birth; *also called* symphysis mandibulae, intermandibular suture.

symptom (*simp'-tom*). Any indication of the presence or course of a disease, either by functional or other change occurring in the patient.

symptomatic (*simp-tom-at'-ik*). Relating to a symptom or set of symptoms.

syn-. Prefix signifying *with, in association with.*

synalgia (*sin-al'-ji-ă*). Pain in one part caused by injury or a lesion in another, distant, part; referred pain.

synarthrosis (*sin-ar-thro'-sis*). A rigid joint with no intervening tissue.

syncheilia (*sin-ki'-li-ă*). Congenital imperforation of the mouth opening.

synchondrosis (*sin-kon-dro'-sis*). The joining of two bone surfaces by means of a cartilagenous band. Synchondroses occur principally in the skull.

syncleisis (*sin-kli'-sis*). Old term for occlusion.

syncope (*sin'-kop-ĕ*). Fainting; temporary unconsciousness caused by cerebral anaemia.

syndrome (*sin'-drōm*). A complex of symptoms, occurring together, which characterize one disease or lesion. For eponymous syndromes *see* under the name of the person first describing or exhibiting the syndrome.

synergist (*sin'-er-jist*). 1. A muscle or other organ which acts together with another. 2. A drug or chemical which aids the action of another.

synodontia (*si-no-don'-shĭ-ă*). The development of one tooth from two distinct tooth follicles.

synovia (*si-no'-vĭ-ă*); **synovial fluid.** A viscid, transparent alkaline and albumen-like fluid contained in joint cavities and tendon sheaths, secreted by the synovial membranes.

synovial (*si-no'-vĭ-al*). Relating to or secreting synovia.

synovial membrane. A membrane secreting synovial fluid, which covers the articulating surfaces and ligaments of a joint.

syphilis (*sif'-il-is*). A contagious venereal disease, manifesting oral and facial lesions.

syringe (*sir-inj'*). An instrument for injecting liquid or gas into the tissues or into a vessel or cavity.

air s. A syringe by means of which compressed air may be blown into a cavity or root canal to dry it or to remove loose debris.

systemic (*sis-tem'-ik*). 1. Relating to or affecting the whole body. 2. Relating to a system.

systole (*sis'-to-lĕ*). The contraction period in each heart beat.

systolic (*sis-tol'-ik*). Relating to the systole.

T

t.d.s. Abbreviation for *ter in die summendus*—to be taken three times a day; used in prescription writing.

t.i.d. Abbreviation for *ter in die*—three times a day; used in prescription writing.

tinct. Abbreviation for *tinctura*—a tincture; used in prescription writing.

tachy-. Prefix signifying *fast, swift.*

tactile (*tak'-tīl*). Relating to touch.

talon (*tal'-on*). A low distal cusp on an upper molar; an extension of the trigon.

talonid (*tal-o'-nid*). A low distal cusp on a lower molar; an extension of the trigonid.

tapinocephalic (*tap"-in-o-sef-al'-ik*). Having a low, flattened top to the cranium.

tapir-mouth. A condition characterized by loose, thickened lips, and caused by atrophy of the orbicularis oris muscle.

tartar (*tar'-tar*). Dental calculus (*q.v.*).

taste (*tāst*). The perception of flavour, a sensation produced by stimulation of the gustatory nerve endings in the tongue with a soluble substance.

taste buds. The end organs of the gustatory nerve, situated at the base of the filiform and vallate papillae on the tongue.

taurodontism (*taw-ro-dont'-izm*). Vertical deepening of the pulp cavity at the expense of the roots.

tectocephalic (*tek"-to-sef-al'-ik*). Having a roof-shaped cranium.

tectonic (*tek-ton'-ik*). Relating to plastic surgery or plastic restoration.

teeth (*tēth*). Plural of tooth (*q.v.*).
  anterior t. The incisors and canines.
  ciliiform t. Very fine, closely set teeth, as found in certain fish.
  cross-pin t. Artificial teeth which are attached by pins running at right-angles to the long axis of the tooth.
  fused t. Teeth, especially incisors, which have become joined together during development and erupt as one large tooth.
  milk t. Deciduous teeth.
  non-anatomical t. Artificial teeth having occlusal surfaces designed functionally rather than carved to reproduce the anatomic forms.

  posterior t. The premolars and molars.
  rake t. Descriptive of widely separated teeth.
  scalpriform t. The chisel-like incisors of a rodent, used for gnawing and cutting.
  sectorial t. The cutting teeth of Carnivora.
  setiform t. Ciliiform teeth (*q.v.*).
  straight-pin t. Porcelain tooth facings having vertical pin attachments.
  succedaneous t. Those teeth in the permanent dentition which replace deciduous teeth.
  tube t. Artificial teeth having a cylindrical hollow running from the occlusal surface to the cervix.

teething (*te'-thing*). The process of eruption of the deciduous teeth.

tegmen (*teg'-men*). A roof.

tegmen tympani. The bony division between the antrum tympanicum and the cranial cavity.

telalgia (*tel-al'-ji-ă*). Referred pain.

telangiectasia, telangiectasis (*tel"-an-ji-ek-ta'-zi-ă; tel"-an-ji-ek'-tas-is*). Dilation of the capillaries and small arteries, forming a type of angioma.

telangiectatic (*tel-an-ji-ek-tat'-ik*). Relating to telangiectasis.

telescope crown. A double metal crown, composed of two tubular or conical crowns, placed one over the other.

temper (*tem'-per*). To render a metal hard and elastic by successive heating and cooling.

temperature (*tem'-per-at-yur*). The degree of intensity of heat or cold.

template (*tem'-plāt*). A mould or pattern.

temple (*tem'-pl*). The flattened part of the head above the zygomatic arch and in front of the ear.

temporal (*tem'-por-al*). Relating to a temple (*anat.*).

temporal artery. Supplies the temporal fascia and zygomatic bone, etc.; three branches: deep, middle, superficial. *See* Table of Arteries—temporalis.

temporal bone. The bone of the temple, at the side and base of the skull.

temporal fossa. The depression on the side of the cranium in which the temporal muscle lodges.

temporal muscle. Retracts protruded mandible and closes mouth. *See* Table of Muscles—temporalis.

temporal process. The posterior angle of the zygomatic bone which articulates with the zygomatic process of the temporal bone.

temporo-. Prefix signifying *temple*.

temporomandibular (*tem"-por-o-man-dib'-yu-lar*). Relating to the temple and the mandible.

temporomandibular fossa. Glenoid fossa (*q.v.*).

temporomandibular joint. The joint between the mandible and the temporal bone; the articulating joint of the jaw.

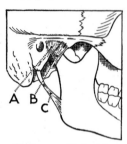

Temporomandibular joint

A Capsule.
B Temporomandibular ligament.
C Stylo-mandibular ligament.

temporomaxillary (*tem"-por-o-maks-il'-ar-ī*). Relating to the temporal bone or region and the maxilla.

temporoparietalis muscle. Tightens the scalp. *See* Table of Muscles.

tender (*ten'-der*). Sensitive; abnormally susceptible to pressure; sore.

tendinous (*ten'-din-us*). Relating to, having the characteristics of, a tendon.

tendon (*ten'-don*). The fibrous connective tissue which attaches muscle fibres to bone or to some other structure.

teno-. Prefix signifying *tendon*.

tenon (*ten'-on*). 1. Any projection fitting into a slot or mortise to make a joint. 2. In dentistry, the pin or post used to attach an artificial crown to a tooth root.

tensor palati muscle. M. tensor veli palatini. *See* Table of Muscles.

tensor tympani muscle. Tenses tympanic membrane. *See* Table of Muscles.

tensor veli palatini muscle. Tightens soft palate and opens pharyngotympanic tube. *Also called* tensor palati. *See* Table of Muscles.

tentorius nerve. Supplies the meninges. *See* Table of Nerves.

ter in die. Latin for *three times a day*; used in prescription writing, and abbreviated *t.i.d.*

ter in die summendus. Latin for *to be taken three times a day;* used in prescription writing, and abbreviated *t.d.s.*

teratoma (*ter-at-o'-mă*). A tumour, sometimes found on the palate, derived from germ cells and containing hair, teeth, etc., in places where these would not normally occur.

teratomatous (*ter-at-o'-mat-us*). Relating to or characteristic of a teratoma.

terminal lingual sulcus. A shallow groove on the

posterior portion of the dorsum of the tongue, dividing it from the root of the tongue.

terminal nerve. Supplies the nasal septum. *See* Table of Nerves—terminalis.

tetanus (*tet'-an-us*). An acute infectious disease, caused by the toxin of *Clostridium tetani*; it is characterized by tonic spasm of the voluntary muscles, and is generally fatal. *Also called* lockjaw.

tetany (*tet'-an-i*). A syndrome caused by abnormal calcium metabolism, and characterized by muscle spasm, cramp, and, occasionally, stridor.

tetarcone (*tet'-ar-kōn*). Tetartocone (*q.v.*).

tetartocone (*tet-ar'-to-kōn*). The distolingual cusp on a maxillary molar or premolar.

tetartoconid (*tet-ar″-to-ko'-nid*). The distolingual cusp on a mandibular molar or premolar.

tetra-. Prefix signifying *four*.

Tetracoccus (*tet″-ră-kok'-us*). A form of coccus in which cell division occurs in two planes, and the cells form into groups of four.

thalamostriate vein. With the choroid veins forms the internal cerebral vein. *See* Table of Veins—thalamostriata.

thecodont (*the'-ko-dont*). Having teeth which are contained in bony sockets or alveoli.

thelium (*the'-li-um*) (*pl.* thelia). A papilla.

therapeutic (*ther-ă-pyu'-tik*). Relating to treatment.

therapy (*ther'-ap-i*). The treatment of disease. *See* treatment.

thermal (*ther'-mal*). Relating to or characterized by heat.

thermocautery (*ther-mo-kaw'-ter-i*). The use of heated points for cauterization.

thermo - hardening material. A plastic material which undergoes a chemical change during processing, so that the material of the finished product is different from the original material; *e.g.* vulcanite.

thermo-plastic material. A plastic material in which the material of the finished product is chemically identical with the original, having undergone no change, except of shape, during processing; *e.g.* celluloid.

thick-necked. Descriptive of a tooth in which the mesiodistal diameter of the cervix is almost as great as that of the crown.

thirst (*thurst*). A desire for water or any other form of drink.

three-quarter crown. A form of shell crown, retained by cement and slotted into the tooth, covering all but the labial or buccal surface; *also called* a Carmichael crown.

throat (*thrōt*). The gullet; the pharynx and the fauces; the anterior part of the neck.

thrombus (*throm'-bus*). A blood clot formed and remaining in a blood vessel or in the heart which may cause serious obstruction to the circulation.

thrush (*thrush*). A type of moniliasis caused by infection with *Candida albicans*, and occurring generally in children and old people; it is characterized by the formation of whitish spots on the tongue and buccal mucous membrane.

thyro-arytenoid muscle. Closes larynx and relaxes vocal cords. *See* Table of Muscles — thyroarytenoideus.

thyrocele (*thi'-ro-sēl*). Goitre (*q.v.*).

thyrocervical trunk. The blood supply for the neck, thyroid gland, oesophagus and trachea. *See* Table of Arteries—truncus thyrocervicalis.

thyro-epiglottic muscle. Closes larynx. *See* Table of Muscles—thyro-epiglotticus.

thyroglossal (*thi-ro-glos'-al*). Relating to the thyroid gland and the tongue.

thyroglossal cyst. A cyst occurring in or arising from the thyroglossal duct.

thyroglossal duct. A duct extending from the thyroid gland to the base of the tongue; found in the embryo and occasionally persisting into adult life.

thyrohyoid (*thi"-ro-hi'-oyd*). Relating to both the thyroid gland and the hyoid bone.

thyrohyoid muscle. Depresses hyoid bone or raises larynx. *See* Table of Muscles—thyro-hyoideus.

thyroid artery. Supplies the thyroid gland, and the muscles of the neck, the oesophagus and the larynx; two branches: inferior and superior. *See* Table of Arteries—thyroidea.

thyroid gland. A large ductless endocrine gland situated in front of the trachea, and consisting of two lateral lobes joined by an isthmus. It is made up of follicles lined with epithelium, and secretes a colloid material.

thyroid veins. The veins draining the thyroid gland. *See* Table of Veins—thyroidea.

thyroidea ima artery. An inconstant branch of the brachiocephalic trunk, supplying the thyroid gland. *See* Table of Arteries.

thyropharyngeal muscle. Part of constrictor pharyngis inferior. *See* Table of Muscles—thyropharyngeus.

tic (*tik*). A spasmodic twitching, particularly of the facial muscles; a habit spasm.

tic douloureux. Spasmodic neuralgia affecting the facial nerves.

tin (*tin*). A silver-white metallic element, chemical symbol Sn. Used especially in metal alloys.

tinctura. Latin for *tincture*; used in prescription writing, and abbreviated *tinct.*

tincture (*tink'-tyur*). A solution of a medicinal substance in alcohol.

tinnitus (*tin'-it-us*). A ringing noise in the ears.

tissue (*tis'-yu*). A mass of similar cells performing a specialized function.

Tomes' fibres (Sir John Tomes, 1815-95. English dentist). Odontoblastic processes (*q.v.*).

Tomes' granular layer (Sir John Tomes, 1815-95. English dentist). The outer layer of interglobular dentine, near to the cemento-enamel junction.

Tomes' processes (Sir Charles Tomes, 1846-1928. English dentist). Ameloblastic processes (*q.v.*).

-tomy. Suffix signifying *cutting*, in surgery.

tone (*tōn*). 1. The state of slight tension maintained in healthy muscle tissue. 2. The quality of a sound.

tongue (*tung*). A muscular body situated in the floor of the mouth, attached to it by the lingual fraenum, and to the hyoid bone, the epiglottis and the soft palate by muscles and membranes; the organ of taste, and also an important adjunct in speech, mastication and deglutition.
adherent t. A tongue which is attached to both the floor and sides of the mouth by folds of mucous membranes.

bald t. A clean, smooth tongue having no prominent papillae on its surface, seen in conditions such as vitamin B deficiency.

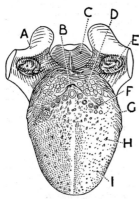

Tongue

A Palatopharyngeal arch.
B Foramen caecum.
C Epiglottis.
D Lingual follicles.
E Palatine tonsil.
F Vallate papillae.
G Foliate papillae.
H Filiform papillae.
I Fungiform papillae.

bifid t. One which is split down the midline from its tip.
black t. Black patches of pigmentation on the tongue, composed of hypertrophied filiform papillae and micro-organisms.

cardinal t. One which has a bright red appearance, being denuded of epithelium.
coated t. One having a whitish covering of the tongue surface containing food particles, epithelial debris and bacteria.
cobblestone t. Hypertrophy of the lingual papillae and a whitish coating, associated with leukoplakia and glossitis.
crocodile t. Scrotal tongue (*q.v.*).
frog t. Ranula (*q.v.*).
furred t. One having the papillae coated, thus giving the mucous membrane a whitish, furry appearance.
geographic t. A tongue having scaly patches, resembling maps, on the dorsal surface.
hairy t. One having hair-like papillae.
magenta t. Glossitis associated with ariboflavinosis, giving the tongue a magenta-coloured hue.
mappy t. Geographic tongue (*q.v.*).
parrot t. A horny, dry tongue, seen in typhus and low fever, which cannot be protruded.
scrotal t. A fissured and deeply furrowed tongue, its appearance being similar to the skin of the scrotum.
smoker's t. Leukoplakia (*q.v.*).
strawberry t. One having prominent red fungiform papillae, seen in scarlet fever.

wooden t. One affected by actinomycosis.

tongue, Clarke's. *See* Clarke's tongue.

tongue-tie. Abnormal shortness of the lingual fraenum, resulting in limited movement of the tongue; ankyloglossia.

tonsil (*ton'-sil*). One of the two almond-shaped bodies situated one on each side of the fauces, between the pillars.
lingual t. The collective term for the nodules, produced by the lingual follicles, and found on the pharyngeal portion of the dorsum of the tongue.

tonsillar (*ton'-sil-ar*). Relating to a tonsil.

tonsillar artery. Branch of the facial artery supplying the faucial tonsil and the base of the tongue. *See* Table of Arteries—tonsillaris.

tonsillectomy (*ton-sil-ek'-tom-i*). Surgical excision of the tonsils.

tonsillith (*ton'-sil-ith*). *See* tonsillolith.

tonsillitis (*ton-sil-i'-tis*). Inflammation of the faucial tonsils.
acute ulcerative t. An acute ulceration of the tonsils in which the predominant infection is fuso-spirochaetal; *also called* Vincent's angina.

tonsillolith (*ton-sil'-o-lith*). A calculus occurring in tonsillar tissue.

tonus (*to'-nus*). Tone (*q.v.*).

tooth (*tūth*) (*pl.* teeth). One of the calcified structures in the maxillary and mandibular alveolar processes in the mouth, retained in its socket by means of a root or roots. The tooth body consists of a central cavity, containing the dental pulp and surrounded by dentine; the exposed portion or crown is covered by enamel, and the root or roots by cementum. *See also* dentition; teeth.

axle t. Azzle tooth (*q.v.*).

azzle t. A molar tooth; obsolete term.

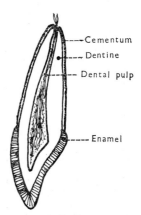

Tooth

canine t. A single-cusped tooth, resembling a dog's,

found between the lateral incisor and the first molar or premolar. There is one in each quadrant in both the deciduous and the permanent dentitions in man.

deciduous t. One of the teeth in the primary dentition in man.

eye t. A maxillary canine.

impacted t. One so placed in the jaw that it cannot erupt.

incisor t. A cutting tooth in the centre of the dental arch. There are two incisors in each quadrant in both the deciduous and the permanent dentitions in man, one *central* and one *lateral*.

malacotic t. A poorly formed tooth with a high susceptibility to dental caries.

molar t. One of the back, grinding teeth. There are two in each quadrant in the deciduous dentition, and three in each quadrant in the permanent dentition in man.

neonatal t. A deciduous tooth present in the mouth at birth or erupting within a few days of birth.

permanent t. A tooth in the second, permanent, dentition in man.

premolar t. A bicuspid, found in front of the molar teeth; there are two in each quadrant in the permanent dentition in man.

scion t. A tooth used for transplantation, to replace one extracted.

supernumerary t. An extra tooth, above the normal number occurring in the mouth.

supplemental t. A supernumerary tooth which is identical in form to the normal teeth in that area of the mouth in which it occurs.

wall t. A molar tooth.

wisdom t. A third molar; obsolete term.

tooth, Turner. *See* Turner tooth.

tooth angle. The angle formed by the surfaces of a tooth, named according to the surfaces which form it.

tooth germ. The enamel organ, dental papilla and sac; the rudiments of the developing tooth.

tooth hood. The flap of mucosa which remains over the occlusal surface of an erupting posterior tooth.

tooth pick. A small pointed implement, of wood or metal, used to remove surplus food from the interdental spaces.

tooth rash. Strophulus (*q.v.*).

tooth socket. An alveolus (*q.v.*).

toothache (*tūth′-āk*). Any pain associated with a tooth.

toothborne (*tūth′-born*). *In prosthetic dentistry:* Descriptive of a restoration which is held in position by the use of abutment teeth only, and is not supported by the tissues.

toothbrush (*tūth′-brush*). A small brush head on a long handle, designed for cleaning the teeth and applying stimulation to the gingival tissues.

toothpaste (*tūth'-pāst*). Paste form of dentifrice.

tophus (*to'-fus*). A calculus (*q.v.*); an obsolete term.

topical (*top'-ik-al*). Local (*q.v.*).

topical anaesthesia. Surface anaesthesia (*q.v.*).

Topinard's line (P. Topinard, 1830-1912. French anthropologist). The line joining the mental point to the glabella.

torque (*tork*). The rotation of a tooth about its long axis.

torsiversion (*tor-si-ver'-shun*). Rotation (*q.v.*).

torso-occlusion (*tor''-so-ok-lu'-zhun*). Rotation (*q.v.*).

torus (*tor'-us*). A rounded projection or swelling; a bony tumour.

torus mandibularis. An exostosis occurring on the lingual aspect of the mandible, between the canines and the molars.

torus palatinus. An exostosis occurring at the junction of the hard palate and the intermaxillary bone.

toxaemia (*toks-e'-mi-ă*). Generalized blood poisoning caused by the absorption of toxins from a local focus of infection into the blood stream.

toxic (*toks'-ik*). Relating to a poison; poisonous.

toxicoid (*toks'-ik-oyd*). Resembling a toxin or poison.

toxicosis (*toks-i-ko'-sis*). Any pathological condition due to poisoning.

toxin (*toks'-in*). A poisonous substance produced by animal or vegetable cells, more particularly by bacteria; if injected into animals or man it causes the formation of specific antibodies or antitoxins.

toxoid (*toks'-oyd*). A detoxified toxin which still retains its antigenic properties.

trabecula (*tră-bek'-yu-lă*). 1. A septum extending from the outer capsule or envelope into an organ. 2. The bony lamellae or spicules found in cancellous bone.

tracer (*tra'-ser*). A mechanical device used to record the pattern of mandibular movement.

trachea (*tră-ke'-ă*). The wind-pipe; a cartilagenous tube which extends from the lower end of the larynx to the bronchi.

tracheal (*tră-ke'-al*). Relating to the trachea.

tracheal artery. Branch of the inferior thyroid artery, supplying the trachea. *See* Table of Arteries—trachealis.

trachelomastoid muscle. M. longissimus capitis. *See* Table of Muscles.

traction (*trak'-shun*). The act of moving by pulling or drawing.

traction screw. A screw used in orthodontics to produce a pulling force sufficient to move a malposed tooth.

tragale (*tra-ga'-lĕ*). The most distal point on the tragus; a cephalometric soft tissue landmark.

tragus (*tra'-gus*). The small cartilagenous prominence over the external meatus of the ear.

transillumination (*trans-il-lu-min-a'-shun*). The illumination of the interior of an object by means of a strong light shining through the walls.

translucent (*trans-lu'-sent*). Capable of partial transmission of light rays, but not of a visual image.

transparent (*trans-par'-ent*). Clear; affording transmission of light rays, and able to be seen through.

transplantation (*trans-plant-a'-shun*). *Of the teeth*: The operation of removing teeth from one site and inserting them into empty sockets, either in the same mouth or in another mouth.

transposition (*trans-po-zish'-un*). *Of the teeth*: The interchange in position of two adjacent teeth.

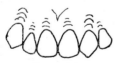

Transposition

transverse facial artery. Supplies the masseter muscle, the parotid gland and the facial skin. *See* Table of Arteries—transversa faciei.

transverse muscle of the tongue. Changes the shape of the tongue. *Also called* lingualis transversus. *See* Table of Muscles—transversus linguae.

transverse sinus. A venous sinus, found in the groove on the occipital bone and the posterior inferior angle of the parietal bone, into which drain the superior sagittal or the straight sinus, the cerebral and cerebellar veins and the superior petrosal sinus. *See* Table of Veins—sinus transversus.

transversion (*trans-ver'-shun*). Transposition (*q.v.*).

transversus colli muscle. M. longissimus cervicis. *See* Table of Muscles.

transversus colli nerve. Supplies the skin of the anterior triangle of the neck. *See* Table of Nerves.

transversus menti muscle. Superficial fibres of M. depressor anguli oris. *See* Table of Muscles.

trapezius muscle. Raises shoulder and draws back scapula. *See* Table of Muscles.

trauma (*traw'-mă*). Any injury or wound.

traumatic (*traw-mat'-ik*). Relating to or produced by trauma.

traumatic cyst. A cyst caused by some traumatic injury.

traumatic occlusion. Any form of malocclusion which causes damage to the teeth or to the periodontal tissues.

traumatism (*traw'-mat-izm*). A condition resulting from a trauma.

periodontal t. Degenerative changes occurring in the periodontium as a result of excessive stress transmitted through the teeth over a prolonged period of time.

traumatogenic (*traw''-mat-o-jen'-ik*). Capable of producing trauma.

tray (*tra*).

impression t. A metal receptacle in which wax or plastic impression material is placed when taking mouth impressions.

Treacher-Collins syndrome (E. Treacher-Collins, 1862-1919. English ophthalmologist). Mandibulo-facial dysostosis (*q.v.*).

treatment (*trēt'-ment*). 1. The means used to combat or cure a disease. 2. The care and management of a sick patient.

trench mouth. 1. Acute ulcerative gingivitis (*q.v.*). 2. Acute ulcerative stomatitis (*q.v.*).

Treponema (*trep-on-e'-mă*). A genus of the Spirochaetaceae family of bacteria, a thread-like, spiral microorganism, pathogenic to man.

tri-. Prefix signifying *three*.

trial plate. A temporary dental plate of soft material or wax, used to hold the artificial teeth for fitting in the mouth.

triangle (*tri'-an-gl*). Any three-sided plane figure.

cephalic t. Formed by lines from the chin to forehead and occiput, and a line joining the occiput to the forehead.

facial t. Formed by lines joining alveolar and nasal points and the basion.

palatal t. Formed by a line across the greatest transverse diameter of the palate, and lines from either end of this base to the alveolar point.

For eponymous triangles *see* under the personal name by which the triangle is known.

triangles of the neck.

anterior. Formed by anterior margin of sternocleidomastoid, anterior median line of neck, base of mandible, continued to the mastoid process; apex at the sternum.

carotid. Formed by sternocleidomastoid, superior belly of omohyoid, styloid, and posterior belly of digastric muscles.

digastric. Formed by base of mandible, continued to mastoid process, posterior belly of digastric and styloid, and anterior belly of digastric muscles.

muscular. Formed by anterior margin of sternocleidomastoid, median line of neck from sternum to hyoid bone, and superior belly of omohyoid.

occipital. Formed by sternocleidomastoid, trapezius, and omohyoid, splenius capitis, levator scapulae, and scalenus medius et posterior muscles.

posterior. Formed by sternomastoid, anterior margin of trapezius and middle third of clavicle. Divided by inferior belly of omohyoid into occipital and supraclavicular triangles.

subclavian. See supraclavicular.

submandibular, or *submaxillary.* See digastric.

submental, or *suprahyoid.* Formed by anterior belly of digastric, hyoid bone, and mylohyoid muscles; apex at mandible.

supraclavicular. Formed by inferior belly of omohyoid, clavicle and lower part of posterior border of sternocleidomastoid.

triangular muscle. M. depressor anguli oris. *See* Table of Muscles.

tribe (*trīb*). An intermediate division in biological classification, coming between the family and the genus.

trichoglossia (*trik-o-glos'-ī-ǎ*). Hairy tongue (*q.v.*).

Trichomonas (*trik-o-mo'-nas*). A genus of flagellate protozoa of the class Mastigophora and having a pear-shaped body and several flagellae.

T. buccalis. A form of Trichomonas found in the mouth.

triconodont (*tri-kon'-o-dont*). A tooth having three cusps in a line.

tricuspid (*tri-kus'-pid*). Having three cusps.

trigeminal nerve. The fifth cranial nerve, which divides into N. ophthalmicus, N. maxillaris, and N. mandibularis. *See* Table of Nerves—trigeminus.

trigon (*tri'-gon*). The three main cusps, in a group, of a trituberculate maxillary molar.

trigonid (*tri-go'-nid*). The first three cusps on a mandibular molar.

trigonodont (*trig'-on-o-dont*). A tooth having three cusps in the form of a triangle.

trilobate (*tri-lo'-bāt*). Having three lobes.

trimmer (*trim'-er*). Any instrument used to trim or shape.

gingival margin t. A type of chisel designed for bevelling gingival enamel margins.

triple-angle. *Of an instrument:* Having three angles in the shank.

trismus (*triz'-mus*). Lockjaw, caused by muscle spasm, and generally associated with tetanus.

tritocone (*tri'-to-kōn*). The distobuccal cusp on a maxillary premolar; not found in man.

tritoconid (*tri-to-ko'-nid*). The distobuccal cusp on a mandibular premolar; not found in man.

tritubercular (*tri"-tu-ber'-kyu-lar*). Having three cusps or tubercles.

triturate (*trit'-yu-rāt*). 1. To rub to a fine powder. 2. Trituration (*q.v.*).

trituration (*trit-yu-ra'-shun*). 1. The reduction of a solid substance to a powder by rubbing. 2. A substance so reduced.

trochlear nerve. The fourth cranial nerve, supplying the obliquus superior muscle of the eyeball. *See* Table of Nerves—trochlearis.

truncus brachiocephalicus. *See* Table of Arteries.

truncus thyrocervicalis. *See* Table of Arteries.

try-in. A preliminary fitting of a restoration, at any stage of its construction, to determine occlusal relationships, etc.

tube (*tyūb*). A hollow cylindrical body open at both ends.
pharyngotympanic t. A canal connecting the upper pharynx with the middle ear.

tube, Eustachian. Pharyngotympanic tube (*q.v.*).

tube teeth. Artificial teeth having a cylindrical hollow running from the occlusal surface to the cervix.

tubercle (*tyu'-ber-kl*). 1. A nodule. 2. A rounded eminence on a bone. 3. The lesion produced by the tuberculosis bacillus.
genial t. One of two elevations on either side of the mental protuberance on the mandible.
maxillary t. A small rough tubercle at the distal end of the maxillary alveolar process.

mental t. One of two small projections of bone on the inner surface of the mandible on either side of the symphysis menti. *Also called* the mental spine.
paramolar t. An additional cusp occurring on the mesiobuccal aspect of a second or third molar; it is thought to be a rudimentary paramolar.

tubercle of Carabelli. *See* Carabelli's tubercle.

tuberculate (*tu-ber'-kyu-lāt*). Having tubercles.

tuberculated (*tu-ber'-kyu-la-ted*). Covered with tubercles.

tuberosity (*tyu-ber-os'-it-ĭ*). A broad protuberance on a bone.

tubule (*tyu'-byūl*). A small tube.
dentinal t. One of the minute tubes in the dentine, radiating from the pulp chamber to the amelodentinal junction.

tufts (*tufts*).
enamel t. Bundles of poorly calcified enamel rods extending into the tooth enamel from the amelodentinal junction.

tumefaction (*tyu-mĕ-fak'-shun*). The state of being or becoming swollen; a swelling.

tumour (*tyu'-mor*). An abnormal mass of tissue, the growth of which exceeds and is uncoordinated with that of the normal tissues, and persists in the same excessive manner after cessation of the stimuli which evoked the change (Willis). It may also be used in the more general sense of any localized swelling.

tumour, Krompecher's. *See* Krompecher's tumour.

turbid (*tur'-bid*). Cloudy.

turgid (*tur'-jid*). Swollen, congested.

Turner tooth (J. G. Turner, 1870-1955. British dentist). A permanent tooth which has been damaged in some way during development because of infection or trauma affecting its deciduous predecessor.

turrecephalic, turricephalic (*tur-ĕ-sef-al'-ik*). Oxycephalic (*q.v.*).

tusk (*tusk*). A very large canine or incisor protruding beyond the lips.

twin wire arch, Johnson. *See* Johnson twin wire arch.

twinning (*twin'-ing*). *In dentistry:* The development of two separate teeth from one follicle; schizodontia.

two-piece crown. A crown made from a contoured metal band joined to a swaged cap.

tylosis linguae (*ti-lo-'sis lin'-gwa*). Lingual leukoplakia (*q.v.*).

tympanic (*tim-pan'-ik*). Relating to the tympanum.

tympanic artery. Supplies the tympanum and tensor tympani muscle; four branches: anterior, posterior, inferior, superior. *See* Table of Arteries—tympanica.

tympanic nerve. Supplies the mucosa of the middle ear and the pharyngotympanic tube. *See* Table of Nerves—tympanicus.

tympanum (*tim'-pan-um*). The middle ear, the eardrum.

tyndallization (*tin-dal-i-za'-shun*). (J. Tyndall, 1820-93. English physicist). A method of sterilizing culture media by exposure to steam at 100°C on three successive days, for about 30 minutes each day.

U

ung. Abbreviation for *unguentum*—an ointment; used in prescription writing.

ula (*yu'-lă*). The gingivae.

ulaemorrhagia (*yu-lem-or-a'-ji-ă*). Bleeding from the gums.

ulaganectesis (*yu-lag-an-ek'-tes-is*). Irritation in the gums.

ulalgia (*yu-lal'-ji-ă*). Pain in the gums.

ulatrophy (*yu-lat'-rof-ĭ*). Gingival recession.

ulcer (*ul'-ser*). A localized lesion on the surface of the skin or mucous membrane, with superficial necrosis and tissue loss resulting in the exposure of the deeper tissues in an open sore.

aphthous u. Aphthae (*q.v.*) which break down into at shallow and painful ulcer.

dental u. An ulcer on the oral mucosa produced by local trauma.

rodent u. A basal-cell carcinoma of superficial origin, arising in the epidermis, and occurring generally on the face or neck.

serpiginous u. One which is constantly spreading in one direction whilst healing in another.

ulcer, Jacob's. *See* Jacob's ulcer.

ulceration *(ul-ser-a'-shun).* The formation of ulcers.

ulcerative *(ul'-ser-at-iv).* Relating to or characterized by ulceration.

ulcerative gingivitis, acute. An acute ulcerative condition of the gingivae in which the predominant micro-organisms are a mixture of Fusiformis fusiformis and Borrelia vincentii; *also called* Vincent's infection.

ulcerative gingivitis, necrotizing. Acute ulcerative gingivitis *(q.v.).*

ulcerative stomatitis, acute. A severe form of stomatitis, characterized by painful shallow ulcers on the lips, and buccal mucosa, and necrosis of the oral tissues.

ulcerative tonsillitis, acute. An acute ulceration of the tonsils in which the predominant infection is fusospirochaetal; *also called* Vincent's angina.

ulceromembranous *(ul''-ser-o-mem'-bran-us).* Characterized by ulceration accompanied by a membranous exudation.

ulceromembranous gingivitis. Acute ulcerative gingivitis *(q.v.).*

ulceromembranous stomatitis. Acute ulcerative stomatitis *(q.v.).*

ulceronecrotic *(ul''-ser-o-nek-rot'-ik).* Characterized by ulceration accompanied by necrosis.

ulcerous *(ul'-ser-us).* Relating to or characterized by ulcers.

ulectomy *(yu-lek'-tom-i).* Gingivectomy *(q.v.).*

ulemorrhagia. *See* ulaemorrhagia.

uletic *(yu-let'-ik).* Relating to the gingiva.

ulitis *(yu-li'-tis).* Generalized inflammation of the gingiva.

ulo-. Prefix signifying 1. *a scar;* 2. *the gingivae.*

ulocace *(yu-lok'-as-ĕ).* Gum ulceration.

ulocarcinoma *(yu''-lo-kar-sin-o'-mă).* Carcinoma affecting the gums.

uloglossitis *(yu''-lo-glos-i'-tis).* Inflammation of both the gums and the tongue.

uloncus *(yu-lon'-kus).* Any tumour or swelling of the gums.

ulorrhagia *(yu-lor-a'-ji-ă).* Bleeding from the gums.

ulorrhoea *(yu-lor-e'-ă).* Oozing of blood from the gums.

ulotomy *(yu-lot'-om-i).* Incision of the gums.

ulotropsis *(yu''-lo-trop'-sis).* The nourishing and revitalizing of the gums by massage.

ultra-. Prefix signifying *excessive* or *beyond.*

unciform (*un'-sĭ-form*). Hook -shaped.

undercut (*un'-der-kut*). That part of a tooth or cavity which provides, by design or fortuitously, an area of resistance to the withdrawal of a clasp or restoration.

underhung bite. A form of malocclusion in which the mandibular anterior teeth occlude with the labial surfaces of their maxillary antagonists.

unerupted (*un-er-up'-ted*). Relating to a tooth which has not come through the gums, either in the normal course or because it lacks the physiological impetus.

unguentum (*un-gwen'-tum*). Latin for *ointment*; used in prescription writing, and abbreviated *ung*.

uni-. Prefix signifying *one*.

unicuspid (*yu-nĭ-kus'-pid*). Unitubercular (*q.v.*).

unicuspidate (*yu-nĭ-kus'-pid-āt*). Unitubercular (*q.v.*).

unilateral (*yu-nĭ-lat'-er-al*). Occurring on or relating to one side only.

unilocular cyst. A cyst having only one cavity.

united enamel epithelium. Reduced enamel epithelium (*q.v.*).

unitubercular (*yu-nĭ-tyu-ber'-kyu-lar*). Having only one tubercle or cusp.

unstriated muscle. Smooth muscle (*q.v.*).

unstriped muscle. Smooth muscle (*q.v.*).

uranal angle. The angle formed at the junction of

lines connecting the highest point on the sagittal curvature of the palate with the premaxillary point and with the posterior nasal spine.

uraniscochasma (*yur'-an-is-ko-kaz'-mă*). Cleft palate.

uraniscolalia (*yur"-an-is-ko-lal'-ĭ-ă*). Defective speech caused by a palatal cleft.

uranisconitis (*yur"-an-is-kon-i'-tis*). Inflammation of the palate.

uraniscoplasty (*yur-an-is'-ko-plast-ĭ*). Uranoplasty (*q.v.*).

uraniscorrhaphy (*yur-an-is-kor'-af-ĭ*). Palatorrhaphy (*q.v.*).

uraniscus (*yur-an-is'-kus*). The palate.

urano-. Prefix signifying *palate*.

uranoplastic (*yur-an-o-plast'-ik*). Relating to uranoplasty.

uranoplasty (*yur-an-o-plast'-ĭ*). Surgical closure of a hard palate cleft.

uranoplegia (*yur-an-o-ple'-jĭ-ă*). Palatal paralysis; paralysis affecting the soft palate muscles.

uranorrhaphy (*yur-an-or'-af-ĭ*). Palatorrhaphy (*q.v.*).

uranoschisis (*yur-an-os'-kis-is*). Cleft palate.

uranoschism (*yur-an'-o-sizm*). Cleft palate.

uranostaphyloplasty (*yur-an-o-staf"-il-o-plast'-ĭ*). Repair of a cleft involving both hard and soft palates, by means of plastic surgery.

uranostaphylorrhaphy (*yur-an-o-staf"-il-or'-af-ĭ*). Closure of a cleft involving both the hard and soft palate with sutures.

uranostaphyloschisis (*yur″-an-o-staf-il-os′-kis-is*). Palatal fissure affecting both the hard and soft palates.

uranosteoplasty (*yur-an-os′-tē-o-plast-ĭ*). Uranoplasty (*q.v.*).

uveal artery. A. ciliaris posterior brevis. *See* Table of Arteries.

uvula (*yu′-vyu-lă*). A small muscular appendage hanging from the posterior border of the soft palate.

uvular (*yu′-vyu-lar*). Relating to the uvula.

uvular muscle. Forms the uvula. *See* Table of Muscles —uvulae.

uvulitis (*yu-vyu-li′-tis*). Inflammation of the uvula.

uvuloptosis (*yu-vyu-lop-to′-sis*). A relaxed condition of the uvula.

V

vaccine (*vak′-sēn*). 1. Lymph obtained from a cowpox vesicle and used in inoculation against smallpox. 2. Any material used for preventive inoculation against a specific disease.

vacuum (*vak′-yu-um*). A space from which the air content has been exhausted.

vacuum chamber. Air chamber (*q.v.*).

vaginate (*vaj′-in-āt*). Within a sheath.

vagus nerve. The tenth cranial nerve, supplying the striate muscles and mucosa of the pharynx and larynx. *See* Table of Nerves.

Valentin's ganglion (G. G. Valentin, 1810-1833. German physiologist). A pseudoganglion occurring at the junction of the posterior and middle branches of the dental nerve.

vallate (*val′-āt*). Having a surrounding wall or rim.

vallate papilla. Any one of the large flat papillae, having a surrounding rim, found in front of the terminal sulcus of the tongue.

Valleix's aphthae (F. L. Valleix, 1807-55. French physician). Bednar's aphthae (*q.v.*).

varnish (*var′-nish*). A solution of resin or resins, which, when painted on thinly, leaves a clear hard coat over the surface treated.
sandarac v. A solution of transparent resin in alcohol, used as a separating fluid and protective coating for plaster casts in dentistry.
separating v. One used to coat a plaster mould and prevent adhesion of fresh plaster poured in to produce a model.

vascular (*vas′-kyu-lar*). Relating to or composed of vessels.

vasoconstrictor (*va-zo-kor-strikt′-or*). A nerve, or some external agent, which causes vascular contraction.

vasodentine (*va-zo-den′-tēn*). Dentine containing blood vessels.

vasodilator (*va-zo-di-la'-tor*). A nerve, or external agent, which causes vascular dilatation.

vasomotor nerve. Any nerve which controls the calibre of blood and lymph vessels; it may be a *vasodilator* or a *vasoconstrictor*.

vault (*vawlt*). Any arch- or dome-like structure; used in dentistry for the roof of the mouth.

Veau's operation (V. Veau, b. 1871. French surgeon). An operation for repair of cleft palate which included dissection and suturing up of the nasal mucosa.

vehicle (*ve'-ikl*). *In medicine:* Any substance employed as a medium for the administration of a medicine.

vein (*vān*). One of the blood vessels which carries de-oxygenated blood to the heart.
pulmonary v. One of the short thick vessels conveying oxygenated blood from the lungs to the heart.

velar (*ve'-lar*). Relating to a velum.

velopharyngeal (*ve"-lo-far-in'-jĕ-al*). Relating to the soft palate and the pharynx.

velosynthesis (*ve-lo-sin'-thes-is*). Repair of a cleft in the soft palate.

velum (*ve'-lum*). Any veil-like structure.
artificial v. An appliance used in prosthetic treatment of a cleft of the soft palate.

velum palatinum. The soft palate.

venous (*ve'-nus*). Relating to a vein.

venter (*ven'-ter*). 1. The stomach or abdomen. 2. Any hollow, belly-shaped part, as the belly of a muscle.

ventral (*ven'-tral*). Relating to a belly, the abdomen or any other venter.

venule (*ven'-yul*). A minute vein.

vermiform (*ver'-mi-form*). Worm-like.

vermilion border. The red margin of the lips.

verrucous crown. A wart-like overgrowth of enamel on a tooth crown.

version (*ver'-shun*). The act of turning, as of teeth during orthodontic treatment.

vertebra (*ver'-teb-rǎ*) (*pl.* vertebrae). One of the bones of the spinal column.

vertebral (*ver'-te-bral*). Relating to a vertebra or to vertebrae.

vertebral artery. Supplies the cerebellum, the cerebrum, spinal cord, meninges and neck muscles. *See* Table of Arteries—vertebralis.

vertebral veins. *See* Table of Veins—vertebralis.

vertical muscle of the tongue. Changes the shape of the tongue. *Also called* lingualis verticalis. *See* Table of Muscles—verticalis linguae.

vertical overlap. Overbite (*q.v.*).

verticomental (*ver-tik-o-men'-tal*). Relating to the crown of the head and the chin.

vertigo (*ver'-tig-o*). A sensation of loss of equilibrium in which the patient either feels the world is revolving round him or that he is revolving in space.

vesicle (*ve'-sikl*). 1. A small bladder or sac containing liquid. 2. A blister.

vesiculation (*ves-ik-yu-la'-shun*). The formation of vesicles.

vessel (*ves'-el*). Any tube or canal conveying fluid especially lymph or blood.

vestibular (*vest-ib'-yu-lar*). Relating to the vestibule.

vestibular lamina. The oral ectoderm in the embryo which later divides to form the vestibule of the oral cavity.

vestibular nerve. *See* Table of Nerves—vestibularis.

vestibule (*vest'-ib-yūl*). A cavity or space serving as the entrance to a canal.

vestibule *of the ear.* The oval cavity in the inner ear leading to the cochlea.

vestibule *of the mouth.* The space between the lips and cheek and the gums and teeth.

vestibulocochlear nerve. The eighth cranial nerve, dividing into N. cochlearis and N. vestibularis. *See* Table of Nerves—vestibulocochlearis.

vestige (*vest'-ij*). A rudimentary part or remnant which at some stage was fully developed and functional.

vestigial (*vest-ij'-ĭ-al*). Relating to a vestige; rudimentary.

viable (*vi'-abl*). Able to live of itself.

viability (*vi-ab-il'-it-ĭ*). Ability to live after birth.

vibration (*vi-bra'-shun*). Any rapid to-and-fro movements; oscillation.

vibrator, oral. A prosthetic appliance designed to provide a method of speaking for those patients who, either from operation or paralysis, have no current of air passing through the mouth. It consists of a flexible diaphragm fitted into the palate of an upper denture and vibrated by means of electric batteries, thus creating the necessary current of air.

Vibrio (*vib'-ri-o*). A genus of the Spirillaceae family of bacteria, seen as short curved rods.

vicarious (*vik-a'-ri-us*). 1. Relating to a normal process occurring in an abnormal position or under abnormal conditions. 2. Acting as a substitute.

Vidius' nerve (V. Vidius [G. Guido], 1500-69. Italian anatomist and physician). N. canalis pterygoidei. *See* Table of Nerves.

Vignal's bacillus (G. Vignal, 19th century French physiologist). Leptotrichia buccalis (*q.v.*).

villiform (*vil'-ĭ-form*). Hair-like, having hairlike projections.

Vincent's angina (J. H. Vincent, 1862-1950. French physician and bacteriologist). Acute ulcerative tonsillitis (*q.v.*).

Vincent's infection (J. H. Vincent, 1862-1950. French physician and bacteriologist). Acute ulcerative gingivitis (*q.v.*).

vinculum (*vin'-kyu-lum*). A ligament or fraenum.

vinculum linguae. The lingual frenum.

Vinson syndrome (P. P. Vinson, b. 1890. American physician). *See* Plummer-Vinson syndrome.

Virchow's angle (R. L. K. Virchow, 1821-1902. German pathologist). The angle formed at the intersection of a line joining the nasofrontal suture and the most prominent point on the lower edge of the maxillary alveolar process with a line joining the lower border of the orbit to the external auditory meatus.

virulence (*vir'-ul-ens*). 1. Malignancy. 2. The infectiousness of a micro-organism.

virulent (*vir'-u-lent*). Toxic, poisonous.

virus (*vi'-rus*). A complex organic particle, of submicroscopic dimensions, capable of growth and reproduction only within the cells of the host organism it infects.

viscera (*vis'-er-ă*). Plural of viscus (*q.v.*).

visceral (*vis'-er-al*). Relating to the viscera.

viscid (*vis'-id*). Sticky, adhesive.

viscous (*vis'-kus*). Sticky, adhesive, viscid.

viscosity (*vis-kos'-it-ĭ*). The property or state of being glutinous or adhesive.

viscus (*vis'-kus*) (*pl.* viscera (*vis'-er-ă*)). Any one of the organs in either the thoracic, abdominal or pelvic cavity; used particularly of those organs in the abdomen.

vital (*vi'-tal*). Living; relating to life.

vitality (*vi-tal'-it-ĭ*). The state of being alive.

vitalometer (*vi-tal-om'-et-er*). A name given to an apparatus used to test for the vitality of tooth pulp.

vitreodentine (*vit"-re-o-den'-tēn*). Vitreous dentine (*q.v.*).

vitreous (*vit'-rĕ-us*). Relating to glass, glassy.

vitreous dentine. A very hard type having few dentinal tubules.

vitro-dentine (*vit"-ro-den'-tēn*). Vitreous dentine (*q.v.*).

Vogt's angle (K. Vogt, 1817-95. German physiologist). The angle formed between the nasobasilar and the alveolonasal lines.

voluntary muscle. Any muscle which is directly under the control of the will.

vomer (*vo'-mer*). The flat bone forming the posterior

and lower portion of the nasal septum.

vomerine (*vo'-mer-īn*). Relating to the vomer.

vomit (*vom'-it*). 1. To cast up from the stomach through the mouth. 2. The substance vomited.

vomiting (*vom'-it-ing*). The forcible expulsion of the contents of the stomach upwards through the mouth.

vomitus (*vom'-it-us*). Vomit (*q.v.*, 2).

von Korff's fibres. Precollagenous fibres of the dental pulp, which pass between the odontoblasts in developing dentine and undergo a collagenous change, becoming incorporated in the dentine matrix.

vulcanite (*vul'-kan-īt*). A thermo-hardening material produced by heating raw rubber with sulphur; the degree of hardness depends on the amount of sulphur used.

vulcanization (*vul-kan-i-za'-shun*). The process of making vulcanite.

vulcanize (*vul'-kan-īz*). To treat rubber with sulphur so as to render it flexible or hard.

W

wall *of a cavity:* One of the sides of a cavity. Cavity walls take the names of the surfaces towards which they face.

wall-tooth. A molar tooth; obsolete term.

Walther's duct (A. F. Walther, 1688-1746. German anatomist). The duct of the sunblingual salivary gland.

wandering *of the teeth:* The vertical or horizontal displacement of teeth due to destruction of the periodontal membrane.

wandering abscess. An abscess which tracks through the tissues and finally comes to a point some distance from its original site.

wandering rash. Geographic tongue (*q.v.*).

wang tooth. A molar tooth; obsolete term.

Wardill's operation (W. E. M. Wardill, 1895-1961. English surgeon). Operation for the repair of cleft palate by dividing the long muco-periosteal flaps obliquely and rotating and sliding them to obtain greater length of the soft palate without loss of continuity.

warp (*worp*). To alter in shape, becoming twisted or bulging; used of the effect on material such as impression plaster or vulcanite left exposed to the air for too long.

watchmaker's broach. A tapered broach, sharp-angled and having four or five sides, used to enlarge root canals.

water fluoridation. The adjustment of the level of fluoride ion in the water supply to an optimum concentration of 1 p.p.m., to reduce the incidence of dental caries in a community. Usually achieved by the addition of small quantities of sodium fluoride in areas where the naturally occurring concentration is below the optimum.

wax (waks). A plastic substance obtained from plants or from deposits of insects. That used for dental impressions is generally beeswax.

waxing up. The construction and contouring of a wax base plate for an artificial denture, and the temporary attachment of teeth to it with wax.

Weber's glands (E. H. Weber, 1795–1878. German anatomist). The lateral lingual glands.

Weil's basal layer (L. A. Weil, 19th century German dentist). A transparent layer of connective tissue cells inside the odontoblast layer of the tooth pulp.

Weisbach's angle (A. W. Weisbach, 1837–1914. Austrian anthropologist). The angle formed at the alveolar point by lines from the basion and the midpoint of the frontal suture.

Weston crown (H. Weston, fl. 1883. American dentist). A porcelain pivot crown attached to the tooth by means of a flat post riveted to the crown before insertion.

whartonitis (wor-ton-i'-tis). Inflammation of Wharton's duct.

Wharton's duct (T. Wharton, 1614–73. English anatomist). The duct through which saliva from the sublingual and submandibular glands flows into the mouth; its openings are on either side of the lingual frenum.

wheel (whēl). A solid round disk or a hollow round frame capable of revolving on a central axis; wheels of different sizes and materials are used in dentistry in the handpiece of a dental engine for polishing or cutting.

Willis's circle (T. Willis, 1621–75. English anatomist and physician). The circular arterial system at the base of the brain, formed by the anterior and posterior cerebral, the anterior and posterior communicating, and the internal carotid arteries.

window crown. An acrylic veneer gold crown, covering all but the labial or buccal surface of the tooth, and frequently used as a bridge abutment.

wing, Ingrassia's. See Ingrassia's wing.

Winter's elevator (G. B. Winter, contemporary American oral surgeon). An elevator for removing lower third molars.

wire (wīr). 1. Fine flexible metal rods or metal thread used in surgery and in dentistry. 2. To immobilize fractures by means of wire. 3. In orthodontics, to apply wire to the teeth in the correction of malocclusion.

wiring (*wi'-ring*). *See* wire 2 & 3.

alveolar w. Immobilization of a jaw fracture by wires passed through the alveolar bone; used in edentulous patients or those with no suitable teeth to support a splint.

circumferential w. A method of immobilization of a jaw fracture in an edentulous mandible where the vulcanite or other splint is held in place by wires passed over the bone and through the soft tissues.

direct w. Immobilization of a jaw fracture by twisting wires round suitable teeth in both the upper and lower jaws and then joining the twisted ends of opposing upper and lower wires to help maintain the occlusion.

eyelet w. A form of direct wiring in which the wires are doubled to form an eyelet and a tail; these are fastened round two teeth at a time and then linked between the jaws with connecting wires or rubber bands.

interdental w. Immobilization of a jaw fracture by means of wires passed round several teeth on each side of the fracture.

intermaxillary w. Any form of wiring used for immobilizing jaw fractures which links the upper to the lower jaw.

wisdom tooth. A third molar.

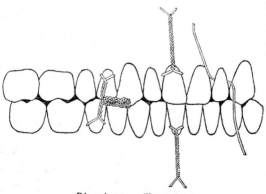

Direct inter-maxillary wiring

wolf jaw. Bilateral cleft extending through the palate, jaw, and lip.

Wood crown. A porcelain crown baked to a platinum cap.

wooden tongue. A tongue affected by actinomycosis.

wormian bones (O. Worm, 1588-1654. Danish anatomist). Small bones in the sutures of the skull.

wound (*wŭnd*). Any injury to the tissues or organs caused by cut, stab, or tear, usually going deeper than the outer skin or integument.

X

X plate. An orthodontic screw-adjusted appliance used to retract protrusive incisors and prevent overbite.

x ray. Radiant energy of short wave lengths, penetrating solid masses impervious to ordinary light rays, and by means of which photographs may be taken of internal body structures.

xanthodont, xanthodontous (*zan'-tho-dont*). Having yellow teeth.

xeno-. Prefix signifying *foreign*.

xero-. Prefix signifying *dry*.

xerocheilia (*zer-o-ki'-li-ă*). Inflammation of the lips marked by excessive dryness.

xerostomia (*zer-o-sto'-mi-ă*). Dryness of the mouth, due to failure of salivary secretion.

Z

Zn Chemical symbol for zinc.

Zagari's disease (G. Zagari, 1863-1946. Italian physician). Xerostomia (*q.v.*).

zinc (*zink*). A bluish-white, crystalline, lustrous metal, chemical symbol Zn. Malleable and ductile at moderately high temperatures, brittle at over 200°C.

Zinn's artery (J. G. Zinn, 1727-59. German anatomist). Central artery of the retina. *See* Table of Arteries —centralis retinae.

Zinn's circle (J. G. Zinn, 1727-59. German anatomist). Circulus arteriosus halleri (*q.v.*).

zona (*zo'-nă*). 1. Herpes zoster (*q.v.*). 2. A band or band-like section.

zoo-. Prefix signifying *animal*.

zoster (*zos'-ter*). Herpes zoster (*q.v.*).

zygion (*zi'-gi-on*). The most lateral point on the surface of the zygoma.

zygoma (*zi-go'-mă*). The cheek-bone; the malar bone.

zygomatic (*zi-go-mat'-ik*). Relating to the zygoma.

zygomatic arch. The arch formed by the zygoma and the zygomatic processes of the maxilla and the temporal bone.

zygomatic bone. The zygoma.

zygomatic fossa. Infratemporal fossa (*q.v.*).

zygomatic muscle. The *greater* zygomatic muscle

raises the corner of the mouth. *See* Table of Muscles—zygomaticus major.

The *lesser* zygomatic muscle is part of M. levator labii superioris. *See* Table of Muscles—zygomaticus minor.

zygomatic nerve. Supplies the skin over the zygoma and the temporal region. *See* Table of Nerves—zygomaticus.

zygomatic process *of the frontal bone.* A thick, strong lateral projection of the frontal bone which articulates with the zygoma.

zygomatic process *of the maxilla.* A rough triangular eminence articulating with the maxillary process of the zygoma.

zygomatic process *of the temporal bone.* A long process from the lower squamous portion of the temporal bone, articulating with the zygoma.

zygomatic reflex. Lateral movement of the mandible to the percussed side in response to a tap over the zygoma with a percussion hammer.

zygomatico-. Prefix signifying *zygoma.*

zygomaticofacial (*zi-go-mat''-ik-o-fa'-shal*). Relating to the zygoma and thd face.

zygomaticofacial nerve. Supplies the skin over the zygoma. *See* Table of Nerves—zygomaticofacialis.

zygomaticomaxillary (*zi-go-mat''-ik-o-maks-il'-ar-i*). Zygomaxillary (*q.v.*).

zygomatico-orbital artery. Supplies the orbicularis oculi muscle. *See* Table of Arteries—zygomatico-orbitalis.

zygomatico-orbital canal. A passage through the orbital process of the zygoma, through which pass the facial and temporal branches of the zygomatic nerve.

zygomaticotemporal nerve. Supplies the skin over the anterior portion of the temporal region. *See* Table of Nerves—zygomaticotemporalis.

zygomaxillare (*zi''-go-maks-il-ar'-ĕ*). A point at the lower end of the zygomatic suture, a craniometric landmark.

zygomaxillary (*zi''-go-maks-il'-ar-i*). Relating to both the zygoma and the maxilla.

TABLE OF ARTERIES OF THE HEAD AND NECK

ARTERIES	ORIGIN	PARTS SUPPLIED
alveolaris inferior [*dentalis inferior*]	Maxillary	Mandibular teeth, floor of mouth, buccal mucous membrane.
alveolaris superior anterior [*dentalis superior anterior*]	Infra-orbital	Maxillary incisors and canines.
alveolaris superior posterior [*dentalis superior posterior*]	Maxillary	Antral mucous membrane, maxillary molars and bicuspids.
angularis	Facial	Inferior portion of orbicularis palpebrum and lacrimal sac.
auditiva interna	Labyrinthi (*q.v.*).	
auditory	Labyrinthi (*q.v.*).	
auricularis anterior	Cervical branch of occipital	External auditory meatus and lateral surface of auricle.
auricularis posterior	External carotid	Digastric and other muscles, parotid gland, middle ear, mastoid cells, auricle.
auricularis profunda	Maxillary	Skin of external auditory meatus and tympanic membrane.
basilaris	Left and right vertebral	Cerebellum and cerebrum.
buccalis [*buccinator*]	Maxillary	Buccal mucous membrane, skin of cheek, buccinator muscle.
buccinator	Buccalis (*q.v.*).	

ARTERIES	ORIGIN	PARTS SUPPLIED
canalis pterygoidii	Maxillary	Levator and tensor veli palatini muscles, pharyngotympanic tube, upper portion of pharynx.
caroticotympanica	Branch of internal carotid	Tympanic cavity.
carotis communis	*right:* Brachiocephalic trunk; *left:* Aortic arch	Divides into internal and external carotid arteries
carotis externa	Common carotid	Meninges, neck, thyroid gland, tongue, tonsils, side of head, face, skin, middle ear.
carotis interna	Common carotid	Parts of brain, orbit, forehead, nose.
centralis retinae	Ophthalmic	Retina.
cerebelli inferior anterior	Basilar	Lower anterior surface of cerebellum.
cerebelli inferior posterior	Vertebral	Medulla, vermiform process and cerebellar cortex.
cerebelli superior	Basilar	Outer rim of cerebellum and superior vermiform process.
cerebri anterior	Internal carotid	Corpus callosum, frontal lobe, optic and olfactory tracts.
cerebri media	Internal carotid	Basal ganglia, island of Reil, frontal, parietal and temporal lobes.
cerebri posterior	Basilar	Temporal and occipital lobes.
cervicalis ascendens	Inferior thyroid	Neck muscles, spinal cord and vertebrae.
cervicalis profunda	Costocervical trunk	Deep muscles at back of neck.

ARTERIES	ORIGIN	PARTS SUPPLIED
cervicalis superficialis	Variable superficial branch of transversa colli.	
choroidea	Choroidea anterior (*q.v.*)	
choroidea anterior [*choroidea*]	Internal carotid	Choroid plexus of lateral ventricle, corpus fibriatum and hippocampus major.
ciliaris anterior	Ophthalmic	Perforating sclera and anastomising with posterior ciliary.
ciliaris posterior brevis [*uveal*]	Ophthalmic	Choroid and ciliary processes of the eye.
ciliaris posterior longa	Ophthalmic	From sclerotic and choroid to iris.
communicans anterior	Anterior cerebral	Forms part of circle of Willis.
communicans posterior	Internal carotid	Uncinate gyrus, thalamus; forms part of circle of Willis.
conjunctivalis anterior	Anterior ciliary	Conjunctiva.
conjunctivalis posterior	Medial palpebral	Conjunctiva and lacrimal caruncle.
cricothyroidea	Branch of superior thyroid	Cricothyroid muscle.
dentalis	Alveolaris (*q.v.*). British terminology.	
dorsalis linguae	Branch of lingual	Pillars of fauces, tonsils, and dorsum of tongue.
dorsalis nasi	Ophthalmic	Skin of dorsum of nose.
episcleralis	Anterior ciliary	Joins greater arterial circle of iris.

ARTERIES	ORIGIN	PARTS SUPPLIED
ethmoidalis anterior	Ophthalmic	Dura mater, frontal sinuses, anterior ethmoid cells, nose, facial skin.
ethmoidalis posterior	Ophthalmic	Dura mater, posterior ethmoid cells, nose.
facialis [*maxillaris externa*]	External carotid	Pharynx, soft palate, tonsil, submandibular gland, part of orbit and lacrimal sac.
Glaserian	Tympanica anterior (*q.v.*).	
gustatoria	Lingualis (*q.v.*).	
hyoidea	Infrahyoidea, suprahyoidea (*q.v.*).	
infrahyoidea	Branch of superior thyroid	Thyrohyoid muscle and membrane.
infraorbitalis	Maxillary	Upper lip, side of nose, lower eyelid and lacrimal sac.
innominate	Truncus brachiocephalicus (*q.v.*).	
labialis inferior	Facial	Lower lip.
labialis superior	Facial	Upper lip and nasal septum.
labyrinthi [*auditiva interna; auditory*]	Anterior inferior cerebellar	Internal ear.
lacrimalis	Ophthalmic	Cheek, eyelids, eye muscle and lacrimal gland.
laryngea inferior	Inferior thyroid	Larynx.
laryngea superior	Superior thyroid	Laryngeal muscles and mucous membrane.
lingualis [*gustatoria*]	External carotid	Sublingual gland, tongue, tonsil, epiglottis.

ARTERIES	ORIGIN	PARTS SUPPLIED
masseterica	Maxillary	Deep surface of masseter muscle.
mastoidea	Branch of occipital	Dura mater, lateral sinuses, mastoid cells.
maxillaris [*maxillaris interna*]	External carotid	Meninges, muscles of cheek, palate, nose, mandibular alveolar process and teeth, ear.
maxillaris externa	Facialis (*q.v.*).	
maxillaris interna	Maxillaris (*q.v.*).	
meningea	Branch of vertebral	Dura mater of posterior cranial fossa.
meningea accessoria	Branch of maxillary or meningea media	Trigeminal ganglion.
meningea anterior	Ophthalmic	Dura mater of middle cranial fossa.
meningea media	Maxillary	Dura mater and cranium.
meningea posterior	Ascending pharyngeal	Dura mater.
mentalis	Inferior alveolar	Lower lip and chin.
nasales posteriores, laterales et septi	Sphenopalatine	Nasal cavity and nasal septum, and the adjacent sinuses.
nasopalatina	Sphenopalatina (*q.v.*).	
occipitalis	External carotid	Neck and scalp muscles.
ophthalmica	Internal carotid	Eyeball, eye muscles, nose, ethmoid sinuses.
palatina ascendens	Facial	Palate, tonsils, and upper portion of pharynx.
palatina desdendens	Maxillary	Hard and soft palates.
palatina major	Descending palatine	Hard palate.

ARTERIES	ORIGIN	PARTS SUPPLIED
palatina minor	Descending palatine	Soft palate.
palpebralis inferior	Ophthalmic	Caruncle, conjunctiva, lacrimal sac, and lower eyelid.
palpebralis lateralis	Lacrimal	Eyelids and conjunctiva.
palpebralis medialis	Ophthalmic	Conjunctiva, lacrimal sac, eyelid.
palpebralis superior	Ophthalmic	Upper eyelid.
parotidea	Branch of superficial temporal	Parotid gland.
petrosa	Branch of middle meningeal	Tympanic cavity.
pharyngea	Branch of pharyngea ascendens	Pharynx.
pharyngea ascendens	External carotid	Membranes of brain, neck muscles and nerves, pharynx, soft palate, tympanum.
pontina	Branch of basilar	Pons.
profunda linguae [*ranine*]	Lingual	Lower surface of tongue.
pterygoidea	Branch of maxillary	Pterygoid muscles.
ranine	Profunda linguae (*q.v.*).	
septi	Maxillary	Nasal mucous membrane.
sphenopalatina [*nasopalatina*]	Maxillary	Lateral nasal wall and septum.
sternocleidomastoidea	1. Branch of occipital; 2. Branch of superior thyroid	Sternocleidomastoid muscle.
stylomastoidea	Posterior auricular	Middle ear.
subclavia	*right:* Brachiocephalic trunk; *left:* Aortic arch	Upper limb, spinal cord, neck, brain, meninges.

ARTERIES	ORIGIN	PARTS SUPPLIED
sublingualis	Lingual	Lower jaw muscles, floor of mouth, side of tongue, sublingual gland.
submentalis	Facial	Tissues below jaw.
suprahyoidea	Branch of lingual	Muscles above hyoid bone.
supraorbitalis	Ophthalmic	Superior orbital muscles, forehead.
supratrochlearis	Ophthalmic	Antero-medial part of forehead.
temporalis media	Superficial temporal	Temporal fascia.
temporalis profunda	Maxillary	Zygomatic bone, temporal muscle and temporal fossa.
temporalis superificialis	External carotid	Temporal fascia.
thyroidea ima (*inconstant*)	Brachiocephalic trunk	Thyroid gland.
thyroidea inferior	Subclavian	Neck muscles, oesophagus, larynx, thyroid gland.
thyroidea superior	External carotid	Thyroid gland, larynx, sternocleidomastoid and infrahyoid muscles.
tonsillaris	Branch of facial	Base of tongue and faucial tonsil.
trachealis	Branch of inferior thyroid	Trachea.
transversa faciei	Superficial temporal	Masseter muscle, parotid gland, facial skin.
truncus brachiocephalicus [*innominate*]	Aortic arch	Right upper limb, right side of head and neck.
truncus linguofacialis	The common trunk and facial arteries the external carotid	by which the lingual frequently arise from artery.

ARTERIES	ORIGIN	PARTS SUPPLIED
truncus thyrocervicalis	Subclavian	Neck, thyroid gland, oesophagus, trachea.
tympanica anterior [*Glaserian*]	Maxillary	Tympanum.
tympanica inferior	Ascending pharyngeal	Tympanum.
tympanica posterior	Posterior auricular	Tympanic membranes.
tympanica superior	Middle meningeal	Tensor tympani muscle.
uveal	Ciliaris posterior brevis (*q.v.*).	
vertebralis	Subclavian	Cerebellum, cerebrum, spinal cord, meninges, neck muscles.
zygomatico-orbitalis	Superficial temporal	Orbicularis oculi.

Head and neck arteries

A Superficial temporal.
C Facial.
D Inferior alveolar.
E Lingual.
F Superior thyroid.
G Common carotid.
H Internal carotid.
I Occipital.
M Maxillary.
N Posterior auricular.
O Superior alveolar.
P External carotid.

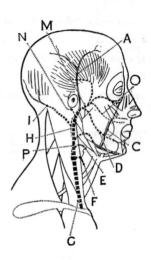

MUSCLE	ORIGIN
alveololabialis	Buccinator (*q.v.*).
alveolomaxillary	Buccinator (*q.v.*).
aponeurosis epicranialis	Galea aponeurotica (*q.v.*).
aryepiglotticus	Inconstant fascicle of oblique arytenoid, from the apex of the arytenoid cartilage
arytenoideus obliquus	Dorsal aspect of muscular process of arytenoid cartilage
arytenoideus transversus	Dorsal aspect of arytenoid cartilage
auricularis anterior	Lateral part of epicranial aponeurosis
auricularis posterior	Lateral part of mastoid process
auricularis superior	Lateral part of epicranial aponeurosis
buccinator [*alveolabialis; alveolomaxillary*]	Maxillary alveolar process, buccinator ridge on mandible, and pterygo-mandibular ligament
buccopharyngeus	Part of constrictor pharyngis superior.
caninus	Levator anguli oris (*q.v.*).
cephalopharyngeus	Constrictor pharyngis superior (*q.v.*).
ceratopharyngeus	Part of constrictor pharyngis medius.
chondroglossus	Lesser horn of hyoid bone
chondropharyngeus	Part of constrictor pharyngis medius.
ciliaris	Sphincter of ciliary body and scleral spur
complexus	Semispinalis capitis (*q.v.*).
compressor naris [*nasalis*]	Maxilla, between nasal notch and canine fossa
constrictor pharyngis inferior	Lateral surface of ala of thyroid cartilage, tendinous arch to cricoid cartilage and side of cricoid cartilage

THE HEAD AND NECK

INSERTION	NERVE SUPPLY	FUNCTION
Lateral margin of epiglottis		
Apex of opposing arytenoid cartilage	Recurrent laryngeal	Closes inlet of larynx.
Opposing arytenoid cartilage	Recurrent laryngeal	Approximates arytenoid cartilages.
Anterior part of helix of auricle	Facial	Draws forward auricle.
Cranial surface of auricle	Facial	Draws auricle back.
Cranial surface of auricle	Facial	Raises auricle.
Orbicularis oris, at angle of mouth	Buccal branch of facial	Closes lips, and compresses cheeks.
Tongue	Hypoglossal	Draws back and depresses tongue.
Ciliary processes	Oculomotor and ciliary ganglion	Accommodation of vision.
By aponeurosis into nasal cartilage	Facial	Compresses nostril.
Posterior median raphe of pharyngeal wall	Pharyngeal plexus	Constriction of pharynx.

MUSCLE	ORIGIN
constrictor pharyngis medius	Lower portion of stylohyoid ligament, and both horns of hyoid bone
constrictor pharyngis superior [*cephalopharyngeus*]	Posterior border and hamulus of medial pterygoid plate, pterygomandibular raphe, upper end of mylohyoid line, and side of tongue
corrugator supercilii	Superciliary arch on frontal bone
cricoarytenoideus lateralis	Lateral part of cricoid cartilage
cricoarytenoideus posterior	Posterior surface of cricoid cartilage
cricopharyngeus	Part of constrictor pharyngis inferior.
cricothyroideus	Front and side of cricoid cartilage
depressor alae nasi	Depressor septi (*q.v.*).
depressor anguli oris [*triangularis*]	Mandible
depressor labii inferioris [*mentolabialis: quadratus labii inferioris*]	Mandible
depressor septi [*depressor alae nasi*]	Maxilla
depressor supercilii	Fibres from orbital part of orbicularis oculi
digastricus, *anterior belly*	Digastric fossa on the base of the mandible
digastricus, *posterior belly*	Mastoid notch
dilatator naris [*nasalis*]	Maxilla
distortor oris	Zygomaticus minor (*q.v.*).
epicranius	Muscular cover of the scalp; it includes the temporoparietal and occipito–frontal muscles and the galea aponeurotica.

INSERTION	NERVE SUPPLY	FUNCTION
Posterior median raphe of pharyngeal wall	Pharyngeal plexus	Constriction of pharynx.
Pharyngeal tubercle, posterior median raphe of pharyngeal wall	Pharyngeal plexus	Constriction of pharynx.
Skin of eyebrow	Facial	Draws eyebrows down and wrinkles forehead, as in frowning.
Muscular process of arytenoid cartilage	Recurrent laryngeal	Narrows glottis.
Muscular process of arytenoid cartilage	Recurrent laryngeal	Opens glottis.
Lamina of thyroid cartilage	Superior laryngeal	Tenses vocal folds.
Skin at angle of mouth	Facial	Pulls down angle of mouth.
Skin about the mouth	Facial	Pulls down lower lip.
Nasal septum	Facial	Assists in widening nostrils.
Eyebrow		Depresses eyebrow.
Lesser horn of hyoid bone	Mylohyoid branch of inferior alveolar	Raises and holds hyoid bone.
Lesser horn of hyoid bone	Facial	Raises and holds hyoid bone.
Bridge of nose	Facial	Assists in widening nostrils.

MUSCLE	ORIGIN
frontalis (*anterior belly of occipito-frontalis*)	Galea aponeurotica
galea aponeurotica [*aponeurosis epicranialis*]	The aponeurosis connecting the separate parts of the occipito-frontal muscle.
genioglossus	Inner surface of mandible near symphysis
geniohyoideus	Inner surface of mandible near symphysis
glossopalatinus	Palatoglossus (*q.v.*).
glossopharyngeus	Part of constrictor pharyngis superior.
hyoglossus	Hyoid bone
levator anguli oris [*caninus*]	Maxillary canine fossa
levator labii superioris [*quadratus labii superioris*]	Inferior margin of orbit
levator labii superioris alaeque nasi	Nasal process of maxilla
levator menti	Mentalis (*q.v.*).
levator palati	Levator veli palatini (*q.v.*).
levator palpebrae superioris	Roof of orbit
levator veli palatini [*levator palati*]	Apex of petrous portion of temporal bone and cartilage of pharyngotympanic tube
lingualis inferior	Longitudinalis inferior (*q.v.*).
lingualis superior	Longitudinalis superior (*q.v.*).
lingualis transversus	Transversus linguae (*q.v.*).
lingualis verticalis	Verticalis linguae (*q.v.*).
longissimus capitis [*trachelomastoideus*]	Articular processes of lower cervical and transverse processes of upper thoracic vertebrae
longissimus cervicis [*transversus colli*]	Transverse process of upper thoracic vertebrae
longitudinalis inferior [*lingualis inferior*]	Root of tongue

INSERTION	NERVE SUPPLY	FUNCTION
Skin of forehead	Facial	Raises eyebrows and draws forward scalp.
Hyoid bone, and under side of tongue	Hypoglossal	Raises hyoid bone, retracts and protrudes tongue.
Anterior surface of hyoid bone above the mylohyoid attachment	1st cervical, via hypoglossal	Raises and draws forward hyoid bone with jaw fixed.
Base and sides of tongue	Hypoglossal	Draws down sides of tongue.
Angle of mouth	Facial	Raises angle of mouth.
Orbicularis oris	Facial	Raises upper lip.
Orbicularis oris and ala	Facial	Dilates nostril and raises upper lip.
Skin of upper eyelid	Oculomotor	Raises upper eyelid.
Aponeurosis of soft palate	Accessory, via pharyngeal plexus	Raises soft palate.
Mastoid process of temporal bone	Posterior branches of spinal	Extends vertebral column.
Transverse processes of cervical vertebrae	Posterior branches of spinal	Extends spinal column.
Tip of tongue	Hypoglossal	Changes shape of tongue.

MUSCLE	ORIGIN
longitudinalis superior [*lingualis superior*]	Root of tongue
longus capitis	Transverse processes of 3rd, 4th, 5th and 6th cervical vertebrae
longus cervicis	Longus colli (*q.v.*).
longus colli [*longus cervicis*]	Lower cervical and upper thoracic vertebrae
masseter	Zygomatic arch
mentalis [*levator menti*]	Incisive fossa of mandible
mentolabialis	Depressor labii inferioris (*q.v.*).
mylohyoideus	Mylohyoid line of mandible
mylopharyngeus	Part of constrictor pharyngis superior.
nasalis	Compressor naris *and* dilatator naris (*q.v.*).
obliquus auriculae (*vestigial*)	Helix
obliquus capitis inferior	Spine of axis
obliquus capitis superior	Lateral mass of atlas
obliquus oculi inferior	Middle of floor of orbit
obliquus oculi superior	Edge of optic foramen
occipitalis (*posterior belly of occipitofrontalis*)	Superior nuchal line of occipital bone
occipitofrontalis	The scalp muscle; consisting connected by the epicranial

INSERTION	NERVE SUPPLY	FUNCTION
Tip of tongue	Hypoglossal	Changes shape of tongue.
Inferior surface of basilar portion of occipital bone	1st and 2nd cervical	Controls movements of head and neck.
Anterior tubercles of cervical vertebrae and atlas	Anterior branches of cervical	Flexes vertebral column.
Lateral surface of ramus of mandible	Mandibular branch of trigeminal	Raises mandible.
Skin of chin	Facial	Protrudes lower lip and wrinkles skin of chin.
Hyoid bone	Mylohyoid branch of inferior alveolar	Assists in raising hyoid bone and depressing mandible during swallowing.
Antihelix	Facial.	
Transverse process of atlas	Posterior branch of 1st cervical	Aids in lateral movements and extension of head.
Between superior and inferior nuchal lines of occipital bone	Posterior branch of 1st cervical	Aids in lateral movements and extension of head.
Sclera	Oculomotor	Elevates and abducts eyeball.
Sclera	Trochlear	Depresses and abducts eyeball.
Galea aponeurotica	Facial	Draws back scalp.

of 4 bellies: 2 frontal (*frontalis*) and 2 occipital (*occipitalis*),
aponeurosis. *See* frontalis and occipitalis muscles.

MUSCLE	ORIGIN
omohyoideus, *inferior belly*	Superior border of scapula and suprascapular ligament
omohyoideus, *superior belly*	Intermediate tendon to *inferior belly*
orbicularis oculi	Sphincter of palpebral fissure
orbicularis oris	Sphincter of mouth
orbitalis (*vestigial*)	Bridges the inferior orbital fissure
palatoglossus [*glossopalatinus*]	Soft palate
palatopharyngeus [*pharyngopalatinus*]	Soft palate and pharyngotympanic tube
pharyngopalatinus	Palatopharyngeus (*q.v.*).
platysma	Fascia of pectoralis major and deltoid muscles
procerus	Skin over nose
pterygoideus	Pterygoideus lateralis (*q.v.*).
pterygoideus externus	Pterygoideus lateralis (*q.v.*).
pterygoideus lateralis [*pterygoideus; pterygoideus externus*]	*Upper head:* Infratemporal crest and infratemporal surface of greater wing of sphenoid *Lower head:* lateral surface of lateral pterygoid plate

INSERTION	NERVE SUPPLY	FUNCTION
Intermediate tendon to *superior* belly	Ansa cervicalis	Depresses hyoid bone and tightens deep cervical fascia in lower part of neck.
Lower border of hyoid bone beside sterno-hyoid	Superior branch of ansa cervicalis	Depresses hyoid bone and tightens deep cervical fascia in lower part of neck.
	Facial	Closes eyelids.
	Facial	Purses lips and puckers up mouth.
	Sympathetic.	
Tongue	Accessory	Raises tongue and constricts anterior fauces.
Aponeurosis of pharynx	Accessory, via pharyngeal plexus	Aids in swallowing.
Skin about chin, oblique line of mandible, and skin and muscles at angle of mouth	Cervical branch of facial	Raises skin from underlying structures and, with risorius, retracts angle of mouth.
Skin of forehead	Facial	Wrinkles skin over nose.
Anterior part of capsule of mandibular joint, anterior border of articular disc and pterygoid fovea on anterior surface of neck of mandible	Mandibular	Draws articular disc down and forward to the articular eminence.

MUSCLE	ORIGIN
pterygoideus medialis	*deep head:* Medial surface of lateral pterygoid plate and posterior surface of pyramid of palate bone. *superficial head:* Lateral surface of pyramid of palatine bone and adjacent part of maxillary tuberosity
pterygopharyngeus	Part of constrictor pharyngis superior.
quadratus labii inferioris	Depressor labii inferioris (*q.v.*).
quadratus labii superioris	Levator labii superioris (*q.v.*).
quadratus menti	Depressor labii inferioris (*q.v.*).
rectus capitis anterior	Lateral mass of atlas
rectus capitis lateralis	Transverse process of atlas
rectus capitis posterior major	Spine of axis
rectus capitis posterior minor	Posterior tubercle of atlas
rectus oculi inferior	Lower margin of optic foramen
rectus oculi lateralis	Lateral margin of optic foramen
rectus oculi medialis	Median margin of optic foramen
rectus oculi superior	Upper edge of optic foramen
risorius	Fascia over masseter and parotid gland
salpingopharyngeus	Part of palatopharyngeus, arising from pharyngotympanic tube.
semispinalis capitis [*complexus*]	4th cervical to 5th thoracic vertebrae
semispinalis cervicis [*semispinalis colli*]	Transverse processes of lower cervical and upper thoracic vertebrae
semispinalis colli	Semispinalis cervicis (*q.v.*).

INSERTION	NERVE SUPPLY	FUNCTION
Deep surface of mandible between angle and groove for mylohyoid nerve	Mandibular	With masseter and temporalis closes mouth; with lateral pterygoid protrudes mandible.
Basilar portion of occipital bone	1st cervical	Aids in support and movement of head.
Jugular process of occipital bone	1st cervical	Aids in support and movement of head.
Occipital bone	1st cervical	Draws head back and rotates it.
Occipital bone	1st cervical	Draws back head and rotates it.
Sclera	Oculomotor	Depresses and adducts eyeball.
Sclera	Abducens	Abducts eyeball.
Sclera	Oculomotor	Adducts eyeball.
Sclera	Oculomotor	Elevates and adducts the eyball.
Skin of angle of mouth	Facial	Draws angle of mouth sideways, as in grinning.
Occipital bone, between the superior and inferior nuchal lines	Posterior branches of spinal	Extends head.
Spinous processes of lower cervical vertebrae	Posterior branches of spinal	Extends vertebral column and rotates it.

MUSCLE	ORIGIN
spinalis capitis (*inconstant*)	Spinous processes of lower cervical and upper thoracic vertebrae
spinalis cervicis (*inconstant*) [*spinalis colli*]	Spinous processes of lower cervical and upper thoracic vertebrae
spinalis colli	Spinalis cervicis (*q.v.*).
splenius capitis	Spinous processes of lowest cervical and upper thoracic vertebrae and nuchal ligament
splenius cervicis [*splenius colli*]	Spinous processes of lowest cervical and upper thoracic vertebrae and nuchal ligament
splenius colli	Splenius cervicis (*q.v.*).
stapedius	Pyramid of tympanum
sternocleidomastoideus [*sternomastoideus*]	Manubrium sterni and clavicle
sternohyoideus	Clavicle and manubrium sterni
sternomastoideus	Sternocleidomastoideus (*q.v.*).
sternothyroideus	Manubrium sterni and 1st costal cartilage
styloglossus	Styloid process of temporal bone
stylohyoideus	Styloid process of temporal bone
stylopharyngeus	Styloid process of temporal bone
temporalis	Temporal fossa
temporoparietalis	Temporal fascia over ear
tensor palati	Tensor veli palatini (*q.v.*).
tensor tympani	Cartilage of pharyngotympanic tube

INSERTION	NERVE SUPPLY	FUNCTION
Occipital bone	Posterior branches of spinal	Extends head.
Spinous processes of 2nd, 3rd and 4th cervical vertebrae	Posterior branches of spinal	Extends vertebral column.
Mastoid process and superior nuchal line	Posterior branches of spinal	Extends head.
Transverse processes of upper cervical vertebrae	Posterior branches of spinal	Extends spinal column.
Neck of stapes	Facial	Retracts stapes.
Mastoid process	Accessory	Flexes head and turns it to the opposite side.
Hyoid bone	Ansa cervicalis	Depresses hyoid bone.
Oblique line of lamina of thyroid cartilage	Ansa cervicalis	Depresses thyroid cartilage and larynx.
Side of tongue	Hypoglossal	Raises tongue.
Hyoid bone	Facial	Raises tongue and hyoid bone, and draws them back.
Lamina of thyroid cartilage and side of pharynx	Glossopharyngeal	Raises and opens pharynx.
Medial surface, apex and anterior border of coronoid process, and anterior border of ramus of mandible	Deep temporal branches of anterior division of mandibular	Retracts protruded mandible and closes mouth.
Galea aponeurotica	Temporal branches of facial	Tightens scalp.
Manubrium mallei	Mandibular	Tenses tympanic membrane.

MUSCLE	ORIGIN
tensor veli palatini [*tensor palati*]	Scaphoid fossa of sphenoid bone and cartilage of pharyngotympanic tube
thyro-arytenoideus	Lamina of thyroid cartilage
thyro-epiglotticus	Lamina of thyroid cartilage
thyrohyoideus	Oblique line of thyroid cartilage
thyropharyngeus	Part of constrictor pharyngis inferior.
trachelomastoideus	Longissimus capitis (*q.v.*).
transversus colli	Longissimus cervicis (*q.v.*).
transversus linguae [*lingualis transversus*]	Median lingual raphe
transversus menti	Superficial fibres of depressor anguli oris.
trapezius	The inion, the superior nuchal line, cervical and thoracic spines and the supraspinous ligament
triangularis	Depressor anguli oris (*q.v.*).
uvulae	Posterior nasal spine
verticalis linguae [*lingualis verticalis*]	Dorsum of tongue
zygomaticus major	Zygomatic bone
zygomaticus minor [*distortor oris*]	Part of levator labii superioris.

INSERTION	NERVE SUPPLY	FUNCTIONS
Aponeurosis of soft palate	Mandibular	Tightens soft palate and opens pharyngo-tympanic tube
Muscular process of arytenoid cartilage	Recurrent laryngeal	Closes larynx and relaxes vocal cords.
Epiglottis	Recurrent laryngeal	Closes larynx.
Lower border of great horn of hyoid bone	1st cervical via hypoglossal	Depresses hyoid bone or raises larynx.
Dorsum and sides of tongue	Hypoglossal	Changes shape of tongue.
Posterior border and upper surface of clavicle, and the spine and acromion of the scapula	Accessory, and anterior branches of cervical	Raises shoulder and draws back scapula.
Aponeurosis of soft palate	Accessory, via pharyngeal plexus.	
Sides and base of tongue	Hypoglossal	Changes shape of tongue.
Skin about the face	Facial	Raises corner of mouth.

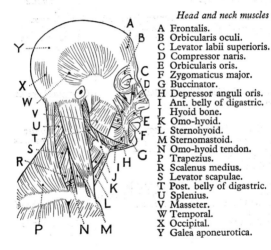

Head and neck muscles

A Frontalis.
B Orbicularis oculi.
C Levator labii superioris.
D Compressor naris.
E Orbicularis oris.
F Zygomaticus major.
G Buccinator.
H Depressor anguli oris.
I Ant. belly of digastric.
J Hyoid bone.
K Omo-hyoid.
L Sternohyoid.
M Sternomastoid.
N Omo-hyoid tendon.
P Trapezius.
R Scalenus medius.
S Levator scapulae.
T Post. belly of digastric.
U Splenius.
V Masseter.
W Temporal.
X Occipital.
Y Galea aponeurotica.

TABLE OF NERVES OF

NAME	ORIGIN
abducens (m) (*6th cranial*)	Brain stem, lower border of pons
accessorius (m) (*11th cranial*)	(a) *bulbar:* Lateral aspect of medulla oblongata (b) *spinal:* Upper segments of cervical cord
acusticus	Vestibulocochlearis (*q.v.*).
alveolaris inferior [*dentalis inferior*]	Mandibular
alveolaris superior anterior [*dentalis superior anterior*]	Infraorbital
alveolaris superior medius (s) [*dentalis superior medius*]	Infraorbital
alveolaris superior posterior (s) [*dentalis superior posterior*]	Maxillary
ampullaris anterior	Vestibular ganglion of vestibulocochlear
ampullaris lateralis	Vestibular ganglion of vestibulocochlear
ampullaris posterior	Vestibular ganglion of vestibulocochlear
ansa cervicalis, *ramus inferior* (m) [*ansa hypoglossi; descendens cervicis; descendens hypoglossi*]	Cervical plexus
ansa cervicalis, *ramus superior* (m)	Cervical plexus
ansa hypoglossi	Ansa cervicalis (*q.v.*).
auditorius	Vestibulocochlearis (*q.v.*).
auricularis (s)	Branch of vagus.
auricularis magnus (s)	Facial
auricularis posterior (m)	Cervical plexus
auriculotemporalis (s)	Mandibular
buccalis (s) [*buccinator*]	Mandibular
buccinator (m)	Facial
buccinator (s)	Buccalis (*q.v.*).
canalis pterygoidei	Union of N. petrosus major and N. petrosus profundus

THE HEAD AND NECK

DISTRIBUTION

Lateral rectus muscle of eye.

Striated muscles of pharynx and larynx.

Sternocleidomastoid and trapezius muscles.

Teeth and gingivae of lower jaw, mylohyoid and anterior belly of digastric muscles.
Maxillary incisors and canines, mucosa of nasal floor.

Maxillary premolars.

Molars and mucosa of maxillary sinus.

Ampulla of anterior semicircular duct.

Ampulla of lateral semicircular duct.

Ampulla of posterior semicircular duct.

Omohyoid, sternohyoid, and sternothyroid muscles.

Omohyoid, sternohyoid and sternothyroid muscles.

Skin of auricle and external auditory meatus.
Occipitalis muscle and intrinsic muscles of auricle.
Skin over angle of mandible and of adjacent part of auricle.
Skin over temple and scalp.
Skin and mucous membrane of cheek.

Buccinator muscle.

Lacrimal gland and glands of nose and palate, via pterygopalatine ganglion.

NAME	ORIGIN
caroticotympanicus [*petrosus profunda minor*]	Internal carotid sympathetic plexus
caroticus externus	Superior cervical ganglion
caroticus internus	Superior cervical ganglion
cervicales (m):	
1st anterior and posterior	1st segment of cervical cord
2nd anterior and posterior	2nd segment of cervical cord
3rd anterior and posterior	3rd segment of cervical cord
4th anterior	4th segment of cervical cord
4th-8th posterior	4th-8th segments of cervical cord
5th-8th anterior	5th-8th segments of cervical cord
chorda tympani (m & s)	Intermedius
ciliaris brevis (m)	Ciliary ganglion
ciliaris longus (s)	Nasociliary
cochlearis (s)	Brain stem, inferior border of pons; part of vestibulo-cochlearis
craniales	
1st=olfactorius 2nd=opticus 3rd=oculomotorius	
8th=vestibulocochlearis 9th=glossopharyngeus 10th=vagus	
cutaneous colli	Transversus colli (*q.v.*).
dentalis inferior	Alveolaris inferior (*q.v.*).
dentalis inferior	Branches of inferior alveolar
dentalis superior	Branches of superior alveolar
dentalis superior anterior	Alveolaris superior anterior (*q.v.*).
dentalis superior medius	Alveolaris superior medius (*q.v.*).
dentalis superior posterior	Alveolaris superior posterior (*q.v.*).
descendens cervicalis	Ansa cervicalis, ramus inferior (*q.v.*).
descendens hypoglossi	Ansa cervicalis, ramus inferior (*q.v.*).
ethmoidalis anterior (s)	Nasociliary
ethmoidalis posterior (s)	Nasociliary
facialis (m) (*7th cranial*)	Brain stem, lower border of pons
frontalis (s)	Ophthalmic

DISTRIBUTION

Tympanic plexus of glossopharyngeal.

Filaments to glands and smooth muscles of head.
Filaments to glands and smooth muscles of head.

Neck muscles.
Neck muscles and skin of neck.
Deep muscles and skin of neck.
Back and neck muscles, skin of neck, diaphragm.
Deep muscles of upper part of back and of neck, skin on upper part of back.
Muscles and skin of arms.

(s): taste buds on anterior two-thirds of tongue, via lingual nerve.
(m): Submandibular and sublingual glands via lingual nerve and submandibular ganglion.
Eyeball, ciliary muscle and constrictor pupillae.
Eyeball.
Spiral organ of cochlea.

4th = trochlearis   5th = trigeminus   6th = abducens   7th = facialis
11th = accessorius   12th = hypoglossus.

Mandibular teeth.
Maxillary teeth.

Mucosa of nasal cavity and anterior ethmoidal sinus, and skin of nose.
Mucosa of posterior ethmoidal and of sphenoidal sinuses.
Muscles of facial expression, posterior belly of digastric muscle, stapedius and stylohyoid.
Skin of scalp, forehead, and upper eyelids.

NAME	ORIGIN
gingivalis inferior	Branches of inferior alveolar
gingivalis superior	Branches of superior alveolar
glossopalatinus	Intermedius (*q.v.*).
glossopharyngeus (m & s) (*9th cranial*)	Medulla oblongata, lateral aspect
hypoglossus (m) (*12th cranial*)	Medulla oblongata
infraorbitalis (s)	Maxillary
infratrochlearis (s)	Nasociliary
intermedius (m & s) [*glossopalatinus*]	Part of facial
jugularis	Communicating branch to vagus
labialis inferior (s)	Branch from inferior dental plexus
labialis superior (s)	Branch of infra-orbital
lacrimalis (s)	Ophthalmic
laryngeus externus (m)	Branch of superior laryngeal
laryngeus inferior (m & s)	Recurrent laryngeal
laryngeus internus (s)	Branch of superior laryngeal
laryngeus recurrens (m & s) [*recurrens*]	Vagus
laryngeus superior (m & s)	Vagus
lingualis (s)	Mandibular
malar	Zygomaticofacialis (*q.v.*).
mandibularis (m & s)	Trigeminal
massetericus (m & s)	Mandibular
maxillaris (s)	Trigeminal
meatus acustici externi (s)	Auriculotemporal
meningeus (s)	Branches of vagus, maxillary, hypoglossal, mandibular
meningeus medius (s)	Branch of maxillary
mentalis (s)	Inferior alveolar
mylohyoideus (m)	Inferior alveolar
nasalis externus (s)	Branches of infraorbital and nasociliary

Mandibular gingivae.
Maxillary gingivae.

(m): Stylopharyngeus and parotid gland.
(s): Mucosa of posterior one-third of tongue and taste buds.
Muscles of tongue.

Lower eyelid, skin and mucosa of the nose, upper lip and maxillary
    teeth.
Skin of bridge of nose.
(m): Nasal and palatal glands, sublingual and submandibular glands.
(s): taste buds of anterior two-thirds of tongue.
from superior cervical ganglion.
    Skin of lower lip.

Skin of cheek and upper lip.
Skin about lateral commissure of eye.
Cricothyroid.
(m): Intrinsic laryngeal muscles.
(s): Larynx below vocal cords.
Larynx above vocal cords.
(m): Constrictor pharyngis inferior, and intrinsic laryngeal muscles.
(s): Larynx below vocal cords.
(m): Cricothyroid (N. laryngeus externus).
(s): Larynx below vocal cords (N. laryngeus internus).
Mucosa of anterior two-thirds of tongue and of floor of mouth.

(m): Mylohyoid, anterior belly of digastric, tensor tympani, tensor
    veli palatini, and muscles of mastication.
(s): Mucosa of cheek, floor of mouth, and anterior two-thirds of
    tongue, skin of lower part of face, mandibular teeth, meninges.
Masseter muscle and temporo-mandibular joint.
Meninges, skin of upper part of face, maxillary teeth, mucosa of
    nose, cheeks, and palate.
Skin lining external auditory meatus, and tympanic membrane.
Meninges.

Meninges.
Skin of chin and lower lip.
Mylohyoid and anterior belly of digastric muscles.
Skin of nose.

NAME	ORIGIN
nasalis internus (s)	Branch of infraorbital
nasalis lateralis (s)	Branch of nasociliary
nasalis medius (s)	Branch of nasociliary
nasalis posterior inferior lateralis (s)	Branch from pterygopalatine ganglion
nasalis posterior superior lateralis (s) [*sphenopalatinus brevis*]	Branch from pterygopalatine ganglion
nasociliaris (s)	Ophthalmic
nasopalatinus (s) [*sphenopalatinus longus*]	Pterygopalatine ganglion
occipitalis major (s)	Posterior branch of 2nd cervical
occipitalis minor (s)	Cervical plexus
occipitalis tertius (s)	Posterior branch of 3rd cervical
oculomotorius (m) (*3rd cranial*)	Brain stem
olfactorius (s) (*1st cranial*)	Olfactory bulb
opthalmicus (s)	Trigeminal
opticus (s) (*2nd cranial*)	Optic tracts
orbitalis (s)	Branch from pterygopalatine ganglion
palatinus anterior	Palatinus major (*q.v.*).
palatinus major (s) [*palatinus anterior*]	Maxillary, via pterygopalatine ganglion
palatinus medius	Palatinus minor (*q.v.*).
palatinus minor (s) [*palatinus medius & palatinus posterior*]	Maxillary via pterygopalatine ganglion
palatinus posterior	Palatinus minor (*q.v.*).
palpebris (s)	Branch of infratrochlear
palpebris inferior (s)	Branch of superior alveolar
petrosus major (s)	Branch of facial
petrosus profundus	Carotid sympathetic plexus
petrosus profundus minor	Caroticotympanicus (*q.v.*).
pharyngeus:	
(1) (s)	Glossopharyngeal
(2) (s)	Pterygopalatine ganglion
(3) (m)	Vagus

DISTRIBUTION

Nasal mucosa.
Nasal mucosa.
Mucosa of nasal septum.
Mucosa of inferior nasal concha.

Mucosa of superior and middle nasal conchae.

Eyeball, skin and mucosa of eyelid, nose, and ethmoidal and sphenoidal air sinuses.
Mucosa of hard palate and nose.

Skin over posterior portion of scalp.
Skin of posterior portion of scalp and posterior aspect of auricle.
Skin over posterior aspect of neck and scalp.
Muscles of eye and upper eyelid.

Olfactory mucosa.

Skin of anterior portion of scalp and forehead, orbit and eyeball, meninges, mucosa of nose, frontal, ethmoidal and sphenoidal air sinuses.
Retina.

Orbit.

Mucosa of palate.

Mucosa of palate and uvula.

Upper eyelid.
Lower eyelid.
Palatal mucosa and glands, via pterygopalatine ganglion.
Palate, via N. canalis pterygoidei.

Pharyngeal mucosa.
Pharyngeal mucosa.
Pharyngeal muscles.

NAME	ORIGIN
pterygoideus lateralis (m)	Mandibular
pterygoideus medialis (m)	Mandibular
pterygopalatinus (s) [*sphenopalatinus*]	Maxillary
recurrens	Laryngeus recurrens (*q.v.*).
saccularis (s)	Vestibulocochlear
sphenopalatinus	Pterygopalatinus (*q.v.*).
sphenopalatinus brevis	Nasalis posterior superior lateralis (*q.v.*).
sphenopalatinus longus	Nasopalatinus (*q.v.*).
stato-acusticus	Vestibulocochlearis (*q.v.*).
sublingualis (s)	Lingual
supraorbitalis (s)	Frontal
supratrochlearis (s)	Frontal
temporalis profundi (m)	Mandibular
tentorius	Branch of ophthalmic
terminalis	Medial olfactory tract
transversus colli (s) [*cutaneous colli*]	Cervical plexus
trigeminus (*5th cranial*)	Brain stem at infero-lateral surface of pons
trochlearis (m) (*4th cranial*)	Dorsal surface of midbrain
tympanicus (s)	Inferior ganglion of glosso-pharyngeal
vagus (*10th cranial*)	Post-olivary sulcus of medulla oblongata
vestibularis (s)	Brain stem; part of vestibulo-cochlearis
vestibulocochlearis (*8th cranial*) [*acusticus, auditorius, stato-acusticus*].	Divides into cochlearis and vestibularis
zygomaticus (s)	Maxillary
zygomaticofacialis (s) [*malar*]	Branch of zygomatic
zygomaticotemporalis (s)	Branch of zygomatic

DISTRIBUTION

Lateral pterygoid muscle.
Medial pterygoid muscle, tensor tympani, tensor veli palatini.
Mucosa of hard palate and nose.

Filaments to macula sacculi.

Area of the sublingual gland.
Mucosa of frontal sinus, skin of forehead and upper eyelid.
Skin of centre of forehead, bridge of nose, and upper eyelid.
Temporal muscles.
Meninges.
Nasal septum.
Skin of anterior triangle of neck.

Divides into ophthalmicus, maxillaris, and mandibularis (q.v.).

Obliquus superior of eyeball.

Mucosa of middle ear and pharyngotympanic tube.

Branches to striate muscles of larynx and pharynx, skin of external
  auditory meatus, meninges, laryngeal and pharyngeal mucosa,
  thoracic and abdominal viscera.
Branches to ampullae of semicircular ducts, maculae of utricle and
  saccule, via vestibular ganglion.
vestibularis (q.v.).

Skin in temporal region and over zygoma.
Skin over zygoma.

Skin over anterior portion of temporal region.

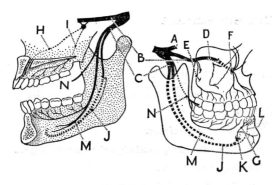

Head and neck
Nerves of maxilla and mandible

A	Ophthalmic division	of	H Long sphenopalatine.
B	Maxilla	„ Trige-	I Greater palatine.
C	Mandibular	„ minal.	J Inferior dental.
D	Infra-orbital.		K Mental foramen.
E	Posterior superior dental.		L Inferior dental to incisors and canine teeth.
F	Infra-orbital foramen.		M Lingual.
G	Mental branches to incisors and to lower lip and skin of chin.		N Buccal.

TABLE OF VEINS OF

This table includes only those veins whose names or courses differ from

NAME	DRAINAGE OR TRIBUTARIES
anonyma	Brachiocephalica (*q.v.*).
basalis	Formed by union of anterior vein.
brachiocephalica (*dextra and sinistra*) [*innominate; anonyma*]	Internal jugular and sub-clavian, vertebral, internal mammary, 1st posterior intercostal, *and left*: thoracic duct
cerebri inferior	Lower part of hemisphere, drain-
cerebri interna	Thalamostriate and choroid veins
cerebri magna	Internal cerebral veins
cerebri media profunda	Insula
cerebri media superificalis	Lower part of lateral surface of hemisphere
cerebri superioris	Upper portion of medial and lateral surfaces of hemisphere
facialis [*facialis anterior*]	Junction of supratrochlear and supra-orbital veins
facialis anterior	Facialis (*q.v.*).
facialis communis	Junction of facial and retro-mandibular veins
facialis posterior	Retromandibularis (*q.v.*).
faciei profunda	Communicating vein to facial
innominate	Brachiocephalica (*q.v.*).
jugularis anterior	Arises in submental region
jugularis externa	Posterior auricular and branch from retromandibular veins
jugularis interna	Brain, face, and neck
nasalis externa	Side of nose
ophthalmica inferior	Tributaries corresponding to branches of ophthalmic artery

THE HEAD AND NECK

the accompanying artery, or which have no accompanying artery.

DESTINATION	LOCATION
cerebral and deep middle cerebral veins, and joins great cerebral	
Superior vena cava	Medial portion of root of neck, to terminate behind 1st right costal cartilage.
ing into adjacent sinus.	
Great cerebral	Below splenium of corpus callosum.
Straight sinus	Behind and beneath splenium of corpus callosum.
Joins anterior cerebral to form basal vein.	
Cavernous sinus	Lateral sulcus.
Superior sagittal sinus.	
Joins retromandibular to form common facial, and ends in internal jugular	Front portion of side of face, from medial angle of eye.
Internal jugular	Below the angle of the mandible.
from pterygoid plexus, between masseter and buccinator muscles.	
External jugular or subclavian	Lateral to midline of neck.
Subclavian	Side of neck, below and behind angle of mandible.
Brachiocephalic	Side of neck, deep to sterno-mastoid muscle.
Facial.	
Pterygoid plexus and cavernous sinus	Near floor of orbit.

NAME	DRAINAGE OR TRIBUTARIES
ophthalmica superior	Tributaries corresponding to those of ophthalmic artery
palatina externa [*paratonsillar*]	Palatal region
paratonsillar	Palatina externa (*q.v.*).
plexus basilaris	Inferior petrosal sinuses
plexus pharyngeus	Plexus in the lateral wall of the
plexus pterygoideus [*plexus venosus pterygoideus*]	Corresponds to branches of maxillary artery
plexus venosus pterygoideus	Plexus pterygoideus (*q.v.*).
plexus venosus suboccipitalis	Occipital vein
retromandibularis [*facialis posterior*]	Superficial temporal and maxillary veins
sinus cavernosus	Superior and inferior ophthalmic veins, cerebral veins, spheno-palatine sinus
sinus intercavernosus	One of two (*anterior* and *posterior*) ring round the pituitary fossa.
sinus occipitalis	Variable anastomosing channel between the transverse and sigmoid sinuses
sinus petrosus inferior	Cavernous sinus
sinus petrosus superior	Cavernous sinus
sinus rectus	Formed by the union of the inferior sagittal sinus and the great cerebral vein.
sinus sagittalis inferior	Dura mater
sinus sagittalis superior	Superior cerebral, diploë of cranium, dura mater
sinus sigmoideus	Continuous with transverse sinus
sinus spheno-parietalis	Dura mater
sinus transversus	Superior sagittal or straight sinus, cerebral and cerebellar veins, superior petrosal sinus
thalamostriata	Caudate nucleus and thalamus

DESTINATION	LOCATION
Cavernous sinus	Near roof of orbit.
Facial.	
Vertebral plexus	Basilar portion of occipital bone.

pharynx, from which the pharyngeal veins arise.

Maxillary vein	Between the pterygoid muscles, in the infra-temporal fossa.
Vertebral vein	Posterior portion of scalp.
Common facial and external jugular	Parotid gland, and side of face by ear.
Divides into superior and inferior petrosal sinuses	At the side of the pituitary fossa.

terior) sinuses joining the two cavernous sinuses and forming a

	Cranial attachment of falx cerebelli.
Internal jugular	Inferior petrosal sulcus.
Junction of transverse and sigmoid sinuses	Upper margin of petrous portion of temporal bone.
Transverse sinus	Junction of tentorium cerebelli and falx cerebri.
Joins great cerebral vein to form straight sinus	Lower free margin of falx cerebri.
Transverse sinus	Cranial attachment of falx cerebri.
Internal jugular	Mastoid portion of temporal bone.
Cavernous sinus.	
Via sigmoid sinus to internal jugular	Groove on occipital bone and postero-inferior angle of parietal bone.
With choroid veins forms internal cerebral	On the floor of the central part of the lateral ventricle.

NAME	DRAINAGE OR TRIBUTARIES
thyroidea inferior	Lower part of thyroid gland, via plexus thyroidea impar
thyroidea media	Lower part of thyroid gland
vertebralis accesoria	Venous plexus on the vertebral artery
vertebralis anterior	Arises from venous plexus

DESTINATION	LOCATION
Left brachiocephalic.	Short vein in front of common carotid artery.
Internal jugular	
Brachiocephalic vein.	
Vertebral	Cervical transverse processes.

Appendix I—Drugs

This appendix includes preparations that are of interest to the dentist and the information is arranged in the following order: name of the drug, form in which it may be prescribed with the dose, a brief indication of its action and use, and proprietary names associated with it.

Wherever possible the information will be found under an 'Official or Approved Name'. Proprietary names (in italics) are also included with cross references. It is not intended to imply that a preparation described by a proprietary name is the same as the drug to which the reader is referred, but that under the official name there will be some information relevant to the constituents of the preparation available under the proprietary name. When a name is not in italics it must not be regarded as implying that it is not subject to proprietary rights.

The following abbreviations are used:

B.P.	British Pharmacopoeia and Supplement 1968
B.P.C.	British Pharmaceutical Codex 1968
B.N.F.	British National Formulary 1971
U.S.P.	Pharmacopoeia of the United States XV
U.S.D.	United States Dispensatory
A.D.R.	Accepted Dental Remedies
U.S.N.F.	United States National Formulary

Abbocillin-DC: see Procaine Penicillin.

Abbocin: see Oxytetracycline Tablets.

Absolute Alcohol: see Alcohol.

Absorbable Gelatin Sponge (B.P.) (U.S.P.) Sponge-like absorbable haemostatic. *Gelfoam, Sterispon.* Impregnated with antiseptic. *Dequaspon.*

Acetaminophen: see Paracetamol Tablets.

Acetomenaphthone Tablets (B.P.) Menadione Capsules (U.S.P.) 2 mg. daily. Action similar to Vitamin K. See Phytomenadione. Administered orally in deficiency. *Prokayvit oral, Vitavel K.*

Acetophenetidin: see Phenacetin.

Acetylsalicylic Acid (B.P.) Syn: Aspirin 0.3–1 G. (U.S.P.) 600 mg. Tablets (B.P.) (U.S.P.) Antipyretic, analgesic. Main use is in mild pain either alone or with other analgesics. *Aspirin, Aspro, Empirin, Genasprin.* Soluble Acetylsalicylic Acid Tablets (B.P.) Syn: Soluble Aspirin Tablets (contain citric acid and calcium carbonate which aid disintegration and solution). *Disprin, Solprin.*

Acetylsalicylic Acid and Phenacetin Tablets (B.P.C.) 1-2 (approx. 230 mg. acetylsalicylic acid and 160 mg. phenacetin). Antipyretic, analgesic.

Acetylsalicylic Acid and Quinine Compound Tablets (Dental Practitioners' Formulary). Syn: Aspirin and Quinine Compound Tablets. (Contain acetylsalicylic acid, phenacetin, caffeine and quinine sulphate.) Analgesic with very small doses of caffeine and quinine sulphate. *Anadin.*

Acetylsalicylic Acid Compound Tablets (B.P.C.) 1-2 (approx. 230 mg. acetylsalicylic acid, 160 mg. phenacetin and 30 mg. caffeine). Syn: A.P.C. Tablets. Antipyretic analgesic.

Acetylsalicylic Acid with Ipecacuanha and Opium Tablets (B.P.C.) 1-2 tablets (approx. 160 mg. acetylsalicylic acid and 160 mg. powder of ipecacuanha and opium). Antipyretic analgesic. Used in mild fevers.

Achromycin: see Tetracycline.

Acriflavine (B.P.C.) (U.S.N.F.) Dye produced from coal tar. Lethal to Gram-positive and Gram-negative organisms. Active in the presence of body fluids and pus. Emulsion Acriflavine (B.P.C. 1934). Antiseptic for local application. Solution of acriflavine in saline 1:1000 used for toilet of contaminated wounds and pre-operative preparation of skin.

Activated 7-Dehydrocholesterol: see Vitamin D.

Actomol: see Monoamine Oxidase Inhibitors.

Adrenaline (B.P.) 0.2-0.5 mg. subcut. Adrenaline Acid Tartrate (B.P.) 0.4-1 mg. subcut. as a single dose (Syn: Epinephrine Bitartrate). Adrenaline Injection (B.P.) 0.2-0.5 ml. subcut. (1:1000). Epinephrine Injection (U.S.P.) 0.5 mg. subcut. (1:1000). Adrenaline is a vaso-constrictor. With local anaesthetics 1:100,000—1:20,000. Haemostatic applied topically 1:50,000-1:1000. Used also in anaphylaxis and bronchospasm of asthma. *Adrenaline, Suprarenin.*

Adrocaine: see Procaine Hydrochloride.

Aerosporin: see Polymyxin B Sulphate.

A.H.G.: see Anti-haemophilic Globulin.

Albamycin: see Novobiocin.

Alcohol (B.P.). Syn: Ethyl Alcohol 95 per cent.: also 90, 80, 70, 60, 50, 45, 25 and 20 per cent. (U.S.P.) 94.5 per cent. Diluted Alcohol (U.S.P.) 49.5 per cent. Dehydrated Alcohol (B.P.C.) Syn: Absolute Alcohol. A strong solution precipitates proteins in dentinal tubules, dries cavities, dissolves fats and is an obtundant. A 70 per cent. solution is used as disinfectant. Systemically, dilute solutions have a hypnotic action.

Aleudrin: see Isoprenaline.

Alkaline Phenol Mouth-wash: see Phenol.

Allobarbitone (B.P.C.) Syn: Diallylmalonylurea. 30-200 mg. Diallylbarbituric Acid (U.S.N.F.) Medium acting barbiturate, see Barbiturates.

Allocaine: see Procaine Hydrochloride.

Alum (B.P.) Potassium or ammonium aluminium sulphate. Precipitates proteins, astringent. 1-4 per cent. in mouth-washes or gargles in stomatitis or pharyngitis.

Amaranth Solution (B.P.C.) Solution of a red culinary dye used for colouring mouth-washes and gargles.

Amethocaine Hydrochloride (B.P.) Nerve block 0.1 per cent., infiltration 0.03-0.1 per cent., topical 0.5-2 per cent. Tetracine Hydrochloride (U.S.P.) infiltration 0.1-0.25 per cent. (A.D.R.) not more than 1 ml. of 2 per cent. for topical anaesthesia in dentistry. Local anaesthetic about ten times more potent than procaine and equally more toxic, onset of action slower but more lasting. Syn: Pantocaine. *Anethaine, Pontocaine.*

Amidone: see Methadone Hydrochloride.

Amidopyrine, 300-600 mg. Aminopyrine Tablets (U.S.N.F.) usual strength 300 mg. Antipyretic analgesic with action and uses like phenazone, but effective in smaller doses. Can cause agranulocytosis.

Aminacrine Hydrochloride (B.P.) Antiseptic produced from coal tar. See Acriflavine. Non-staining.

Aminophylline Tablets (B.P.) 100-300 mg. (U.S.P.) 200 mg. Also injections. Syn: Theophylline Ethylenediamine. Smooth muscle relaxant. Relieves bronchial spasm. *Cardophyllin, Delaminoph.*

Amphetamine Sulphate Tablets (B.P.) 5-10 mg., (U.S.P.) 10 mg. Sympathomimetic. Locally, vasoconstriction. Systemically, central nervous system stimulation, notably cerebrum and medullary centres. *Benzedrine, Raphetamine.*

Aminopyrine: see Amidopyrine.

Amobarbital: see Amylobarbitone Tablets.

Amosan: see Sodium Perborate.

Amphotericin (B.P.C.): Anti fungal agent. Preparations—Ointment 3 per cent. in aqueous base—Lozenges 10 mgs.—Tablets 100 mgs. *Fungilin.*

Ampicillin Capsules (B.P.) (B.N.F.): Antibiotic 1—6G daily (divided) Semi-synthetic penicillin with broad spectrum of activity. *Penbritin.*

Amyl Nitrite (B.P.C.) 0.12-0.3 ml. by inhalation (U.S.P.) 0.3 ml. by inhalation. Vasodilator used in angina pectoris.

Amylobarbitone Tablets (B.P.) 100-200 mg. Amobarbital Tablets (U.S.P.) 100 mg. Amylobarbitone Sodium Capsules and Tablets (B.N.F.) 100-200 mg. Amobarbital Sodium

Capsules (U.S.P.) 100 mg. Medium acting. See Barbiturates. *Sodium Amytal, Dorminal.*
Amytal: see Amylobarbitone Tablets.
Anacobin: see Cyanocobalamin Injection.
Anadin: see Acetylsalicylic Acid and Quinine Compound Tablets.
Anaesthesin: see Benzocaine.
Anaesthetic Ether: see Ether.
Ancolan: see Meclozine Hydrochloride.
Anectine: see Suxamethonium.
Anethaine: see Amethocaine Hydrochloride.
Aneurine Compound Tablets, Strong: see Vitamin B Compound Tablets, Strong.
Ansolysen: see Pentolinium Tartrate.
Antazoline Hydrochloride (B.P.) 50-100 mg. (U.S.P.) 100 mg. Antihistamine. *Antistin, Histostab.*
Anthisan: see Mepyramine Maleate.
Antihaemophilic Globulin (Syn : A.H.G.). Plasma fraction from human, bovine or porcine source, as an alternative to large volumes of human plasma in haemophilia. Reactions to animal antigens are common.
Antiphlogistine: see Kaolin Poultice.
Antipyrin: see Phenazone.
Antistin: see Antazoline Hydrochloride.
Antrenyl: see Oxyphenonium Bromide.
A.P.C. Tablets: see Acetylsalicylic Acid Compound Tablets.
Aquamephyton: see Phytomenadione.
Aromatic Cascara Sagrada Fluid Extract: see Cascara Elixir.
Aromatic Sodium Perborate: see Sodium Perborate.
Arsenic Trioxide (B.P.C.) Protoplasmic poison. Was used locally as a devitalising agent, but leakage caused necrosis of gum or bone.
Ascorbic Acid Tablets: see Vitamin C.
Ascorvel: see Vitamin C.
Ascoxal: see Vitamin C.
Aspirin: see Acetylsalicylic Acid.
Aspirin and Dovers Powder Tablets: see Acetylsalicylic Acid with Ipecacuanha and Opium Tablets.
Aspirin and Quinine Compound Tablets: see Acetylsalicylic Acid and Quinine Compound Tablets.
Aspro: see Acetylsalicylic Acid.
Ataractic: see Tranquillizers.
Atropine Sulphate (B.P.) 0.25-1 mg. (U.S.P.) 0.5 mg. Block post-ganglionic parasympathetic nerve endings. Stimulant followed by depressant central action. Antispasmodic. Mydriatic. Pre-operatively it reduces salivary and bronchial secretions.

Aureomycin: see Chlortetracycline.
Aventyl: see Tricyclic Antidepressants.
Avomine: see Promethazine Theoclate.

Bacitracin (B.P.). Antibiotic with an antibacterial range like penicillin. Used for topical application.
Bactrim: see Trimethoprim and Sulphamethoxazole.
Banthine: see Methantheline Bromide.
Barbiturates. Hypnotic and sedative drugs obtained by combination of derivatives of malonic acid and urea. May be classified as long acting (over 8 hours), used as sedatives and in epilepsy, medium (6-8 hours) and short acting (2-3 hours), used as hypnotics and in pre-operative and post-operative medication, and ultra short acting used as intravenous anaesthetics and for induction.
Bemigride, *Megimide*, 50 mg. i.v. repeated. Analeptic used in barbiturate poisoning.
Benactyzine Hydrochloride (B.P.C.) 1-2 mg. Tranquilizer. Relieves nervous tension and anxiety without producing drowsiness. Some anticholinergic properties. *Suavitil*.
Benadryl: see Diphenhydramine.
Benzalkonium Chloride Solution (B.P.C.) 50 per cent. (U.S.P.) topically as 0.1-0.01 per cent. Cationic surface active antiseptic. Benzalkonium Lozenges (B.P.C.) 0.5 mg. in each with menthol, thymol, eucalyptus oil and lemon oil. *Drapolene*, *P.R.Q. Antiseptic, Roccal, Zephiran*.
Benzathine Penicillin (B.P.) Benzathine Penicillin G. (U.S.P.) See also Penicillin. Available: Tablets (B.P.) 300,000-600,000 units. Sterile Benzathine Penicillin G Suspension (U.S.P.) 600,000 U.S.P. units i.m. *Bicillin, Megacillin, Penidural, Permapen*.
Benzedrine: see Amphetamine Sulphate Tablets.
Benzethonium Chloride Solution (U.S.P.) Skin 0.1 per cent. Surface active antiseptic. Bactericidal and fungicidal. *Phemerol*.
Benzocaine (B.P.) 5-10 per cent. topical. Syn: Ethyl Aminobenzoate. Local anaesthetic. *Anaesthesin*. Benzocaine Lozenges (Dental Practitioners' Formulary) 10 mg. in each. Benzocaine Compound Lozenges (B.P.C.) 97.2 mg. with menthol and borax.
Benzoic Acid (B.P.) Bacteriostatic and fungistatic properties. Usually used as a preservative of medicinal preparations.
Benzylpenicillin (B.P.) Potassium Penicillin G (U.S.P.) Sodium Penicillin G (U.S.P.) The soluble Sodium or Potassium salt of benzylpenicillin. See Penicillin. Preparations available: Injection (B.P.) 250,000-1,000,000 units i.m., Tablets (B.P.),

Buffered Crystalline Penicillin G (U.S.P.) 200,000 U.S.P. units oral; 50,000 units i.m., Tablets (U.S.P.) 200,000 U.S.P. units. *Crystapen, Eskacillin, Falapen, Penevan, Peniset, Penisol, Purapen G, Solupen, Tabillin.*

Berkmycen: see Oxytetracycline Tablets.

Bicillin: see Benzathine Penicillin.

Biocetab: see Cetrimide Solution.

Biotexin: see Novobiocin.

Bishydroxycoumarin Tablets: see Ethyl Biscoumacetate.

Bi-Stabillin: see Procaine Penicillin.

Bitevan: see Cyanocobalamin Injection.

Bocasan: see Sodium Perborate.

Bocosept: see Sodium Perborate.

Borax: see Boric acid.

Boric Acid (B.P.) (U.S.P.). Borax (B.P.). Sodium Salt of boric acid. Mild bacteriostatic and fungistatic action. Used in solution in glycerin, e.g. Borax Glycerin (B.P.C.) 12 per cent. as a paint for the mouth or diluted as a mouth-wash.

Bradosol: see Domiphen Bromide.

Brevidil M: see Suxamethonium.

Brietal Sodium: see Methohexitone Sodium.

Brilliant Green (B.P.) Syn: Viride Nitens. Antiseptic with persistant action when used on skin or mucous membrane. Constituent of Brilliant Green and Crystal Violet Paint (B.P.C.) Syn: Pigmentum Tinctorum.

Bromadal: see Carbromal.

Bubal: see Butobarbitone Tablets.

Buffered Crystalline Penicillin: see Benzylpenicillin.

Butazolidin: see Phenylbutazone.

Butethal: see Butobarbitone Tablets.

Butethamine Hydrochloride (U.S.N.F.). Local anaesthetic about one third more potent and about one third more toxic than procaine. Used by injection in 1 per cent. solution. *Monocaine.*

Butobarbitone Tablets (B.P.) 100-200 mg. Medium acting, see Barbiturates. Syn: Butethal, *Bubal, Butomet, Sonabarb, Soneryl.*

Butomet: see Butobarbitone Tablets.

Calciferol: see Vitamin D.

Calcipen V: see Phenoxymethylpenicillin.

Calcium Alginate (B.P.C.) Absorbable material supplied as a wool or gauze for use as haemostatic. *Calgitex.*

Calcium Gluconate Tablets (B.P.C.). 1-6 tablets (each contains 650 mg. in chocolate basis). Used in calcium replacement therapy. Less irritant to stomach than other forms of calcium.

Calcium Lactate Tablets (B.P.) 1-4 G. Used in calcium replacement therapy.

Calcium Sodium Lactate Tablets (B.P.C.) 0.3-2 G. Soluble salt of calcium used orally in calcium deficiency.

Calcium with Vitamin D Tablets (B.P.C.) 1-2 tablets. Calciferol Compound Tablets. Contain calcium sodium lactate and calcium phosphate with calciferol (approx. 500 units of antirachitic activity or Vitamin D). For augmentation of calcium intake during Vitamin D therapy.

Calcium Peroxide. Similar action and uses to Magnesium Peroxide *q.v.*

Calgitex: see Calcium Alginate.

Calomel: see Mercurous Chloride Tablets.

Calpol: see Paracetamol Tablets.

Camphor (B.P.) (U.S.P.) Crystalline volatile substance. Externally it has a mild analgesic and rubifacient action. Liquifies with menthol or thymol and such mixtures are used as obtundents.

Carbachol Injection (B.P.) 0.25-0.5 mg. subcut. Has actions like acetylcholine at parasympathetic nerve endings and also autonomic ganglia. Main use in urinary retention.

Carbamazepine Tablets (B.P.). 200—1200 mgs. daily. Used in gradually increasing dosage. Trigeminal Neuralgia. *Tegretol.*

Carbolic Acid: see Phenol.

Carboxymethylcellulose Gelatin Paste: Adheres to oral mucosa and provides mechanical protection. *Orabase.*

Carbromal (B.P.) 0.3-1 G. Syn: Uradal, Bromadal. Mild hypnotic. Tablets (B.P.).

Cardiamide: see Nikethamide Injection.

Cardiazol: see Leptazol Injection.

Cardiazole: see Leptazol Injection.

Cardophyllin: see Aminophylline Tablets.

Cascara Compound Tablets (B.P.C.) 1-2 tablets (contain cascara, rhubarb, nux vomica, ginger oleoresin and podophyllum resin). Purgative.

Cascara Elixir (B.P.) 2-4 ml. Aromatic Cascara Sagrada Fluid Extract (U.S.P.) 2 ml. Sweetened and flavoured liquid with the activity of cascara an anthraquinone purgative.

Cascara Tablets (B.P.) 120-250 mg. Anthracene purgative.

Celin: see Vitamin C.

Cephalexin Capsules (B.N.F.). 1—4 G daily (divided) Broad Spectrum antibiotic. *Ceporex, Keflex.*

Cephaloridine Injection (B.P.) 0.5—1 G Antibiotic. Alternative to penicillin with similar spectrum. *Ceporin.*

Ceporex: see Cephalexin Capsules.

Ceporin: see Cephaloridine Injection.

Cetal: see Paracetamol Tablets.

Cetavlon: see Cetrimide Solution.

Cetrimide Solution (B.N.F.) 1 per cent. Antiseptic and detergent with cationic surface action. Used to clean skin or instruments. *Biocetab, Cetavlon, Savlon.*

Cevalin: see Vitamin C.

Chloral Draught: see Chloral Hydrate.

Chloral Elixir for Infants: see Chloral Hydrate.

Chloral Hydrate (B.P.) 0.3-2 G. (U.S.P.) 600 mg. Chloral Hydrate Mixture (B.N.F.) 15 ml. (1.5 G). Chloral Draught (Dental Practitioners' Formulary). Freshly prepared solution containing 20 grains of chloral hydrate flavoured with liquorice. Chloral Elixir for Infants (B.N.F.) 4 ml. (approx. 120 mg.). Hypnotic lasting six to eight hours.

Chloramphenicol (B.P.); Capsules (B.P.) 1.5-3 G. daily, divided; (U.S.P.) 250 mg. Broad spectrum antibiotic, now synthesized. Given systemically as bacteriostatic against Gram-positive and Gram-negative organisms. Effective against rickettsiae. *Chloromycetin, Clocetin, Enicol, Kemecetine.*

Chorbutol (B.P.) Sedative when given orally. Preservative for solutions for injection. Ingredient of *Dentalone* which has uses similar to those of oil of cloves.

Chlorcyclizine Hydrochloride (B.P.) 50-150 mg. (U.S.P.) 50 mg. Antihistamine. *Di-Paralene, Histantin.*

Chlordiazepoxide Tablets: (B.P.) 10—100 mgs. daily. Tranquilizer less toxic than barbiturates. *Librium.*

Chlorhexidine. Wide range antibacterial action. Used as a general antiseptic. *Hibitane.* Lozenges contain the dihydrochloride 5 mg. and benzocaine 2 mg. Used for bacterial and fungal infections of the mouth.

Chlorinated Soda Surgical Solution: see Chlorine.

Chlorine. Several antiseptic and disinfectant solutions containing chlorine are used as cleansing solutions, e.g. Surgical Chlorinated Soda Solution (B.P.): Syn: Dakins Solution; Solution of Chlorinated Lime with Boric Acid (B.P.C.). Syn: Eusol; Sodium Hypochlorite Solution (U.S.N.F.) and Diluted Sodium Hypochlorite Solution (U.S.N.F.). They are bacteriostatic for a wide range of organisms and disintegrate protein debris. Used to clean instruments and dentures. *Milton, Chloros, Deosan.*

Chlorocresol (B.P.). Halogenated cresol. More bactericidal than cresol. General antiseptic. Constituent of Chlorocresol Gargle.

Chloroform (B.P.) (U.S.P.). Trichloromethane. Liquid, the vapour of which was used as a general anaesthetic. Used as a solvent for gutta percha and acrylics. Chloroform Emulsion

(B.P.C.) 0.3-2 ml. (1:20). Chloroform Water (B.P.) 15-30 ml.
(1:400), Carminative and flavouring agent.

Chloroform Emulsion: see Chloroform.

Chloroform Water: see Chloroform.

Chloromycetin: see Chloramphenicol.

Chloros: see Chlorine.

Chloroxylenol Solution (B.P.) Syn: Roxenol. Contains chloroxylenol, a non-irritant bactericide. Used as a general disinfectant. Main action on Gram-negative organisms. The following are commercial preparations containing chlorinated
phenols: *C.M.X. Antiseptic, Clearsol, Cresantol* 15, *Dettol,
G.P. Germicide, Ibcol, Jeypine, Prinsyl, Sterillium, Supersan,
T.C.P., Zal, Zant.*

Chlorpheniramine Maleate (B.P.C.) 6-16 mg. orally daily, 10-
20 mg. subcut. i.m. or slow i.v. (U.S.P.) 4 mg. Syn: Chlorprophenpyridamine. Anti-histamine, rarely produces side
effects. *Chlor-Trimeton, Haynon, Histafen, Piriton.*

Chlorpromazine Injection (B.P.) 25-50 mg. i.m. Tablets (B.P.)
25-50 mg. Many actions. Used as tranquillizer in major
psychiatric disorders, to potentiate the action of analgesics,
and as antiemetic. *Largactil, Thorazine.*

Chlorprophenpyridamine: see Chlorpheniramine Maleate.

Chlortetracycline Capsules (B.P.) 1-3 G. daily (divided), (U.S.P.)
250 mg. Chlortetracycline Injection (B.P.) 250-500 mg. i.v.,
(U.S.P.) 250 mg. see Tetracyclines for uses. *Aureomycin.*

Chlor-Trimeton: see Chlorpheniramine Maleate.

Choovit: see Vitamin C.

Chromic Acid: see Chromium Trioxide.

Chromium Trioxide (B.P.C.) (Chromic Acid) Caustic. Used in
Vincent's infections for its oxidising properties.

Cinchocaine Hydrochloride (B.P.). Nerve block 0.1 per cent.,
infiltration 0.03-0.1 per cent., topical 0.5-2 per cent. Dibucaine
Hydrochloride Injection (U.S.P.) infiltration 1-50 ml. of 0.1
per cent. Local anaesthetic about forty times the potency of
procaine. To give mild local anaesthesia of the mucosa the
following is available: Cinchocaine Hydrochloride Lozenges
(B.P.C.) each containing 1 mg. *Nupercaine Hydrochloride.*

Clearsol: see Chloroxylenol Solution.

Clinimycin: see Oxytetracycline Tablets.

Clinitetrin: see Tetracycline Capsules.

Clocetin: see Chloramphenicol.

Clove Oil (B.P.) (U.S.P.) Protoplasmic poison. Antiseptic and
analgesic action in carious tooth or on exposed pulp. With
zinc oxide forms a temporary filling. On skin it is rubifacient.

Cloxacillin (B.P.) (B.N.F.) 1—3 G orally or 1M on divided doses.

Antibiotic used for infections caused by pencillin resistant Staphylococci. *Orbenin.*

C.M.X. Antiseptic: see Chloroxylenol Solution.

Cobalin: see Cyanocobalamin Injection.

Cobastab: see Cyanocobalamin Injection.

Cocaine Hydrochloride (B.P.) The first local anaesthetic, an alkaloid. Now replaced in dentistry by safer synthetic drugs.

Codeine Compound Tablets: see Compound Codeine Tablets.

Codeine Phosphate Tablets (B.P.) 10-60 mg. (U.S.P.) 30 mg. Mild analgesic and hypnotic. Less constipating than morphine. Used to allay an irritating unproductive cough and also in mild pain usually with other analgesics.

Cod Liver Oil: see Vitamin D.

Compocillin V: see Phenoxymethylpenicillin.

Compound Acetylsalicylic Acid Tablets: see Acetylsalicylic Acid Compound Tablets.

Compound Cascara Tablets: see Cascara Compound Tablets.

Compound Codeine Tablets (B.P.) 1-2 (approx. 260 mg. each acetylsalicylic acid and phenacetin and 8 mg. codeine phosphate). Antipyretic, analgesic. *Veganin.*

Compound Glycerin of Thymol (B.P.C.). Contains borax, sodium bicarbonate, sodium benzoate, several aromatic flavouring principles and glycerin. Mouthwash when diluted with 3 parts of water. Of limited antiseptic value. Refreshing.

Compound Iodine Paint: see Iodine.

Compound Paint of Iodoform (B.P.C.) Syn: Whitehead's Varnish. Iodoform 10 per cent. with benzoin, storax and balsam of tolu in solvent ether. Iodoform releases iodine slowly but the main value of the paint is to seal incisions in tongue or lips.

Compound Sodium Chloride Mouth-Wash (B.P.C.) (Sodium chloride 1.71 per cent. sodium bicarbonate 0.86 per cent.) Diluted with an equal quantity of warm water before use. Mildly stimulant and cleaning.

Compound Tartrazine Solution (B.P.C.) Solution of culinary dyes giving a yellow concentrate. Used to colour mouthwashes and gargles.

Compound Thymol Glycerin: see Compound Glycerin of Thymol.

Compound Thymol Solution-tablets: see Thymol Compound Solution-Tablets.

Coramine: see Nikethamide Injection.

Corlan Pellets: see Hydrocortisone Pellets.

Cormed: see Nikethamide Injection.

Corvotone: see Nikethamide Injection.

Cream of Magnesia: see Magnesium Hydroxide Mixture.

Cresantol 15: see Chloroxylenol Solution.

Cresol (B.P.) (U.S.P.). Protoplasmic poison. Caustic. Used only to disinfect articles owing to its tarry odour and pungent taste. Constituent of Cresol and Soap Solution (B.P.) Syn: Lysol.

Crystacillin A.S.: see Phenoxymethylpenicillin.

Crystal Violet (B.P.) Syn: Medicinal Gentian Violet. Crystal Violet Paint (B.N.F.) 0.5 per cent., Methylrosanaline Chloride Solution (U.S.P.) 1 per cent. Antiseptic. Persistent action on Gram-positive organisms and various moulds and fungi.

Crystapen: see Benzylpenicillin.

Crystapen V: see Phenoxymethylpenicillin.

Cyanocobalamin Injection (B.P.) 50-100 μg i.m. (U.S.P.) 1-15 m.c.g. i.m. Syn: Vitamin B_{12} Injection. Essential factor in treatment of pernicious anaemia. *Anacobin, Bitevan, Cobalin, Cobastab, Cytacon, Distavit B_{12}, Hydroxycobalamin, Neo-Cytamen, Rubramin.*

Cyclizine Hydrochloride (B.P.C.) 25-50 mg. Antihistamine. *Marzine, Marezine, Valoid.*

Cyclobarbital: see Cyclobarbitone.

Cyclobarbitone Tablets (B.P.) 200-400 mg. Cyclobarbital. Short acting, see Barbiturates. *Phanodorm. Phanodorn, Rapidal.*

Cyclopropane (B.P.) (U.S.P.) Syn: Trimethylene. Powerful anaesthetic gas in concentration of 10-20 per cent. Rapid induction and recovery. Of special value in chest surgery and in severely shocked patients. Inflammable.

Cytacon: see Cyanocobalamin Injection.

Dakin's Solution: see Chlorine.

d-Amfetasul: see Dexamphetamine.

Davitamon C: see Vitamin C.

Debenox: see Dicyclomine Hydrochloride.

Dehydrated Alcohol: see Alcohol.

Delaminoph: see Animophylline.

Demerol: see Pethidine Injection.

Democracin: see Tetracycline Capsules.

Dentalone. Uses similar to clove oil.

Deosan: see Chlorine.

Dequaspon: see Absorbable Gelatin Sponge.

Dettol: see Chloroxylenol Solution.

Dexamphetamine Tablets (B.P.) 5-10 mg. Dextro Amphetamine Sulfate Tablets (U.S.P.) 5 mg. Sympathomimetic. Like amphetamine but central effects predominate. *d-Amfetasul, Dexedrine.*

Dexedrine: see Dexamphetamine Tablets.

Dextro Amphetamine: see Dexamphetamine.

D.F. 118: see Dihydrocodeine Tablets.

Diallylbarbituric Acid: see Allobarbitone.

Diallylmalonylurea: see Allobarbitone.

Diazepam Tablets (B.P.): 5-30 mgs. orally. Tranquillizer with similar effect to barbiturates. Also used I.V. as sedative for dental treatment in doses of 5-30 mgs. *Valium.*

Dibucaine: see Cinchocaine Hydrochloride.

Dicoumarol: A long acting anticoagulant.

Dicyclomine Hydrochloride. 10-20 mg. Atropine substitute. *Debenox, Merbentyl, Wyovine.*

Diethyl Ether: see Ether.

Digoxin Tablets (B.P.) initial 1-1.5 mg. maintenance 0.25 mg. (U.S.P.) initial 1.5 mg.; 3 mg. over 24 hours, maintenance 0.5 mg. Also injections. Digitalis glycoside. Shorter acting than digitoxin. Used in cardiac insufficiency. *Lanoxin.*

Digitoxin Tablets (U.S.P.) initial 1.5 mg. divided over 24-48 hours. Maintenance 0.1 mg. Also injection. The most potent digitalis glycoside. Long acting. Used in cardiac insufficiency.

Dihydrocodeine Tablets (B.P.) 30-60 mgs. Analgesic of moderate potency. *D.F. 118, Paracodin.*

Dihydrostreptomycin: see Streptomycin Sulphate Injection.

Dilantin Sodium: see Phenytoin Tablets.

Dimenhydrinate (B.P.C.) 25-50 mg. (U.S.P.) 50 mg. Antihistamine. Said to be of special value for motion sickness. *Dramamine, Gravol.*

Dindevan: see Phenindione Tablets.

Dioloxol: see mephenesin injection.

Di-Paralene: see Chlorcyclizine Hydrochloride.

Diphenhydramine Hydrochloride (B.P.) 25-75 mg. (U.S.P.) 25 mg. Antihistamine. *Benadryl.*

Diphenylhydantoin Sodium Capsules: see Phenytoin Tablets.

Disprin: see Acetylsalicylic Acid.

Distaquaine: see Procaine Penicillin.

Distaquaine V: see Phenoxymethylpenicillin.

Distivit B₁₂: see Cyanocobalamin Injection.

Divinyl Oxide: see Vinyl Ether.

Dolantal: see Pethidine Injection.

Dolantin: see Pethidine Injection.

Dolophine: see Methadone Hydrochloride.

Domiphen Bromide (B.P.C.) Cationic surface active antiseptic for use on wounds (0.02 per cent.) skin and surgical instruments (0.5 per cent. in alcohol). Lozenges containing 0.5 per cent. Bactericidal or bacteriostatic depending on concentration. Also antifungal action. *Bradosol.*

Doriden: see Glutethimide.

Dorminal: see Amylobarbitone Tablets.

Dormison: see Methylpentynol.

379

Dramamine: see Dimenhydrinate.
Drapolene: see Benzalkonium Chloride Solution.
Dromoran: see Levorphanol Tartrate.
Duracillin: see Procaine Penicillin.

Economycin: see Tetracycline Capsules.
Econopen V: see Phenoxymethylpenicillin.
Effervescing Mouth-wash Tablets: see Mouth-wash Solution—tablets.
Eff-vit-C: see Vitamen C.
Efroxine: see Methylamphetamine.
Elorine: see Tricyclamol Methylsulphate.
Empirin: see Acetylsalicylic Acid.
Enicol: see Chloramphenicol.
Epanutin: see Phenytoin Tablets.
Ephedrine Hydrochloride Tablets (B.P.) 16-60 mg. Ephedrine Sulfate Capsules, Injection and Tablets (U.S.P.) 25 mg. oral and subcut. Potentiates adrenaline. Central nervous system stimulant, vasoconstrictor and bronchodilator.
Epinephrine: see Adrenaline.
Epontol: see Propanidid.
Epsom Salts: see Mangesium Sulphate.
Equanil: see Meprobamate.
Erythrocin: see Erythromycin Tablets.
Erythromycin Tablets (B.P.) 1-2 G daily (divided) (U.S.P.) 300 mg. Bactericidal and bacteriostatic antibiotic. Active against Gram-positive organisms and may be used when the patient is allergic to penicillin. *Erythrocin, Erythroped, Ilotycin, Ilosone, Retcin.*
Erythroped: see Erythromycin Tablets.
Eserine Salicylate: see Physostigmine Salicylate.
Eskacillin: see Benzylpenicillin.
Eskacillin 200: see Procaine Penicillin.
Eskacillin V: see Phenoxymethylpenicillin.
Ether (U.S.P.), Anaesthetic Ether (B.P.). Diethyl Ether, Ethyl Ether. Liquid, the vapour of which is a moderately powerful anaesthetic. Unsuitable for ambulant patients and when used to supplement nitrous oxide anaesthesia delays recovery. Inflammable.
Ethocaine: see Procaine Hydrochloride.
Ethocaine Hydrochloride: see Procaine Hydrochloride.
Ethyl Alcohol: see Alcohol.
Ethyl Aminobenzoate: see Benzocaine.
Ethyl Biscoumacetate Tablets (B.P.) initial 1.2 G. maintenance 150-900 mg. Bishydroxycoumarin Tablets (U.S.P.) initial 200-300 mg. maintenance 100-200 mg. Syn: Ethyldicoumarol,

Pelentan.   Oral anticoagulant with shorter action than di-
    coumarol. Treatment of thrombosis. *Tromexan, Peletan.*
Ethyl Chloride (B.P.) (U.S.P.)   Very potent anaesthetic gas
    stored in liquid form under pressure. The cooling effect of
    evaporation of the liquid from the skin produces mild analgesia.
    Inflammable.
Ethyldicoumarol: see Ethyl Biscoumacetate.
Ethylene (U.S.P.)   Anaesthetic gas, more potent than nitrous
    oxide and with similar uses. Unpleasant smell. Inflammable.
Ethyl Ether: see Ether.
Eugenol (B.P.C.) (U.S.P.)   Principle constituent of Clove Oil.
    Action and uses of Clove Oil.
Eusol: see Chlorine.

Falapen: see Benzylpenicillin.
Fastocain: see Lignocaine Hydrochloride.
Febrillix: see Paracetamol Tablets.
Felypressin: Vasoconstrictor used in local anaesthetic solution
    as an alternative to adrenaline.
Ferric Chloride Solution (B.P.C.)   An acid solution containing
    ferric chloride. Used in gargles for its powerful astringent
    action. Painful when used as a styptic. Gargle of Ferric Chlor-
    ide (B.P.C.) 3.13 per cent. with potassium chlorate 3.43 per
    cent.
Ferrous Gluconate Tablets (B.P.) 300-600 mg. (U.S.P.) 300 mg.
    Used in oral replacement therapy in iron deficiency.
Ferrous Sulphate Tablets (B.P.) 60-200 mg. (U.S.P.) 200 mg.
    Used in oral replacement therapy in iron deficiency.
Flagyl: see Metronidazole Tablets.
Flaxedil: see Gallamine Injection.
Flo-cillin: see Procaine Penicillin.
Fluoride: see Sodium Fluoride and Stannous Fluoride.
Fluothane: see Halothane.
Formaldehyde Lozenges (B.P.C.) contain paraformaldhyde
    9.7 mg., menthol 2.6 mg. and flavouring agents. Syn: Form-
    alin Throat Tablets, Formamint Tablets. *See* Formaldehyde
    Solution. *Formalin,* and *Formamint* tablets and lozenges are
    available.
Formaldehyde Solution (B.P.)   Formalin (34-38 per cent.)
    Precipitates proteins. Astringent, germicidal towards a very
    wide range of organisms. Desensitizes dentine. Used as a
    mummifying agent for residual pulp.
Formalin Throat Tablets (B.P.C.): see Formaldehyde Lozenges.
Fortral: see Pentazocine Tablets.
Fungilin: see Amphotericin.

Gallamine Injection (B.P.) Neuromuscular blocking drug. Use is similar to tubocurarine. *Flaxedil.*

Gallamine Triethiodide: see Gallamine Injection.

Gamophen: see Hexachlorophane.

Gardenal: see Phenobarbitone Tablets.

Gargle of Ferric Chloride: see Ferric Chloride Solution.

Gargle of Phenol: see Phenol.

Gargle of Potassium Chlorate and Phenol: see Potassium Chlorate.

Gelatin Sponge: see Absorbable Gelatin Sponge.

Gelfoam: see Absorbable Gelatin Sponge.

Genasprin: see Acetylsalicylic Acid.

Gentian Violet: see Crystal Violet.

Glutethimide 250-500 mg. Hypnotic, rapid acting and lasting about 6 hours. *Doriden.*

Glycerin (B.P.) (U.S.P.) Syn: Glycerol. An alcohol. Dehydrating properties. Diluted with water it is emollient, demulcent and a mild antiseptic.

Glycerin of Borax: see Boric Acid.

Glycerin of Thymol Compound: see Compound Glycerin of Thymol.

Glyceryl Trinitrate Tablets (B.P.) 0.5-1 mg. (U.S.P.) 0.4 sublingual. Syn: Trinitrin, Nitroglycerin. Vasodilator used in angina pectoris.

G.P. Germicide: see Chloroxylenol Solution.

Gravol: see Dimenhydrinate.

Halibut Liver Oil: see Vitamin A.

Halothane (B.P.C.) Liquid, the vapour of which is a potent anaesthetic. Highly volatile. Induction 1-3 per cent. Maintenance 0.5-1.5 per cent. *Fluothane.*

Haynon: see Chlorpheniramine Maleate.

Heparin Injection (B.P.) 5,000-15,000 units i.m., i.v. Heparin sodium Injection (U.S.P.) 5,000-20,000 U.S.P. units. Anticoagulant with a rapid brief action. *Pularin.*

Hexachlorophane. Hexachlorophene (U.S.P.) Non-irritant bactericide most active against Gram-positive organisms. Incorporated in soaps and creams. *Gamophen, Surofene.*

Hexachlorophene: see Hexachlorophane.

Hexamethonium Tartrate. Ganglion blocking drug available as Tablets (B.P.) and Injection (B.P.) Used in hypertension. *Vegolysen T.*

Hibitane: see Chlorhexidine.

Histafen: see Chlorpheniramine Tablets.

Histantin: see Chlorcyclizine Hydrochloride.

Histostab: see Antazoline Hydrochloride.

Howe's Solution: see Silver Nitrate.

Human Fibrin Foam (B.P.) Absorbable sponge-like material used as a pack or cover for bleeding areas.

Human Thrombin: see Thrombin.

Hyaluronidase. An enzyme which causes depolymerisation of interstitial ground substance of tissues. Sometimes added to injections of local anaesthetics to increase the area of spread.

Hydrocortisone Lozenges (B.N.F.) (Hydrocortisone Sodium Succinate Lozenges, Hydrocortisone Pellets) 2.5 mg. Used to suppress inflammatory reactions locally. Does not influence infection but may disguise its progress. *Corlan Pellets.*

Hydrogen Peroxide Solution (B.P.) 6 per cent. (U.S.P.) 3 per cent. Releases nascent oxygen on contact with organic matter. Mild antibacterial and mechanical cleaning properties. 6 per cent. is used as a mouth-wash in Vincent's infection and septic sockets.

Hydroxycobalamin: see Cyanocobalamin Injection.

Hyoscine Hydrobromide (B.P.) 0.3-0.6 mg. Scopolomine Hydrobromide (U.S.P.) Action and uses like atropine sulphate except that the central action is uniformly depressant.

Ibcol: see Choroxylenol Solution.

Icipen: see Phenoxymethylpenicillin

Ilosone: see Erythromycin Tablets.

Ilotycin: see Erythromycin Tablets.

Imferon: see Iron Dextran Complex.

Impericin: see Oxytetracycline Tablets.

Industrial Methylated Spirit (B.P.) Alcohol 19, approved wood naphtha 1.

Injection of Papaveretum (B.P.C.) Contains the natural alkaloids of opium. Action and uses similar to those of Morphine Sulphate *q.v. Omnopon.*

Insomnol: see Methylpentynol Capsules.

Intraval Sodium: see Thiopentone Injection.

Inversine: see Mecamylamine Hydrochloride.

Iodine (B.P.) (U.S.P.) Wide bactericidal, fungicidal and amoebicidal action in low concentrations. Inactivated by organic matter. Stains the skin and hypersensitivity reactions may occur. Counter Irritant. Weak Iodine Solution (B.P.) 2.5 per cent. Syn: Tincture of Iodine. Iodine Tincture (U.S.P.) (2 per cent.). Iodine Compound Paint (B.P.C.). Syn: Mandl's Paint (1.25 per cent. in glycerin).

Iodine Compound Paint: see Iodine.

Iodine Tincture: see Iodine.

Iron Dextran Complex (*Imferon*) 50-100 mg. i.m. For iron

replacement therapy by injection when oral administration is too slow or ineffective.

Isoniazid Tablets: (B.P.): 100-300 mgs. daily (divided) (U.S.P.) 100 mgs. Potent antituberculous drug with no action against other micro-organisms. *Nicetal, Pycazide.*

Isoprenaline Tablets (B.P.) 5-20 mg. Isoproterenol Hydrochloride Tablets (U.S.P.) 10 mg. sublingual. Syn: Isopropylnoradrenaline. Sympathomimetic amine with mainly bronchodilator and peripheral vasodilator actions. *Aleudrin, Isupren, Neo-Epnine, Norisodrone.*

Isopropylnoradrenaline: see Isoprenaline.

Isoproterenol: see Isoprenaline.

Isupren: see Isoprenaline.

Jeypine: see Chloroxylenol Solution.

Kaolin Poultice (B.P.) Cataplasma Kaolini. Counter irritant. *Antiphlogistine.*

Kavosan: see Sodium Perborate.

Keflex: see Cephalexin Capsules.

Kemecetine: see Chloramphenicol.

Kemithal: see Thialbarbitone Sodium.

Konakion: see Phytomenadione.

Lanoxin: see Digoxin Tablets.

Largactil: see Chlorpromazine.

Laudanum: see Opium Tincture.

Leptazol Injection (B.P.) 50-100 mg. subcut. Pentylenetetrazol Injection (U.S.P.) 100 mg. subcut. i.v. Respiratory and vasometer centre stimulant. *Cardiazol. Metrazol.*

Lethidrone: see Nalorphine Injection.

Levallorphan Tartrate (B.P.C.) 0.2-2 mg. i.v. Antagonist of levorphanol and other morphine like analgesics. *Lorphan.*

Levarterenol Bitartrate: see Noradrenaline Acid Tartrate.

Levo-Dromoran Tartrate: see Levorphanol Tartrate.

Levophed: see Noradrenaline Acid Tartrate.

Levorphanol Tartrate (B.P.C.) 1.5-3 mg. oral, 2-4 mg. subcut., i.m. 1-1.5 mg. i.v. Potent analgesic with effects similar to those of morphine. *Dromoran, Levo-Dromoran Tartrate.*

Librium: See Chlordiazepoxide Tablets.

Lidocaine: see Lignocaine Hydrochloride.

Lidothesin: see Lignocaine Hydrochloride.

Lignocaine Hydrochloride (B.P.) Nerve block 2 per cent., infiltration 0.5-2 per cent topical 1-2 per cent., Lignocaine and Adrenaline Injection (B.P.) 2 per cent. with adrenalin 1:60,000. Local anaesthetic. Twice as potent as procaine on injection but only equally toxic, longer duration. Active when applied topically to mucous membrane. *Fastocain, Lidocaine, Lidothesin, Lignostab, Nurocain, Xylocaine, Xylotox.*

Lignostab: see Lignocaine Hydrochloride.

Liquified Phenol: see Phenol.

Lorfan: see Levallorphan Tartrate.

Lozenges of Potassium Chloride: see Potassium Chlorate.

Luminal: see Phenobarbitone Tablets.

Lysol: see Cresol.

Magnesium Hydroxide Mixture (B.P.) 4-16 ml. (16 ml. contains the equivalent of 0.9 G of magnesium oxide). Syn: Cream of Magnesia. Antacid. Given in gastric hyperacidity and peptic ulcer. Mild laxative action. Used also as a mouth-wash. *Milk of Magnesia.*

Magnesium Sulphate (B.P.) 2-16 G. Syn: Epsom Salts. Saline purgative. Rapid action when given orally in dilute solution. Magnesium Sulphate Mixture (B.P.C.) 15-30 ml. (15 ml. contains approx. 4.11 G with approx. 0.69 G light magnesium carbonate).

Magnesium Peroxide. Liberates oxygen on contact with saliva Constituent of dentifrice preparations.

Mandl's Paint: see Iodine.

Marezine: see Cyclizine Hydrochloride.

Marsilid: see Monoamine Oxidase Inhibitors.

Marzine: see Cyclizine Hydrochloride.

Mecamylamine Hydrochloride 5-25 mg. Ganglion blocking drug. Used in hypertension. *Inversine.*

Meclozine Hydrochloride (B.P.C.) 25-50 mg. daily. Long acting antihistamine. *Ancolan.*

Megacillin: see Benzathine Penicillin.

Megapen: see Procaine Penicillin.

Megimide: see Bemigride.

Menadiol Sodium Diphosphate (U.S.P.) 5 mg. daily oral or parenteral. For actions see Menaphthone Sodium Bisulphite Injection.

Menadione: see Menaphthone Sodium Bisulphite Injection.

Menaphthone Sodium Bisulphite Injection (B.P.) 1-2 mg. daily subcut. or i.v. In emergencies 10-50 mg. every 4 hours subcut. or i.v. Menadione Sodium Bisulfite Injection (U.S.P.) 2 mg. daily. In emergencies up to 100 mg. subcut. or i.v. Water soluble analogue of Vitamin K. Used in Hypo-prothrombin-aemia of anticoagulant therapy. Estimations of prothrombin activity are necessary during therapy.

Menthol (B.P.) (U.S.P.). Aromatic crystalline principle from the volatile oils of species of Mentha. Carminative. Mild obtundent. Added to mouth washes and other dental preparations it adds a strong odour and warm taste.

Menthol and Benzoin Inhalation (B.P.C.) 2 per cent. menthol in benzoin inhalation. When added to water at 65°C the vapour is inhaled for the relief of sinusitis, bronchitis and tracheitis.

Menthol and Eucalyptus Inhalation (B.P.C.) contains menthol 2 per cent. and eucalyptus oil 12.5 per cent. with light magnesium carbonate in water. Added to water at 65°C the vapour relieves congestion in sinusitis.

Mepadin: see Pethidine Injection.

Mepavlon: see Meprobamate.

Meperidin: see Pethidine Injection.

Mephenesin Injection (B.P.) 1-10 ml. (10 per cent.) Blocks polysynaptic transmission in brain stem and cord. Muscle relaxant. Used as antagonist in strychnine poisoning, for relaxation during surgery and electro-convulsive therapy and in spastic states. *Dioloxol, Myanesin, Tolserol.*

Mephyton: see Phytomenadione.

Meprate: see Meprobamate.

Meprobamate (B.P.C.) 400-800 mg. Tranquillizer. Relieves nervous tension and anxiety without producing drowsiness. Slight muscle relaxant properties. *Equanil, Mepavlon, Meprate, Miltown.*

Mepyramine Maleate (B.P.) 300-800 mg. daily. Pyrilamine Maleate (U.S.P.) 25 mg. Antihistamine. *Anthisan.*

Merbentyl: see Dicyclomine Hydrochloride.

Mercurous Chloride Tablets (B.P.C.) 30-200 mg. Purgative. Syn: Calomel.

Merthiolate: see Thiomersal.

Mesantoin: see Methoin Tablets.

Mesontoin: see Methoin Tablets.

Methadone Hydrochloride (B.P.) 5-10 mg. Syn: Amidone. Injection (B.P.) 5-10 mg. subcut. (U.S.P.) 7.5 mg. subcut. Tablets (B.P.) 5-10 mg. (U.S.P.) 7.5 mg. Morphine like analgesic with less sedative action. Tolerance and addiction with repeated use. *Amidone, Dolophine, Physeptone.*

Methamphetamine: see Methylamphetamine Injection.

Methantheline Bromide (U.S.P.) 25-100 mg. Atropine substitute. *Banthine.*

Methedrine: see Methylamphetamine Injection.

Methoin Tablets (B.P.) 50-100 mg. Anticonvulsant with actions similar to those of phenytoin. Little or no hypnotic effect. Used in treatment of *grand mal.* epilepsy. *Mesantoin, Mesontoin.*

Methylamphetamine Injection (B.P.), 10-30 mg. i.m. or i.v. Tablets (B.P.) 2.5-10 mg. Methamphetamine Hydrochloride

Tablets (U.S.P.) 5 mg. Like amphetamine but more prolonged effect in hypotension. *Efroxin, Methedrine, Pervitin, Syndrox.*

Methohexitone Sodium (B.P.): 30-100 mgs. i.v. Very short acting barbiturate used for induction of anaesthesia. *Brietal Sodium.*

Methylparafynol: see Methylpentynol.

Methylpentynol Capsules (B.N.F.) 0.25-1 G. Methylparafynol (U.S.D.) Hypnotic. Used in small doses 0.25 G. for the relief of apprehension prior to minor operations. Its action is potentiated by other central nervous system depressants. *Dormison, Insomnol, Oblivon.*

Methyl Rosanaline Chloride: see Crystal Violet.

Metrazol: see Leptazol Injection.

Metronidazole Tablets (B.P.) 600 mgs. daily for treatment of Vincent's Injection. *Flagyl.*

Midarine: see Suxamethonium.

Milk of Magnesia: see Magnesium Hydroxide Mixture.

Milton: see Chlorine.

Miltown: see Meprobamate.

Monoamine Oxidase Inhibitors: Antidepressants—potentiate action of pethidine and morphine. Also react with certain tyramine rich food stuffs leading to severe hypertension and subarachnoid haemorrhage. *Actomol, Marsilid, Nardil, Niamid, Parnate.*

Monocaine: see Butethamine.

Morphine Sulphate Injection (B.P.) 8-20 mg. subcut. and i.m. Morphine Injection (U.S.P.) 15 mg. (10, 15, 20 or 30 mg. of morphine salt in 1 ml.) Central nervous system depressant. Potent analgesic and modifies reaction to pain. Produces drowsiness and depression of reasoning powers. Used in severe pain, surgical shock and as pre-operative and post-operative treatment. Addictable.

Mouth-wash Solution-tablets (B.P.C.). Syn: Effervescing Mouth-wash Tablets. Contain Sodium benzoate, menthol, thymol and eucalyptus oil. Similar action and use to Compound Glycerin of Thymol. One tablet dissolved in half a pint of warm water for use.

Myanesin: see Mephenesin Injection.

Mycifradin: see Neomycin Sulphate.

Myciguent: see Neomycin.

Mysoline: see Primidone Tablets.

Nalline: see Nalorphine Injection.

Nalorphine Injection (B.P.) 5-10 mg. i.v. (1 per cent.), Nalorphine

Hydrochloride Injection (U.S.P.) 5 mg. (0.5 per cent.) Morphine antagonist. Used in morphine poisoning and to identify morphine addiction. *Nalline, Lethidrone.*

Nardil: see monoamine oxidase inhibitors.

Nembutal: see Pentobarbitone Sodium Tablets.

Neo-Cytamen: See Cyanocobalamin injection.

Neo-Epnine: see Isoprenaline.

Neomin: see Neomycin Sulphate.

Neomycin Sulphate (B.P.) Neomycin Sulfate Tablets (U.S.P.) 1 G. (base) Antibiotic. Bactericidal against Gram-positive and some Gram-negative organisms. Often used topically. *Mycifradin, Myciguent, Neomin, Nivemycin.*

Neostigmine Bromide (B.P.) 15-30 mg. (U.S.P.) 15 mg. Parasympathomimetic effects due to blocking of cholinesterase. Used in myasthenia gravis, paralytic ileus and urinary retention. Available also as official Injections. *Prostigmin.*

Neo-synephrine: see Phenylephrine Hydrochloride.

Niamid: see monoamine oxidase inhibitors.

Nicetal: see Isoniazid Tablets.

Nikethamide Injection (B.P.) 0.25-1 G. subcut., i.m., i.v. (U.S.P.) 1 ml. i.m., i.v. (25 per cent.). Medullary stimulant in respiratory failure. Used in barbiturate poisoning. *Cardiamide, Coramine, Cormed, Corvotone Nikorin.*

Nikorin: see Nikethamide Injection.

Nitacin: see Nystatin.

Nitrogen Monoxide: see Nitrous Oxide.

Nitroglycerin: see Glyceryl Trinitrate Tablets.

Nitrous Oxide (B.P.) (U.S.P.) Nitrogen Monoxide. Anæsthetic gas, weak narcotic, powerful analgesic. Used in high concentrations with oxygen to produce analgesia for cavity preparation, anæsthesia for short operations and induction. Rapid recovery.

Nivemycin: see Neomycin.

Noradrenaline Acid Tartrate (B.P.) 5-25 μg per minute i.v. Levarterenol Bitartrate Injection (U.S.P.) 5 mcg. per minute i.v. Vasoconstrictor with local anaesthetics 1:50,000-1:80,000. Topical haemostatic 1:1000. *Levophed.*

Norisodrone: see Isoprenaline.

Novobiocin: Syn: Streptonivicin. Antibiotic with activity similar to penicillin. Bactericidal and bacteriostatic. Used when organisms are resistant to penicillin or erythromycin. *Albamycin, Biotexin.*

Novocain: see Procaine Hydrochloride.

Novutox: see Procaine Hydrochloride.

Nupercaine Hydrochloride: see Cinchocaine Hydrochloride.

Nurocain: see Lignocaine Hydrochloride.

Nystan: see Nystatin.
Nystatin: Antifungal agent used for treatment of Candidal Infections, Preparations. Nystatin Ointment (B.N.F.) 100,000 units per G. Nystatin Tablets (B.P.) (B.N.F.) 500,000 units *Nitacin, Nystan.*

Oblivon: see Methylpentynol Capsules.
Oleandomycin. Antibiotic with activity similar to penicillin.
Omnopon: see Injection of Papaveretum.
Opium Tincture (B.P.) 0.3-2 ml. (U.S.P.) 0.6 ml. Syn: Laudanum. Contains the natural alkaloids of opium, for oral administration. Action and uses similar to those of morphine sulphate.
Oppacyn: see Tetracycline Tablets.
Orabase: see Carboxymethyl Cellulose Gelatin Paste.
Orbenin: see Cloxacillin.
Oxidised Cellulose (B.P.) (U.S.P.) An absorbable gauze for application to bleeding parts to encourage formation of a clot. *Oxycel, Surgicel.*
Oxycel: see Oxidised Cellulose.
Oxymycin: see Oxytetracycline Tablets.
Oxyphenonium Bromide, 5 mg. Atropine substitute. *Antrenyl.*
Oxytetracycline Tablets (B.P.) 1-3 G. daily divided. Capsules (U.S.P.) 250 mg. Oxytetracycline Injection (B.P.) 1-2 G. i.v. (0.1 per cent.) (U.S.P.) 500 mg. i.v. daily. Oral Oxytetracycline for Suspension (U.S.P.) 250 mg. Oxytetracycline and Procaine Injection (B.P.) 200-400 mg. daily i.m. (5 per cent.). See tetracyclines for uses. *Abbocin. Berkmycen, Climimycin, Impericin, Oxymycin, Oxytetrin, Terramycin.*
Oxytetrin: see Oxytetracycline Tablets.

Pamol: see Paracetamol Tablets.
Panadol: see Paracetamol Tablets.
Panok: see Paracetamol Tablets.
Pantocaine: see Amethocaine Hydrochloride.
Papaveretum: see Injection of Papaveretum.
Paracetamol Tablets (B.N.F.) 0.5-1 G. Acetaminophen (U.S.N.F.). Syn: p-acetamidophenol. Chemically allied to phenacetin. Has similar actions. *Calpol, Cetal, Febrillix, Pamol, Panadol, Panok, Salzone, Tabalgin, Tempra, Tetmal, Tylenol.*
Paracodin: see Dihydrocodeine Tablets.
Paraformaldehyde (B.P.C.) Decomposes to formaldehyde which is a protein precipitant. Used as a slow obtundent and mummifying drug. *See also* Formaldehyde Lozenges.
Paraldehyde (B.P.) 2-8 ml. (U.S.P.) 12 ml/day. **Paraldehyde**

Draught (B.P.C.) 45 ml. (4 ml.). Hypnotic lasting about six hours. Unpleasant taste and smell.

Parnate: see Monoamine Oxidase Inhibitors.

P.A.S.: see Sodium Aminosalicylate Tablets.

Pelentan: see Ethyl Biscoumacetate Tablets.

Peletan: see Ethyl Biscoumacetate Tablets.

Pempidine Tartrate 10-60 mg. Ganglion blocking drug used in hypertension. *Perolysen.*

Penbritin: see Ampicillin Capsules.

Penevan: see Benzyl Penicillin.

Penicillin. Antibiotic produced by strains of *Penicillin notatum.* Mainly bacteriostatic towards Gram-positive organisms, gonococcus and meningococcus and spirochaetes. Action not interfered with by pus or serum. Non toxic but can cause sensitisation. Reactions can vary from mild erythema to severe serum sickness and sometimes death from anaphylactic shock. The soluble form known as Benzylpenicillin *q.v.* or Penicillin G. is commonly used by injection for immediate action. The Procaine salt (see Procaine Penicillin) is sparingly soluble and when injected gives a prolonged effect. Phenoxymethylpenicillin *q.v.* or Penicillin V is resistant to destruction by gastric juice and is given orally. Benzathine Penicillin *q.v.* is long acting when given orally or by injection. Non Official Preparations are Chewing gum and Dental Cones.

Penicillin Lozenges (B.P.C.) 1,000 units. See Penicillin. Their use is not recommended. Liable to cause sensitivity to penicillin.

Penicillin V: see Phenoxymethylpenicillin.

Penidural: see Benzathine Penicillin.

Peniset: see Benzyl Penicillin.

Penisol: see Benzyl Penicillin.

Pentazocine Tablets (B.N.F.) 25-100 mgs. Strong analgesic for the relief of moderate and severe pain. Low incidence of addiction. *Fortral.*

Pentobarbital: see Pentobarbitone Tablets.

Pentobarbitone Tablets (B.P.) 100-200 mg. Pentobarbitone Capsules (B.N.F.) Pentobarbital Sodium Capsules (U.S.P.) 100 mg. Short acting, see Barbiturates. *Nembutal.*

Pentolinium Tartrate. Ganglion blocking drug available as Tablets (B.P.) and Injection (B.P.) used in hypertension. *Ansolysen.*

Pentothal: see Thiopentone Injection.

Pentylenetetrazol: see Leptazol Injection.

Pen-Vee: see Phenoxymethylpenicillin.

Peppermint Emulsion: see Peppermint Water.

Peppermint Water (B.P.) An aromatic water made by dissolving a very small amount of essential oil of peppermint in water.

Peppermint Emulsion (B.P.C.) 0.3-2 ml. (10 per cent.). Carminative and flavouring agent.

Permapen: see Benzathine Penicillin.

Perolysen: see Pempidine Tartrate.

Pervitin: see Methylamphetamine.

Pethidine Injection (B.P.) 25-100 mg. subcut., i.m., 25-50 mg. i.v. Meperidine Hydrochloride Injection (U.S.P.) 100 mg. Tablets (B.P.) 25-100 mg. Tablets (U.S.P.) 100 mg. Potent analgesic. Like morphine but better absorption when given orally, less relief of anxiety. *Dolantal, Dolantin, Demerol, Mepadine, Pethoid.*

Pethoid: see Pethidine Injection.

Phanodorm: see Cyclobarbitone.

Phanodorn: see Cyclobarbitone Tablets.

Phemerol: see Benzethonium Chloride Solution.

Phenacetin (B.P.) 300-600 mg. Acetophenetidin (U.S.P.) 300 mg. Tablets (B.P.C.) (U.S.P.) Antipyretic analgesic. Prolonged use may lead to renal damage.

Phenacetin and Caffeine Tablets (B.P.C.) 1-2 tablets (phenacetin 260 mg. caffeine 65 mg.) Antipyretic analgesic used to relieve headache or toothache.

Phenazone (B.P.C.) 300-600 mg. Syn: Antipyrin. Analgesic, antipyretic. For headache, toothache and mild pain generally. Can cause rashes and blood changes. *Antipyrin.*

Phenergan: see Promethazine Hydrochloride.

Phenindamine Tartrate Tablets (B.P.) 25-50 mg. (U.S.P.) 25 mg. Antihistamine with no central depressant action. *Thephorin.*

Phenindione Tablets (B.P.) initial 200-300 mg., maintenance 25-100 mg. Syn: Phenylindanedione. Oral anticoagulant. Action shorter than dicoumarol and longer than ethyl biscoumacetate. *Dindevan, Theradione.*

Phenobarbital: see Phenobarbitone Tablets.

Phenobarbitone Tablets (B.P.) 30-120 mg. Phenobarbital Tablets (U.S.P.) 30 mg. Long acting. *See* Barbiturates. Anticonvulsant and sedative. *Gardenal, Luminal.*

Phenol (B.P.) (U.S.P.) Syn: Carbolic Acid [Liquified Phenol (B.P.) is phenol with 20 per cent. water]. Protoplasmic poison, caustic. Disinfectant. Used as an obtundent in cavities. Constituent of Phenol and Alkali Mouth-wash (B.P.C.) (3.13 per cent. with potassium hydroxide solution 3.13 per cent.). Phenol Gargle (B.P.C.) (5 per cent. Phenol Glycerin) and Thymol Compound Solution-tablets (B.P.C.).

Phenoxymethylpenicillin B.P.) (U.S.P.) Syn: Penicillin V. See also Penicillin. Preparations available: Tablets (B.P.) and Capsules (B.N.F.) 125-250 mg. *Calcipen V., Compocillin V.,*

Crystapen V., Distaquaine V., Econopen V., Eskacillin V., Icipen, Pen-Vee, Stabilin V-K, Tonsillin, V-Cil-K.

Phenylbutazone Tablets (B.N.F.) 200-400 mg. daily (divided). Analgesic, antipyretic. Chemically related to amidopyrine. Many toxic side effects. *Butazolidin.*

Phenylephrine Hydrochloride (B.P.) 5 mg. subcut., i.m., 0.5 mg. i.v. (U.S.P.) 5 mg. subcut., i.m.; 0.3 ml. of 0.25 or 0.5 per cent. topical. Sympathomimetic. Like noradrenaline but longer action. *Neo-Synephrine.*

Phenylindanedione: see Phenindione Tablets.

Phenylmercuric Nitrate (B.P.) Anti-bacterial and antifungal properties. On skin (1:1,500), mucous membranes (1:15,000 to 1:25,000) and as bacteriostatic in injections (1:100,000).

Phenytoin Tablets (B.P.) 50-100 mg. Diphenylhydantoin Sodium Capsules (U.S.P.) 100 mg. Anticonvulsant. Used to prevent *grand mal* attacks. *Dilantin sodium, Epanutin.*

Physeptone: see Methadone Hydrochloride.

Physostigmine Salicylate (B.P.) Syn: Eserine Salicylate 0.6-1.2 mg. subcut. (U.S.P.) 2 mg. oral. Blocks cholinesterase resulting in parasympathomimetic effects. Topical in glaucoma.

Phytomenadione (B.P.C.) 5-50 mg. oral or i.v. Phytonadione (U.S.P.) 2 mg. subcut. or i.v. Syn: Vitamin K_1. Given intravenously for rapid raising of the prothrombin output of the liver particularly in patients on anti-coagulant therapy. *Aquamephyton, Konakion, Mephyton.*

Phytonadione: see Phytomenadione.

Picrotoxin Injection (B.P.) 3-6 mg. i.v. Medullary stimulant in respiratory failure. Given in barbiturate poisoning, with amphetamine.

Pigmentum Tinctorum: see Brilliant Green.

Piriton: see Chlorpheniramine Maleate.

Polymyxin B Sulphate (B.P.) (U.S.P.). Polypeptide antibiotic for Gram-negative organisms. Topical, often mixed with other antibiotics. *Aerosporin.*

Pontocaine: see Amethocaine Hydrochloride.

Potassium Bromide (B.P.) 0.3-1.2 G. Central nervous system depressant. Sedative, taking several days to act when given in normal therapeutic doses.

Potassium Chlorate (B.P.C.) Sialogogue. Included in gargles and lozenges. Potassium Chlorate Lozenges (B.P.C.) (approx. 0.13 G. in each) Potassium Chlorate and Phenol Gargle, (B.P.C.) (potassium chlorate 3.43 per cent., liquified phenol 1.563 per cent.).

Potassium Permanganate Solution (B.N.F.) 0.1 per cent. Potassium Permanganate Tablets (U.S.P.) Solution of 0.02 per cent. as a mouth-wash or gargle is astringent and briefly antibacterial.

Primidone Tablets (B.P.) 0.5-1.5 G. daily, divided. Anticonvulsant. Actions and side actions similar to phenobarbitone. Used to prevent *grand mal* arracks. *Mysoline.*

Prinsyl: see Chloroxylenol Solution.

Pro-Banthine: see Propantheline Bromide.

Procainamide Hydrochloride (B.P.) Quinidine like action on the myocardium and has same uses as quinidine. Available as Procainamide Injection (B.P.) and *Pronestyl Hydrochloride.*

Procafin: see Procaine Hydrocholoride.

Procaine Hydrochloride (B.P.) nerve block 2 per cent., infiltration 0.5-2 per cent. (U.S.P.) subcut. 1-2 per cent. Syn: Allocaine, Ethocaine, Syncaine. Local anaesthetic by injection. Action usually prolonged by the addition of adrenaline. Procaine and Adrenaline Injection (B.P.) (2 per cent. with adrenaline 1:50,000). Procaine Hydrochloride and Epinephrine Injection (U.S.P.) (2 per cent. with adrenaline 1-25,000). *Adrocaine, Ethocaine, Novocaine, Novutox, Procafin, Ruticain.*

Procaine Penicillin (B.P.), Procaine Penicillin G (U.S.P.) see also Penicillin. Preparations available: Procaine Penicillin Injection (B.P.) 500,000-1,000,000 units i.m., Fortified Procaine Penicillin Injection (B.P.) (Procaine Penicillin 300,000 units and Benzylpenicillin 100,000 units in 1 ml.), Sterile Procaine Penicillin G Suspension (U.S.P.) 300,000 U.S.P. units i.m., Sterile Procaine Penicillin G with Aluminium Stearate Suspension (U.S.P.) 300,000 U.S.P. units i.m., Sterile Procaine Penicillin G and Buffered Crystalline Penicillin G for Suspension (U.S.P.) 400,000 U.S.P. units i.m. *Abbocillin DC, Bi-Stabillin, Crysticillin AS, Distaquaine, Duracillin, Eskacillin 200, Flo-cillin, Megapen, Procillin, Pro-Stabillin, Wycillin.*

Proflavine Hemisulphate (B.P.) Proflavine Solution (B.N.F.) (1:1000). Proflavine Tablets (B.N.F.) one tablet dissolved in two ounces of water forms approximately 1:1000 solution of proflavine hemisulphate in saline. See acriflavine.

Procillin: see Procaine Penicillin.

Prokayvit Oral: see Acetomenaphthone.

Promethazine Chlorotheophyllinate: see Promethazine Theoclate.

Promethazine Hydrochloride Tablets (B.P.) 25-75 mg. Antihistamine. *Phenergen.*

Promethazine Theoclate (B.P.C.) Syn: Promethazine Chlorotheophyllinate. Antihistamine with a prolonged anti-emetic action. *Avomine.*

Pronestyl Hydrochloride: see Procainamide Tablets.

Propanidid: 6-8 mgs. per kg. i.v. Short acting i.v. anaesthetic with rapid recovery time *Epontol.*

Propantheline Bromide, 15-30 mg. Atropine substitute. *Pro-Banthine*.

Proscorbin: see Vitamin C.

Pro-Stabillin: see Procaine Penicillin.

Prostigmin: see Neostigmine Bromide.

P.R.Q. Antiseptic: see Benzalkonium Chloride Solution.

Pularin: see Heparin Injection.

Purapen G. See Benzyl penicillin.

Pycazide: see Isoniazid.

Pyrethrum Tincture (B.P.C. 1934). Alcoholic solution of constituents of pyrethrum root. Sialagogue. Applied on cotton wool or rubbed along the gums in toothache.

Pyribenzamine: see Tripelennamine Hydrochloride.

Pyrilamine Maleate: see Mepyramine Maleate.

Quinalbarbitone Tablets (B.P.), 100-200 mg. and Capsules (B.N.F.). Secobarbital Sodium Capsules (U.S.P.), 100 mg. Short acting, see Barbiturates. *Seconal*.

Quinidine Sulphate Tablets (B.P.) Depressant of myocardium. Used in atrial fibrillation and paroxysmal tachycardia.

Quinine Sulphate (B.P.) 300-600 mg. Protoplasmic poison. Toxic to malarial trophozoites. Antipyretic.

Raphetamine: see Amphetamine Sulphate Tablets.

Rapidal: see Cyclobarbitone Tablets.

Redoxon: see Vitamin C.

Reserpine Tablets (B.P.) 0.25-1 mg. Central depressant. Produces lowering of blood pressure and sedation without hypnotic effects. Used in anxiety states and in hypertension, usually with other hypotensive drugs, the actions of which it potentiates. *Alserin, Reserpoid, Serpasil*.

Reserpoid: see Reserpine Tablets.

Retcin: see Erythromycin Tablets.

Roccal: see Benzalkonium Chloride Solution.

Roxenol: see Chloroxylenol Solution.

Rubramin: see Cyanocobalamin Injection.

Russell's Viper Venom. Local haemostatic for use in haemophilia. *Stypven*.

Ruticain: see Procaine Hydrochloride.

Salzone: see Paracetamol Tablets.

Savlon: see Cetrimide Solution.

Scoline: see Suxamethonium.

Scopolomine: see Hyoscine Hydrobromide.

Secobarbital: see Quinalbarbitone Sodium Tablets.

Seconal: see Quinalbarbitone Sodium Tablets.

Septrin: see Trimethoprin and Sulphamethoxazole.

Serpasil: see Reserpine Tablets.

Silver Nitrate (B.P.) (U.S.P.). Caustic, astringent and bactericidal due to formation of silver proteinates. Howe's Solution: Silver nitrate 3 G. water 1 ml. and strong solution of ammonia 2.5 mg. (sufficient to redissolve the precipitate). Obtundent and mummifying agent.

Sodium Aminosalicylate Tablets (B.P.) 10–15 G. daily (divided), (U.S.P.) 3 G. (Aminosalicylic acid is known as P.A.S.) Bacteriostatic action against strains of M. tuberculosis. Used in conjunction with other anti-tuberculosis drugs.

Sodium Amytal: see Amylobarbitone Tablets.

Sodium Bicarbonate (B.P.) 1–4 G. Antacid. Often given with other antacids in hyperacidity. Dissolves mucous.

Sodium Chloride Solution-tablets (Dental Practitioners' Formulary). Each tablet contains 40 grains of sodium chloride and when dissolved in 10 fluid ounces of water forms a solution of about 0.9 per cent. w/v.

Sodium Fluoride Tablets. *F-Tabs.* Each contains the equivalent of 1 mg. of fluorine. Under 2 years, ½ tablet daily; over 2 years 1 tablet daily. One tablet dissolved in 1 quart of water is equivalent to about 1 part of fluoride per million. Imparts to teeth a resistance to caries. Used where fluoride content of water is deficient.

Sodium Hypochlorite Solution: see Chlorine.

Sodium Perborate (B.P.C.). Aromatic Sodium Perborate (U.S.N.F.). Dissolves in water and liberates oxygen slowly. More rapid on contact with saliva. Mild antiseptic used in mouthwashes and dentifrice powders. *Amosan, Bocasan, Bocosept, Kavosan, Vince.*

Sodium Sulphite (B.P.C.). Antiseptic action is made use of in mouthwashes (1:16) in water or as a paint (1:8) in glycerin in aphthous ulcers. Used with boric acid as a bleaching agent for teeth.

Solprin: see Acetylsalicylic Acid.

Soluble Acetylsalicylic Acid Tablets: see Acetylsalicylic Acid.

Soluble Aspirin Tablets: *see* Acetylsalicylic Acid.

Solupen: see Benzylpenicillin.

Solution of Chlorinated Lime with Boric Acid: see Chlorine.

Sonabarb: see Butobarbitone Tablets.

Soneryl: see Butobarbitone Tablets.

Spreading Factor: see Hyaluronidase.

Stabilin V-K: see Phenoxymethylpenicillin.

Stannous Fluoride. Incorporated in a dentifrice it is said to reduce the incidence of caries (A.D.R. list it in Group B).

Steclin: see Tetracycline Capsules.

Sterile Benzathine Penicillin G. Suspension: see **Benzathine** Penicillin.

Sterile Procaine Penicillin Preparations: see Procaine Penicillin.

Sterillium: see Choroxylenol Solution.

Sterispon: see Absorbable Gelatin Sponge.

Streptoduocin: see Streptomycin Sulphate Injection.

Streptomycin Sulphate Injection (B.P.) 0.5-1 G. (base) daily i.m. (U.S.P.) 500 mg. (base) daily i.m. Dihydrostreptomycin Sulphate Injection (B.P.) 0.5-1 G. (base) daily i.m. (U.S.P.) 500 mg. (base) daily i.m. Streptoduocin for Injection (U.S.P.) 500 mg. i.m. Antibiotic with activity against Gram-negative organisms, in particular M. tuberculosis.

Streptonivicin: see Novobiocin.

Strong Compound Aneurine Tablets: see Vitamin B Compound Tablets, Strong.

Stypven: see Russell's Viper Venom.

Suavitil: see Benactyzine Hydrochloride.

Succinylcholine: see Suxamethonium.

Sulphadimidine Tablets (B.P.) 0.5 G. A sulphonamide *q.v.* given every 4 to 6 hours to maintain a therapeutic concentration.

Sulphan Blue Solution (B.P.C.) A blue dye used to colour medicines and foodstuffs.

Sulphonamides. Systemic bacteriostatic drugs which are capable of producing severe toxic reactions. The antibiotics have almost replaced them in dentistry. Of the many preparations the following are examples: Succinylsulphathiazole Tablets (B.P.) 10-20 G. daily, (U.S.P.) 2 G. 4 hourly in intestinal infections. Sulphamerazine Tablets (B.P.) initial 3 G., maintenance 1-1.5 G. 8 hourly, (U.S.P.) initial 4 G., maintenance 1 G. 6 hourly for systemic infections. Sulphacetamide Sodium (B.P.) (U.S.P.) for topical use.

Suprarenin: see Adrenaline.

Surgical Chlorinated Soda Solution: see Chlorine.

Surgicel: see Oxidised Cellulose.

Surmontil: see Tricyclic Antidepressants.

Surofene: see Hexachlorophane.

Suxamethonium. Syn: Succinylcholine. Suxamethonium Chloride Injection (B.P.) 5 per cent. Succinylcholine Chloride Injection (U.S.P.) 20 mg. i.v. Neuromuscular blocking drug. Brief depolarisation. Used as a muscle relaxant. *Anectine, Brevidil M, Midarine, Scoline.*

Syncaine: see Procaine Hydrochloride.

Syndrox: see Methylamphetamine.

Tabalgin: see Paracetamol Tablets.

Tabillin: see Benzylpenicillin.

Tannic Acid (B.P.) Coagulates proteins and used as an astringent and mummifying agent. Tannic Acid Glycerin (B.P.) (15 per cent.).

T.C.P.: see Chloroxylenol Solution.

Tegretol: see Carbemazepine Tablets.

Telotrex: see Tetracycline Tablets.

Tempra: see Paracetamol Tablets.

Terramycin: see Oxytetracycline.

Tetmal: see Paracetamol Tablets.

Tetracaine Hydrochloride: see Amethocaine Hydrochloride.

Tetracycline Capsules and Tablets (B.P.) 1-3 G. daily (U.S.P.) 250 mg. Tetracycline Injection (B.P.) 250-500 mg. i.v. Tetracycline and Procaine Injection (B.P.) 200-400 mg. daily (divided) i.m. Oral Tetracycline Suspension (U.S.P.) 250 mg. *See* Tetracyclines for uses. *Achromycin, Ambramycin, Clinitetrin, Democracin, Economycin, Oppacyn, Steclin, Telotrex, Tetracyn, Tetrex.*

Tetracyclines. Generic name which includes chlortetracycline, oxytetracycline and tetracycline *q.v.* Wide spectrum antibiotics used in systemic infection with organisms resistant to penicillin. Have been used topically.

Tetracyn: see Tetracycline.

Tetrex: see Tetracycline.

Theophylline Ethylenediamine: see Aminophylline Tablets.

Thephorin: see Phenindamine Tartrate.

Theradione: See Phenindione Tablets.

Thialbarbitone Sodium (B.P.C.) 0.2-1 G. i.v. Ultra-short acting, see Barbiturates. *Kemithal.*

Thimerosal: see Thiomersal.

Thiomersal (B.P.), Thimerosal (U.S.N.F.) Antibacterial and antifungal properties. On skin (1:1000) in alcohol, and instruments (1:1000 aqueous). *Merthiolate.*

Thiopentone Injection (B.P.) 100-500 mg. i.v. Thiopental Sodium for Injection (U.S.P.) 2-3 ml. of a 2.5 per cent. solution in 10-15 sec., repeated in about 30 sec. as required. Ultrashort acting, see Barbiturates. *Intraval Sodium, Pentothal.*

Thorazine: see Chlorpromazine.

Thrombin (U.S.P.) Human Thrombin (B.P.). Used locally with or without fibrinogen to arrest capillary bleeding.

Thymol (B.P.). Crystalline volatile substance from Oil of Thyme. Bactericidal. Hartman's Formula consists of thymol 5, ethyl alcohol 4 and ether 8. Used in cavity preparation.

Thymol Compound Solution-tablets (B.P.C.) Compound Thymol Solution-tablets. Similar action and use to Compound Glycerin of Thymol. Contains sodium bicarbonate, borax, phenol, thymol and amaranth. One tablet dissolved in 2 fluid ounces of warm water for use.

Tincture of Iodine: see Iodine.

Tofranil: see Tricyclic Antidepressants.

Tolserol: see Mephenesin.

Tonsillin: see Phenoxymethylpenicillin.

Tranquillizers or Ataractics. Drugs which produce calmness of mind, e.g. Benactyzine, Chlorpromazine, Meprobamate *q.v.*

Trethylene: see Tricholoroethylene.

Trichloroethylene (B.P.) (U.S.P.) Liquid, the vapour of which produces anaesthesia. Used for short dental operations, rapid induction or to supplement nitrous oxide. Potentiates the action of adrenaline. Usually coloured blue. *Triethylene, Trichloroethylene, Trilene.*

Trichloromethane: see Chloroform.

Tricyclamol Chloride (B..P) 50 mg.   Atropine substitute. *Elorine.*

Tricyclic Antidepressants: Severe hypertension may follow the use of small doses of noradrenaline in patients on these drugs and local anaesthetic solutions containing adrenalin or noradrenaline should be avoided. *Aventyl, Tofranil, Tryptizol, Surmontil.*

Tridione: see Troxidone Capsules.

Trilene: see Trichloroethylene.

Trimethadione: see Troxidone Capsules.

Trimethoprim and Sulphamethoxasole (B.P.C.): Broad spectrum antibacterial drug containing Trimethoprin (80 mgs.) and Sulphamethoxasole (400 mgs.) in each tablet. Dose 2-6 tablets daily. The combination acts synergistically and is bactericidal. *Bactrim, Septrin.*

Trimethylene: see Cyclopropane.

Trinitrin: see Glyceryl Trinitrate Tablets.

Tripelennamine Hydrochloride (U.S.P.) 50 mg. Antihistamine. *Pyribenzamine.*

Tromexan: see Ethyl Biscoumacetate.

Troxidone Capsules (B.P.) 1-2 G., child 250-500 mg. daily. Trimethadione (U.S.P.) 300 mg. Anticonvulsant used to prevent attacks of *petit mal. Tridione.*

Tryptizol: see Tricyclic Antidepressants.

Tubarine: see Tubocurarine Injection.

Tubocurarine Injection (B.P.) 1 per cent. Tubocurarine Chloride Injection (U.S.P.) 6-9 mg i.v. followed in 5 minutes by 3-5 mg. more if necessary. Neuromuscular blocking drug. Used to give relaxation with a minimal dose of general anaesthetic, also in tetanus and electroconvulsive therapy. *Tubarine.*

Uradal: see Carbromal.

Valium: see Diazepam Tablets.

Valoid: see Cyclizine Hydrochloride.

V-Cil-K: see Phenoxymethylpenicillin.

Veganin Tablets: see Compound Codeine Tablets.

Vegolysen T: see Hexamethonium Tartrate.

Vince: see Sodium Perborate.

Vinesthene: see Vinyl Ether.

Vinethene: see Vinyl Ether.

Vinyl Ether (B.P.) (U.S.P.)   Divinyl Oxide.   Liquid.   4 per cent. dehydrated alcohol and a stabiliser is added. Vapour is a powerful anaesthetic. Used for induction, short operations and to supplement nitrous oxide anaesthesia. Inflammable. *Vinesthene, Vinethene.*

Viride Nitens: see Brilliant Green.

Vitamin A, Preparations containing. Halibut Liver Oil Capsules (B.P.) 1–3 (approx. 4,500 units/capsule);   (U.S.P.) 5,000 or 25,000 units/capsule.   Oleovitamin A Capsules (U.S.P.) prophyl. 1.5 mg. (5,000 units); therapeutic 7.5 mg. (25,000 units).   Vitamin A capsules, Strong (B.N.F.) 1-2 (50,000-100,000 units). For A and D see Vitamin D. Indicated in deficiency.

Vitamin B Complex includes Aneurine (Thiamine,-B_1), Riboflavine (Lactoflavine), Nicotinic Acid, Pyridoxine (B_6), Panthothenic Acid, Biotin and Folic acid.   Deficiency of several of these may lead to changes in the mouth and lips. Treatment is usually started after investigation of the cause of the deficiency.

Vitamin B Compound Tablets, Strong (B.P.C.) 1-2 tablets. Syn: Aneurine Compound Tablets, Strong. (Each contains aneurine hydrochloride 5 mg., riboflavine 2 mg., nicotinamide 20 mg., and pyridoxine hydrochloride 2 mg.) See Vitamin B Complex.

Vitamin B_{12}: see Cyanocobalamin Injection.

Vitamin C.   Ascorbic Acid Injection (B.P.C.) 2-5 ml. daily, (U.S.P.) 75 mg. required daily, therapeutic 150 mg. subcut. Ascorbic Acid Tablets (B.P.) prophylactic 25-75 mg. daily, therapeutic 200-500 mg. daily.   (U.S.P.) 75 mg. required daily, therapeutic 150 mg.   Indicated in deficiency, i.e. scurvy. *Ascorvel, Ascoxal, Celin, Cevalin, Choovit, Davitamon C, Eff-Vit-C, Proscorbin, Redoxon.*

Vitamin D, Preparations containing. Calciferol Tablets (B.P.) 1-4 daily. (50,000-200,000 units); (U.S.P.) 10 mcg.-5 mg. (400-200,000 units).   Calciferol Solution (B.P.) prophylactic 0.13-0.3 ml. (approx. 400-1,000 units), therapeutic 1.6-16 ml. (approx. 5,000-50,000 units).   Concentrated Vitamin D Solution (B.P.) prophylactic 0.04-0.1 ml. (approx. 400-1,000

units), therapeutic 0.5-5 ml. (approx. 5,000-50,000 units).
Activated 7-Dehydrocholesterol (U.S.P.) 10 mcg.-5 mg. (400-
200,000 units). Concentrated Vitamins A and D Solution
(B.P.) 0.06-0.6 ml. (approx. 2,500-25,000 units A and 250-
2,500 units D). Cod liver Oil (B.P.) 4-16 ml. daily (approx.
600 units A and 85 units D per G), (U.S.P.) 4 ml. (approx.
3,000 units A and 300 units D). Prophylactic in nursing mothers
and infants and in deficiency, i.e. rickets.
Vitamin K₁: see Phytomenadione.
Vitavel K: see Menaphthone Sodium Bisulphite Injection and
Acetomenaphthone.

Weak Iodine Solution: see Iodine.
Whitehead's Varnish: see Compound Paint of Iodoform.
Wycillin: see Procaine Penicillin.
Wyovine: see Dicyclomine Hydrochloride.

Xylocaine: see Lignocaine Hydrochloride.
Xylotox: see Lignocaine Hydrochloride.

Zal: see Chloroxylenol Solution.
Zant: see Chloroxylenol Solution.
Zephiran: see Benzalkonium Chloride Solution.
Zinc Chloride (B.P.C.) Caustic and astringent. More so than
zinc sulphate. Used to desensitise dentine.
Zinc Peroxide. Yields oxygen slowly on contact with enzymes
present in saliva. Insoluble. Used as a suspension (20 per
cent.) to treat anaerobic oral infections.
Zinc Sulphate (B.P.) (U.S.P.) Caustic and astringent. 5-10 per
cent. may be applied to aphthous ulcers. Constituent of Zinc
Sulphate and Zinc Chloride Mouth-Wash (B.P.C.).

Appendix II—Dental Periodicals

Appendix of Dental Periodicals, giving country of origin and frequency of publication where this is known.

Those titles marked * are included in the 1972 *Index to Dental Literature*

*ADM. Revista de la Asociacion dental mexicana. Bi–M. Mexico.

AO (Atualidades odontologicas). Bi–M. Brazil.

Academia ondontológica. Q. Colombia.

Academy review of the California Academy of Periodontology. *Now in* Periodontology and Academy Review. U.S.A.

*Acta odontologica scandinavica. Bi–M. Sweden.

*Acta odontologica venezolana. 3 a year. Venezuela.

*Acta stomatologica belgica. Q. Belgium.

*Acta stomatologica croatica. Q. Yugoslavia.

*Acta stomatologica hellenica. Stomatologika chronika. Bi–M. Greece.

Acta stomatologica Patavina. Italy.

*Actualités odonto-stomatologiques. Q. France.

*Advances in oral biology. Biennial. U.S.A.

*American journal of orthodontics. M. U.S.A.

Anais da Faculdade de farmácia e odontologia do Estado do Rio de Janeiro. Brazil.

Anais da Faculdade de farmácia e odontologia da Universidade de Sao Paulo. A. Brazil.

Anais da Faculdade nacional de odontologia da Universidade do Brasil. A. Brazil.

Anais da Faculdade de odontologia e farmácia da Universidade de Minas Gerais. A. Brazil.

Anais da Faculdade de odontologia da Universidade Federal do Rio de Janiero. Brazil.

Anais da Faculdade de odontologia da Universidade do Parana. Brazil.

Anais da Faculdade de odontologia da Universidade do Recife. Brazil.

Anales argentinos de odontología. Q. Argentina.

*Anales españoles de odontoestomatologia. Bi–M. Spain.

*Anales de la Facultad de odontología, Universidad de la Republica Oriental del Uruguay. 2 a year. Uruguay.

*Anales: Instituto de investigaciones odontologicas. Venezuela.

*Anesthesia progress: journal of the American Dental Society of Anesthesiology. Bi-M. U.S.A.

*Angle orthodontist. Q. U.S.A.

*Anglo-Continental Dental Society journal. 2 a year. Great Britain.

*Annales odonto-stomatologiques. Bi-M. France.

Annali di odontologia. Dead. Italy.

*Annali di stomatologia. Bi-M. Italy.

*Annals of the Australian College of Dental Surgeons. A. Australia.

*Annals of dentistry. Q. U.S.A.

Année odonto-stomatologique et maxillo-faciale. A. France.

Annuaire dentaire. A. France.

Annual publications. Royal Dental School, Malmö, Sweden. *Now called* Annual publications. School of Dentistry, Malmö, Sweden, University of Lund. Sweden.

Annual publications. School of Dentistry, Malmö, Sweden, University of Lund. A. Sweden.

Anuário da Faculdade de farmácia e odontologia de Natal. A. Brazil.

*Apex: the journal of the UCH Dental Society. Bi-M. Great Britain.

*Apollonia. Australia.

*Apollonia. Sweden.

Archives of clinical oral pathology. Dead. U.S.A.

*Archives of oral biology. M. Great Britain.

Archives de stomatologie. Q. Belgium.

Archivio italiano di biologia oral. *Supplement to* Rassegna trimestriale di odontoiatria. Q. Italy.

*Archivio stomatologico. Q. Italy.

Argentina odontológica. Q. Argentina.

*Arizona dental journal. Bi-M. U.S.A.

*Arkansas dental journal. Q. U.S.A.

*Arquivo: orgão da Sociedade Brasileire de implantologia bucal. Brazil.

*Arquivos do Centro de Estudos da Faculdade de odontologia da U.F.M.G. 2 a year. Brazil.

Art dentaire liberal. Bi-M. France.

*Australian dental journal. Bi-M. Australia.

Australian journal of dentistry. *Now in* Australian dental journal. Australia.

*Australian orthodontic journal. Australia.

Bahia odontologica. Brazil.

Baurú odontológico. Brazil.

*Bayerisches Zahnärzteblatt. M. W.Germany.
*Baylor dental journal. Q. U.S.A.
*Begg journal of orthodontic theory and treatment. U.S.A.
Belgisch blad voor tandheelkunde. *See* Journal dentaire
  belge: Belgisch blad voor tandheelkunde.
*Berichte aus der Bonner Universitätsklinik und Poliklinik
  für Mund-, Zahn- und Kieferkrankheiten. W.Germany.
*Blätter für Zahnheilkunde. Bulletin dentaire. 2 a year.
  Switzerland.
Boletim da Associação brasileria de ondontologia. Bi-M.
  Brazil.
Boletim. Curso de odontologia de Santa Maria. Centro
  de Estudos Antonio Pimenta: Universidade Feder
  de Santa Maria. 2 a year. Brazil.
*Boletim de dentistica operatoria. Brazil.
*Boletim da Faculdade de farmacia e odontologia de
  Ribeiras Preto. Brazil.
*Boletim da Faculdade de odontologia de Piracicaba.
  Brazil.
*Boletim de materiais dentarios. Brazil.
*Boletim do servico de odontologia sanitaria da Secretaria
  da Saude do Rio Grande do Sul. Q. Brazil.
Boletín. Academia de estomatología del Perú. Q.
  Peru.
*Boletín de la Asociación argentina de odontología para
  niños. Argentina.
Boletín de la Asociación dental del Estado de Puebla.
  Mexico.
Boletín de la Asociación odontológica argentina. M.
  Argentina.
Boletín de la Catedrá de protesis estomatológica. Spain.
*Boletín del Circulo argentino de odontología. Argentina.
Boletín del Circulo odontológica de Rosario. Dead?
  Brazil.
Boletín del Colegio estomatológica de Guatemala. *After-
  wards called* Revista del Colegio estomatológico de Guatemala.
  Guatemala.
Boletín del Colegio estomatológica de La Habana. Cuba.
Boletín: Confederación odontológica inter-americana.
  Mexico.
Boletín dental argentino. Argentina.
Boletín dental chileno. Bi-M. Chile.
Boletín dental uruguayo. M. Uruguay.
Boletín Dentalcoblan. Colombia.
*Boletín de la dirección general de odontología. Argentina.

Boletín de la Escuela de odontología. **Universidad central de Ecuador.** Ecuador.

Boletín de la Escuela de odontología de la Universidad **Nacional.** Q. Colombia.

Boletín de la Escuela de odontología, **Universidad de San Marco.** *Now called* Boletín de la Facultad de odontología, Universidad de San Marco. Peru.

Boletín de la Facultad de odontología. Argentina.

Boletín de la Facultad de odontología, **Universidad de San Marco.** Peru.

*Boletín de información dental. Bi-M. Spain.

*Boletín de información, illustre Colegio oficial de odontológos y stomatológos (segunda region). Spain.

*Boletín de odontología. Bi-M. Colombia.

*Boletín odontológico. Argentina.

Boletín odontológico. Bolivia.

Boletín odontológico mexicano. Mexico.

*Boletín de protestis. Argentina.

*Boletín de la Sociedad dental de Guatemala. Guatemala.

*Boletín de la Sociedad estomatologica argentina. Argentina.

*Bollettino A.M.D.I.: Organo ufficiale dell'Associazione Medici Dentisti Italiani. M. Italy.

*Bollettino metallografico e di odonto-stomatologia. Q. Italy.

Bollettino odonto-implantologico. Italy.

Brasil odontológico. Brazil.

*British dental journal. 2 a month. Great Britain.

*British dental surgery assistant. M. Great Britain.

British journal of dental science. Dead. Great Britain.

*British journal of oral surgery. 3 a year. Great Britain.

*Bulletin de l'Académie dentaire. France.

Bulletin. Academy of Dentistry for the Handicapped. U.S.A.

Bulletin of the Academy of General Dentistry. *Now called* Journal of the Academy of General Dentistry. U.S.A.

Bulletin of the Alabama Dental Association. Q. U.S.A.

*Bulletin of the American Association of Dental Editors. U.S.A.

*Bulletin of the American Association of Hospital Dentists. U.S.A.

Bulletin of the American Association of Public Health Dentists. Q. U.S.A.

Bulletin des chirurgiens-dentistes independants. *Now in* Revue d'odonto-stomatologie. France.

Bulletin dentaire. *See* Dental bulletin.

Bulletin of dental education. Bi-M. U.S.A.

*Bulletin of the Dental Guidance Council for Cerebral Palsy. 3 a year. U.S.A.

*Bulletin du groupement international pour la recherche scientifique en stomatologie. Q. Belgium.

*Bulletin of the history of dentistry. 2 a year. U.S.A.

Bulletin of the Illinois Dental Hygienists' Association. 3 a year. U.S.A.

Bulletin of the International Academy of Oral Pathology. U.S.A.

*Bulletin of the International Federation of Dental Technicians. Yugoslavia.

Bulletin of the Manitoba Dental Association. Q. Canada.

*Bulletin of the Massachusetts Dental Hygienists Association. U.S.A.

*Bulletin of the Michigan (State) Dental Hygienists' Association. U.S.A.

Bulletin of the National Dental Association. Q. U.S.A.

*Bulletin: National Medical and Dental Association and National Advocates Society. U.S.A.

*Bulletin of the New Jersey College of Medicine and Dentistry. U.S.A.

*Bulletin of the New Jersey Society of Dentistry for Children. U.S.A.

*Bulletin of the New York State Dental Society of Anesthesiology. 2 a year. U.S.A.

*Bulletin of the New York State Society of Dentistry for Children. 2 a year. U.S.A.

*Bulletin officiel du Conseil national de l'ordre des chirurgiens-dentistes. Q. France.

Bulletin of the Oklahoma State Dental Society. Q. U.S.A.

*Bulletin, Pacific Coast Society of Orthodontists. Q. U.S.A.

*Bulletin of stomatology, Kyoto University. Q. Japan.

*Bulletin of Tokyo Dental College. Q. Japan.

*Bulletin of Tokyo Medical and Dental University. Q. Japan.

Bulletin trimestriel de la Société d'odonto-stomatologie de l'Ouest. Q. France.

Bulletin of the Virginia State Dental Association. 3 a year. U.S.A.

Bulletin: Washington State Dental Association. *Now called* Washington State dental journal. U.S.A.

*Bur. 3 a year. U.S.A.

*Caementum. 2 a year. U.S.A.
*Cahiers d'odonto-stomatologie de Touraine. France.
 Cahiers odonto-stomatologiques. Dead. France.
 Calcified tissue abstracts. M. Great Britain.
 Calcified tissue research. Q. W. Germany & U.S.A.
*Canadian dental hygienist. 2 a year. Canada.
 Canadian Forces Dental Services quarterly. Q. Canada.
*Caries research: journal of the European Organization
  for Caries Research. Q. Switzerland.
*Československá stomatologie. Bi-M. Czechoslovakia.
*Ceylon dental journal. A. Ceylon.
*Chirurgia maxillofacialis et plastica. Yugoslavia.
*Chirurgien-dentiste de France. W. France.
 Ciencia arte docencia odontología. 2 a year. Uruguay.
*Cirugia bucal. Mexico.
*Cleft palate journal. Q. U.S.A.
 Clinica odontoiatrica e ginecologia. M. Italy.
 Clinica odonto-protesia. Q. Italy.
*Conector: organo oficial del Instituto de Implant-
  odontologia. Argentina.
*Contact point. 8 a year. U.S.A.
 Cooperador dental. Argentina.
*Czasopismo Stomatologiczne. M. Poland.

*DDZ—Das Deutsche Zahnärzteblatt. *Now in* Z.W.R.
  W. Germany.
*DE: journal of dental engineering. Japan.
*Dens. Denmark.
 Dens. Dead? Japan.
*Dens sapiens. 10 a year. Denmark.
*Dentago. New Zealand.
*Dental abstracts. M. U.S.A.
*Dental anaesthesia and sedation. Journal of the
  Australian Society for the Advancement of Anaesthesia
  and Sedation in Dentistry. Australia.
*Dental assistant. M. U.S.A.
 Dental bulletin. (Bulletin dentaire). Canada.
 Dental bulletin of Osaka University. *Now called* Journal
  of Osaka University School of Dentistry. Japan.
*Dental cadmos. M. Italy.
*Dental clinics of North America. 3 a year. U.S.A.
*Dental concepts. Q. U.S.A.
 Dental cosmos. *Now in* Journal of the American Dental
  Association. U.S.A.
 Dental delineator. Dead. Great Britain.
*Dental Dienst. M. Germany.

Dental digest. *Now in* Quintessence international: dental digest. U.S.A.

*Dental Echo.** 9 a year. W. Germany.

*Dental economics—oral hygiene.** M. U.S.A.

*Dental health: the journal of the British Dental Hygienists' Association.** Q. Great Britain.

*Dental hygienist: journal of the Northern California State Dental Hygienists' Association.** U.S.A.

Dental items of interest. Dead. U.S.A.

Dental journal of Australia. *Now in* Australian dental journal. Australia.

*Dental journal of Malaysia and Singapore.** 2 a year. Malaysia.

Dental journal of Nihon University. *Now called* Journal of Nihon University School of Dentistry. Japan.

*Dental-Labor.** M. Germany.

Dental Laboratorie Bladet. *Now called* Dens. Denmark.

Dental laboratory yearbook and directory. A. Great Britain.

Dental magazine and Oral topics. *Now in* British dental journal. Great Britain.

Dental mirror: journal of Philippine dentistry. 2 a year. Philippines.

Dental outlook. Australia.

*Dental outlook [Shikai Tenbo].** M. Japan.

*Dental practice.** M. Great Britain.

Dental practitioner and Dental record. Dead. Great Britain.

*Dental press.** Italy.

Dental progress. Dead. U.S.A.

*Dental radiography and photography.** Q. U.S.A.

Dental record. *Continued in* Dental practitioner and Dental record. Great Britain.

Dental review. U.S.A.

Dental-Revue. M. Austria.

Dental spectrum. U.S.A.

*Dental survey.** M. U.S.A.

*Dental technician.** M. Great Britain.

*Dental world.** Q. U.S.A.

Dentiste de France. 2 a month. France.

Dentiste militaire. Q. France.

Dentistische Reform. M. W.Germany.

Dentistische Rundschau. *Now called* Zahnärztliche Praxis. Germany.

Dentistry. A digest of practice. U.S.A.

*Dentistry in Japan.** Japan.

Dento-maxillo-facial radiology. Q. Great Britain.
*Dentoral. Turkey.
*Dentoscope. France.
Deutsche Monatsschrift für Zahnheilkunde. Dead. Germany.
*Deutsche Stomatologie. M. Germany.
Deutsche zahnärztliche Wochenschrift. *Continued in* Zahnärztliche Zeitschrift. Germany.
Das Deutsche Zahnärzteblatt. *See* DDZ - Das Deutsche Zahnärzteblatt.
*Deutsche zahnärztliche Zeitschrift. M. Germany.
*Deutsche Zahn-, Mund- und Kieferheilkunde mit Zentralblatt fur die gesamte Zahn-, Mund- und Kieferheilkunde. M. E. Germany.
*Diastema. South Africa.
*Divulgación cultural odontológica. Spain.
Dundee dental journal. Great Britain.

*Edinburgh Dental Hospital gazette. 3 a year. Great Britain.
*Educación dental. 2 a year. Peru.
*Egyptian dental journal. Q. Egypt.
Estomatológia. 2 a year. Mexico.
*Estomatológia e cultura. 2 a year. Brazil.
*European Orthodontic Society reports. A. Great Britain.

Farmacodonto. Brazil.
Farmacodontologia. Brazil.
Finska Tandlälarsällskapets Forhandlingar. *See* Suomen Hammaslääkäriseuran Toimituksia.
*Florida dental journal. M. U.S.A.
*Fogorvosi szemle [Dental review]. M. Hungary.
Folia stomatologica. Q. Yugoslavia.
*Fortnightly review of the Chicago Dental Society. F. U.S.A.
*Fortschritte der Kieferorthopaedie. Q. E.Germany.
*Fortschritte der Kiefer- und Gesichtschirurgie. Biennial. W.Germany.
*Freie Zahnarzt: Monatsschrift deutscher Zahnärtze. M. W.Germany.

Gaceta dental. Venezuela.
Gaceta odontológica. Bi-M. Venezuela.
*Georgetown dental journal. 2 a year. U.S.A.
Giornale di stomatologie delle Venezia. Bi-M. Italy.
*Glasgow dental journal. 2 a year. Great Britain.

*Helvetica odontologica acta. 2 a year. Switzerland.
Heraldo dental. Colombia.
Hygie: Revue française de médecine, d'hygiène et de santé bucco-dentaire. Q. France.

*Illinois dental journal. M. U.S.A.
Index to dental literature. Q. U.S.A.
Index to orthodontic literature of the world. A. Spain.
Indian dental review. M. India.
Indonesian dental journal. Indonesia.
Información dental. Bi-M. Spain.
*Information dentaire. W. France.
*Informationen aus Orthodontie und Kieferorthopaedie. Q. W.Germany.
Informatore odonto-stomatologico. Q. Italy.
*International dental journal. Q. Netherlands.
International dental review. *Now called* Dental review. U.S.A.
International dentistry. M. Egypt.
*International journal of oral surgery. Q. Denmark.
International journal of orthodontia. *Continued as* American journal of orthodontics *and* Oral surgery. U.S.A.
*International journal of orthodontics. Q. U.S.A.
*Iowa dental bulletin. 2 a year. U.S.A.
*Iowa dental journal. U.S.A.
Ipse odontológico. Bi-M. Brazil.
Irish dental journal. *Continued as* Journal of the Irish Dental Association. Eire.
*Irish dental review. M. Eire.
*Israel journal of dental medicine. 2-3 a year. Israel.
Items of interest. *Continued as* Dental items of interest. U.S.A.

Japan oral topics. Japan.
Japanese dental journal. A. Japan.
*Japanese journal of dental health. *Now called* Journal of dental health. Japan.
*Japanese journal of oral surgery. Bi-M. Japan.
*Jornal das auxiliares odontologicas. Brazil.
Jornal de estomatologia. 2 a year. Portugal.
Jornal odontológico. M. Brazil.
*Journal of the Academy of General Dentistry. U.S.A.
*Journal of the Alabama Dental Association. Q. U.S.A.
Journal of the All-India Dental Association. *Now called* Journal of the Indian Dental Association. India.

Journal of the Allied Dental Societies. *Now called* Journal of dental research.   U.S.A.

*Journal of the American Academy of Gold-Foil Operators. 2 a year.   U.S.A.

*Journal of the American College of Dentists.   Q.   U.S.A.

*Journal of the American Dental Association.   M.   U.S.A.

*Journal of the American Dental Hygienists' Association. Q.   U.S.A.

Journal of the American Dental Society of Anesthesiology. *Now called* Anesthesia progress.   U.S.A.

*Journal of the American Society for Geriatric Dentistry. Q.   U.S.A.

*Journal of the American Society for Preventive Dentistry. U.S.A.

*Journal of the American Society of Psychosomatic Dentistry (- and Medicine).   Q.   U.S.A.

Journal of the American Society for the Study of Orthodontics.   2 a year.   U.S.A.

Journal de l'Association Dentaire Canadienne. *See* Journal of the Canadian Dental Association.

*Journal of the Baltimore College of Dental Surgery.   2 a year.   U.S.A.

Journal of the British Dental Association. *Now called* British dental journal.   Great Britain.

*Journal of the British Endodontic Society.   Q.   Great Britain.

*Journal of the California (State) Dental Association (and Nevada State Dental Association).   2 a year.   U.S.A.

*Journal of the Canadian Dental Association. (Journal de l'Association Dentaire Canadienne).   M.   Canada.

*Journal of clinical orthodontics.   M.   U.S.A.

*Journal of the Colorado Dental Association.   Q.   U.S.A.

*Journal of the Connecticut State Dental Association.   Q. U.S.A.

Journal de la Corps dentaire.   France.

Journal dentaire belge: Belgisch blad voor tandheelkunde.   Bi-M.   Belgium.

*Journal dentaire de Quebec.   M.   Canada.

*Journal of the Dental Association of South Africa.   M. South Africa.

*Journal of the Dental Association of Thailand.   Thailand.

*Journal of the dental auxiliaries.   China.

*Journal of dental education.   Q.   U.S.A.

*Journal of dental health.   Japan.

Journal of dental medicine. *Now called* Journal of oral medicine.   U.S.A.

*Journal of dental research. Bi-M. U.S.A.
*Journal of the Dental School, National University of Iran.
   2 a year. Iran.
Journal of dentistry. M. Great Britain.
*Journal of dentistry for children. Bi-M. U.S.A.
*Journal of the District of Columbia Dental Society. Q.
   U.S.A.
Journal of the Florida State Dental Society. M. U.S.A.
*Journal français d'oto-rhino-laryngologie, audio-phono-
   logie et chirurgie maxillo-faciale. France.
*Journal of the Georgia Dental Association. Q. U.S.A.
*Journal of the Hawaii Dental Association. Q. Hawaii.
*Journal of Hiroshima University Dental Society. Japan.
*Journal of the Hokkaido Dental Association. Japan.
*Journal of hospital dental practice. Q. U.S.A.
Journal of implant dentistry. 2 a year. U.S.A.
*Journal of the Indian Academy of Dentistry. 2 a year.
   India.
*Journal of the Indian Dental Association. M. India.
Journal of the Indian Orthodontic Society. Q. India.
*Journal of the Indiana (State) Dental Association. M.
   U.S.A.
Journal of the International Association of Dentistry for
   Children. 2 a year. Great Britain.
*Journal of the Iranian Dental Association. Iran.
Journal of the Irish Dental Association. *Now called* Irish
   dental review. Eire.
*Journal of the Japan Dental Association. M. Japan.
*Journal of Japan Orthodontic Society. 2 a year. Japan.
*Journal of the Japan Research Society of Dental Materials
   and Appliances. Japan.
*Journal of the Japan Society for Dental Apparatus and
   Materials. Japan.
*Journal of the Japan Stomatological Society [Kokubyo
   Gakkai Zasshi]. Japan.
*Journal of the Japanese Stomatological Society [Nippon
   Kokuka Gakkai Zasshi]. Q. Japan.
*Journal of the Kansas State Dental Association. Q.
   U.S.A.
*Journal of the Kentucky (State) Dental Association. Q.
   U.S.A.
*Journal of the Korea Research Society for Dental
   Materials. Q. Korea.
Journal of the Korean Academy for the History of
   Dentistry. A. Korea.
*Journal of the Korean Dental Association. Korea.

*Journal of the Louisiana (State) Dental Association. Q. U.S.A.

*Journal of the Maryland State Dental Association. 3 a year. U.S.A.

*Journal of the Massachusetts Dental Society. Q. U.S.A.

*Journal of maxillofacial orthopedics. Q. U.S.A.

*Journal of the Michigan (State) Dental Society. M. U.S.A.

Journal of the Mississippi Dental Association. Q. U.S.A.

Journal of the Missouri (State) Dental Association. M. U.S.A.

Journal of the National Dental Association. *Now called* Journal of the American Dental Association. U.S.A.

*Journal of the Nebraska (State) Dental Association. Q. U.S.A.

*Journal of the New Jersey Dental Association. Bi-M. U.S.A.

*Journal of the New Jersey Dental Hygienists' Association. 2 a year. U.S.A.

Journal of the New Jersey State Dental Society. *Now called* Journal of the New Jersey Dental Association. U.S.A.

*Journal of Nihon University School of Dentistry. Q. Japan.

*Journal of the North Carolina Dental Society. Q. U.S.A.

Journal of the Ohio State Dental Association. Q. U.S.A.

*Journal of the Oklahoma State Dental Association. Q. U.S.A.

Journal of the Ontario Dental Association. *Now called* Ontario dentist. Canada.

Journal of oral implant and transplant surgery. A. U.S.A.

*Journal of oral medicine. Q. U.S.A.

Journal of oral pathology. Q. Denmark.

*Journal of oral surgery. M. U.S.A.

Journal of oral therapeutics and pharmacology. Dead. U.S.A.

*Journal of the Oregon Dental Association. 10 a year. U.S.A.

*Journal of the Osaka Odontological Society. Bi-M. Japan.

*Journal of Osaka University School of Dentistry. 2 a year. Japan.

*Journal of periodontal research. Q. Denmark.

*Journal of periodontology (- periodontics). M. U.S.A.

Journal of the Philadelphia Dental Laboratory Association. Bi-M. U.S.A.

*Journal of the Philippine Dental Association. Q. Philippines.

Journal of practical orthodontics. Dead. U.S.A.

*Journal of prosthetic dentistry. M. U.S.A.

*Journal of public health dentistry. Q. U.S.A.

*Journal: Rhode Island State Dental Society. Q. U.S.A.

Journal of the Society for Dental Research of the New York University College of Dentistry. A. U.S.A.

Journal of the Southern California Dental Hygienists' Association. Q. U.S.A.

Journal of the Southern California (State) Dental Association. M. U.S.A.

Journal de stomatologie. Dead? Belgium.

Journal de stomatologie. France.

*Journal of the Tennessee (State) Dental Association. Q. U.S.A.

*Journal of the Texas Dental Hygienists' Association. Q. U.S.A.

*Journal of the Tokyo Dental Association. Japan.

Journal of the Western Society of Periodontology. *Now in* Periodontal abstracts: journal of the Western Society of Periodontology. U.S.A.

*Journal of the Wisconsin State Dental Society. M. U.S.A.

*Junior dental. Italy.

Korean dental press. Korea.

Lebanese dental journal. *See* Revue dentaire libanaise.

Leeds dental journal. Dead. Great Britain.

*McGill dental review. Q. Canada.

Malaysian dental journal. *Now called* Dental journal of Malaysia and Singapore. Malaysia.

Massachusetts Dental Society journal. Q. U.S.A.

Mécanicien-dentiste. *See* Zahntechniker: Le mécanicien dentiste.

Mécanicien en prothèse dentaire. France.

Meditsinskii referativnyi zhurnal. Stomatologiya. *Now part of* Meditsinskii referativnyi zhurnal. Razd. VIII. Otorinolaringologiya. Stomatologiya. Oftalmologiya. M. U.S.S.R.

Memoria de la Facultad de odontología, Universidad de Montevideo. A. Uruguay.

*Mentalis: journal of the UCLA School of Dentistry. U.S.A.

*Midwestern dentist. M. U.S.A.
 Minas odontológica. Brazil.
*Minerva stomatologica. M. Italy.
 Mois dentaire. M. France.
 Momento odontológico. Argentina.
 Monatsschrift deutscher Zahnärzte. *Now called* Freie Zahn-
     arzt: Monatsschrift deutscher Zahnärzte. W. Germany.
*Monde dentaire. Canada.
*Mondo odontostomatologico. Bi-M. Italy.
*Munnpleien. Norway.

*Nauchni trudove na Nauchnoizshedoratelskiia Stom-
     atologichen Institut. Bulgaria.
*Nederlands tandartsenblad. F. Netherlands.
*Nederlands Tijdschrift voor Tandheelkunde. Netherlands
     dental journal. M. Netherlands.
*New Mexico (State) dental journal. Q. U.S.A.
*New York journal of dentistry. 10 a year. U.S.A.
*New York State dental journal. 10 a year. U.S.A.
 New York University journal of dentistry. Q. U.S.A.
*New Zealand dental journal. Q. New Zealand.
 New Zealand orthodontic journal. New Zealand.
*New Zealand school dental service gazette. Bi-M. New
     Zealand.
*New Zealand Society of Periodontology bulletin. 2 a year.
     New Zealand.
*Nicaragua odontologica. Nicaragua.
*Niedersachsisches Zahnärzteblatt. W. Germany.
 Nippon Dental College, annual publications. A. Japan.
 Nippon dental review. Japan.
*Norske Tannlægeforenings Tidende. 10 a year. Norway.
*North-west dentistry. Bi-M. U.S.A.
*Northwestern University Bulletin, dental research and
     graduate study. 2 a year. U.S.A.
 Notices signaletiques des travaux orginaux d'odontostom-
     atologie de langue française. A. France.
 Nova acta stomatologica. Bi-M. Italy.

*Odont. Denmark.
 Odontes. M. Italy.
 Odonto post. Brazil.
 Odontoestomatologia portuguesa. Q. Portugal.
*Odontoiatria. M. Spain.
*Odontoiatria pratica. Italy.
 Odontoiatria e protesi dentaria. M. Italy.
*Odontoiatrike. Greece.

Odontoiatriki epitheorisis. Greece.
Odontología: revista de la Facultad de odontología de la Universidad nacional de Colombia. Q. Colombia.
*****Odontología: revista de la Facultad de odontología de la Universidad nacional mayor de San Marcos.** 2 a year. Peru.
Odontología de América. Argentina.
Odontología argentina. Argentina.
*****Ondotologia atual.** Brazil.
*****Odontología chilena.** Bi-M. Chile.
*****Odontología dinamica.** Brazil.
Odontología infantil. Cuba.
*****Odontología peruana.** Peru.
Odontología universitária. Brazil.
*****Odontología uruguaya.** 2 a year. Uruguay.
Odontologica. 3 a year. Switzerland.
*****Odontological bulletin of Western Pennsylvania.** 10 a year. U.S.A.
Odontologie. *Now in* Revue d'odonto-stomatologie. France.
*****Odontologisk revy.** Q. Sweden.
Odontologisk tidskrift. *Now in* Scandinavian journal of dental research/Odontologisk tidskrift. Sweden.
*****Odontologiska Föreningens tidskrift.** Q. Sweden.
Odontologiste des hôpitaux. Bi-M. France.
Odontólogo. Bi-M. Brazil.
Odontólogo. Cuba.
*****Odontology: journal of Nippon Dental College.** Q. Japan.
Odontopediatría. Argentina.
Odontopediatria. M. Brazil.
*****Odontoprotesi.** M. Italy.
Odontoscopio. Brazil.
Odontostomatological progress. Bi-M. Greece.
*****Odontostomatologike proodos.** Greece.
Odontotecnica. *See* Zahntechnik: La technique dentaire: L'odontotecnica.
*****Österreichische Dentisten-Zeitschrift.** M. Austria.
*****Österreichische Zahnärztezeitung.** M. Austria.
*****Österreichische zahntechniker Handwerk.** Austria.
*****Österreichische Zeitschrift für Stomatologie.** M. Austria.
Österreichische Zeitschrift für Zahnheilkunde. M. Austria.
*****Ohio dental journal.** Bi-M. U.S.A.
*****Ontario dentist.** 11 a year. Canada.
*****Oral health.** M. Canada.

Oral hygiene. Q. Taiwan.
Oral hygiene. *Now called* Dental economics-oral hygiene. U.S.A.
Oral implantology. U.S.A.
Oral research abstracts. 13 a year. U.S.A.
Oral sciences reviews. Denmark.
Oral surgery. Japan.
*****Oral surgery, oral medicine and oral pathology.** M. U.S.A.
Oregon State dental journal. 10 a year. U.S.A.
*****Orthodontie française.** A. France.
*****The Orthodontist.** 2 a year. Great Britain.
*****Ortodoncia.** 2 a year. Argentina.
Ortodoncia clinica. 2 a year. Argentina.
*****Ortodontia.** Q. Brazil.
*****Ortopedia maxilar.** Argentina.

*****Pakistan dental review.** Q. Pakistan.
Paradentium: Zeitschrift für die Grenzgebieten der Medizin und Odontologie. W. Germany.
Paradentología. 2 a year. Argentina.
Paraiba odontológica. Q. Brazil.
Parodontologie. *Now called* Parodontologie and Academy Review. Switzerland.
*****Parodontologie and Academy Review.** *Supplement to* Schweizerische Monatsschrift für Zahnheilkunde. Q. Switzerland.
*****Parodontopathies: Association pour les Recherches sur les Parodontopathies.** Switzerland.
*****Pedodontie française.** France.
*****Penn dental journal.** 3 a year. U.S.A.
*****Pennsylvania dental journal.** 9 a year. U.S.A.
Periodontal abstracts: journal of the Western Society of Periodontology. Q. U.S.A.
Periodontics. *Now in* Journal of periodontology-periodontics. U.S.A.
Periodontology today. 2 a year. U.S.A.
Pernambuco odontológico. Q. Brazil.
*****Pharmacology and therapeutics in dentistry.** Q. U.S.A.
Philippines medical-dental journal. M. Philippines.
Plomjo. Bi-M. E. Germany.
*****Plugger: Iowa dental assistants journal.** U.S.A.
Postepy stomatologii. A. Poland.
Practical dental monographs. Dead. U.S.A.
*****Practice in prosthodontics.** Japan.
*****Prakticke Zubni Lekarstvi.** 10 a year. Czechoslovakia.

Pratique odonto-stomatologique. Switzerland.

*Proceedings of the British Paedodontic Society. Great Britain.

Proceedings of the British Society for the Study of Prosthetic Dentistry. A. Great Britain.

Proceedings of the British Society of Periodontology. A. Great Britain.

Proceedings of the Finnish Dental Society. Bi-M. Finland.

*Proceedings of the International Academy of Oral Pathology. U.S.A.

Proceedings of the International Conference on Oral Surgery. Denmark.

*Progrès odonto-stomatologique. France.

*Promotion dentaire. Q. France.

Protesis dental. Spain.

*Protesista dental. Argentina.

*Protetyka stomatologiczna. Bi-M. Poland.

Punjab dental journal. Q. India.

Quarterly dental review. Q. Great Britain.

*Quarterly of the National Dental Association. Q. U.S.A.

Queensland dental journal. *Now in* Australian dental journal. Australia.

*Quintessence international: dental digest. M. W. Germany.

*Quintessenz: die Monatszeitschrift für den praktizierenden Zahnarzt. M. W.Germany.

*Quintessenz journal: Zeitschrift für die Zahnarzthelferin. M. W.Germany.

Quintessenz der zahnärztlichen Literatur. M. Germany.

*Quintessenza. Italy.

Radiodoncia. Argentina.

*Rassegna internazionale di stomatologia pratica. Italy.

Rassegna della letteratura odontoiatrica. 3 a year. Italy.

Rassegna di odontoiatria. Q. Italy.

*Rassegna di odontotechnica. Italy.

*Rassegna trimestrale di odontoiatria. Q. Italy.

Refuat Hashinaim. *Now called* Refuat Hape Vehashinaim. Israel.

Refuat Hape Vehashinaim. Q. Israel.

Reseñas odontológicas. Paraguay.

Resúmenes de la Facultad de odontología. Cuba.

Review of dentistry for children. *Now called* Journal of dentistry for children. U.S.A.

*Revista de ALAFO: Asociacion latinoamericana de Facultades de odontología. 2 a year. Guatemala.

*Revista de la Agrupación odontológica argentina. Q. Argentina.

Revista de la Agrupación odontológica de la Capital federal. *Now called* Revista de la Agrupación odontológica argentina. Argentina.

Revista argentina para la defusion de la anestesia general en odontología. Bi-M. Argentina.

*Revista Asociación odontológica argentina. M. Argentina.

Revista de la Asociación odontológica de Costa Rica. *Now called* Revista odontológica de Costa Rica. Costa Rica.

Revista de la Asociación odontológica del Cuba. Cuba.

Revista de la Asociación odontológica del Perú. Q. Peru.

Revista de la Asociación odontológica uruguaya. Uruguay.

*Revista da Associacão paulista de cirurgioes dentistas. Bi-M. Brazil.

*Revista del Ateneo de la Catedrá de tecnica de operatória dental. Argentina.

Revista bahiana de odontologia. Bi-M. Brazil.

*Revista de biologia oral. Brazil.

*Revista brasileira de odontologia. Bi-M. Brazil.

*Revista Centro America Odontológica. El Salvador.

*Revista del Circulo argentino de odontología. Argentina.

*Revisto del Circulo odontológico de Córdoba. M. Argentina.

Revista del Circulo odontológico correntino. Argentina.

Revista del Circulo odontológico del Oeste. Q. Argentina.

Revista del Circulo odontológico de Rosario. Dead. Argentina.

Revista del Circulo odontológico santafesino. Argentina.

*Revista del Circulo odontológico del Sur. 2 a year. Argentina.

Revista del Circulo odontológico de Tucumán. Bi-M. Argentina.

Revista o cirurgião dentista. Brazil.

Revista del Colegio estomatológico du Guatemala. *Now called* Revista guatemalteca de estomatologia. Guatemala.

Revista cubana de estomatología. 3 a year. Cuba.

Revista dental. Q. Dominican Republic.

*Revista dental. El Salvador.

*Revista dental de Chile. Bi-M. Chile.

Revista dental de Puerto Rico. Puerto Rico.

*Revista de la Escuela de Odontología, Universidad nacional de Tucumán, Facultad de Medicina. Argentina.

*Revista española de estomatología. Bi-M. Spain.
*Revista española de parodoncía. Spain.
Revista estomatológica de Cuba. Cuba.
Revista estomatológica de La Habana. Cuba.
*Revista da Faculdade de Farmacia e Odontologia de
Araraquara. Brazil.
Revista da Faculdade de Odontologia de Pelotas. M.
Brazil.
*Revista da Faculdade de Odontologia de Porto Alegre.
A. Brazil.
*Revista da Faculdade de Odontologia da Universidade
de Pernambuco. Brazil.
*Revista da Faculdade de Odontologia da Universidade de
Sao Paulo. 2 a year. Brazil.
*Revista de la Facultad de Odontología, Universidad de
Buenos Aires. Argentina.
*Revista de farmácia e odontologia. M. Brazil.
Revista de la Federación odontológica argentina. Q.
Argentina.
*Revista de la Federación odontológica colombiana. 2 a
year. Colombia.
*Revista de la Federación odontológica ecuatoriana.
Ecuador.
*Revista gaucha de odontologia. Q. Brazil.
*Revista guatemalteca de estomatologia. Bi-M. Guate-
mala.
Revista latino-americana de periodoncia. Argentina.
Revista mineira de odontologia. Brazil.
Revista naval de odontologia. Q. Brazil.
*Revista odonto-estomatologia. Brazil.
*Revista de odontologia da Universidade Federal da
Santa Catarina. Brazil.
*Revista odontológica. Bolivia.
Revista odontológica. Dominican Republic.
*Revista odontológica del Circulo de odontólogos del
Paraguay. Q. Paraguay.
*Revista odontológica de Concepción. Q. Chile.
*Revista odontológica de Costa Rica. Costa Rica.
*Revista odontológica ecuatoriana. Ecuador.
*Revista odontológica, Facultad de Odontología, Univer-
sidad nacional de Cordoba. Q. Argentina.
Revista odontológica de Merida. Q. Venezuela.
Revista odontológica de México. Mexico.
Revista odontológica de Paraiba. Q. Brazil.
*Revista odontológica de Puerto Rico. Puerto Rico.
Revista odontológica del Zulia. Venezuela.

Revista passofundenese de odontologia. Brazil.
*__Revista paulista de odontologia.__ Brazil.
*__Revista portuguesa de estomatologia e cirurgia maxilo-facial.__ Q. Portugal.
Revista seára odontológica brasileira. M. Brazil.
Revista do Sindicato dos odontologistas do Rio de Janeiro. Q. Brazil.
Revista Sociedad colombiana de ortodoncia. Q. Colombia.
Revista de la Sociedad de estudios de ortodoncia Tweed de México. 2 a year. Mexico.
*__Revista de la Sociedad odontologica de Atlantico.__ Colombia.
Revista da Sociedade portuguesa de estomatologia. *Now called* Revista portuguesa de estomatologia e cirurgia maxilofacial. Portugal.
Revista da União odontológica brasileira. Brazil.
*__Revue belge de médecine dentaire.__ Q. Belgium.
Revue belge d'odontologie. Belgium.
Revue belge de science dentaire. *Now called* Revue belge de médecine dentaire. Belgium.
Revue belge de stomatologie. *Continued in* Acta stomatologica belgica *and* Revue belge de science dentaire. Belgium.
Revue du Cercle odontologique douaisien. France.
Revue dentaire de France. *Now in* Revue d'odonto-stomatologie. France.
*__Revue dentaire libanaise.__ (Lebanese dental journal.) Q. Lebanon.
Revue dentaire de Syrie. Syria.
Revue française d'odonto-stomatologie. *Now in* Revue d'odonto-stomatologie. France.
*__Revue française de la prothèse dentaire.__ Bi-M. France.
Revue d'histoire de l'art dentaire. France.
Revue de l'Institut d'odonto-stomatologie d'Alger. Q. Algeria.
Revue mensuelle suisse d'odonto-stomatologie. *See* Schweizerische Monatsschrift für Zahnheilkunde: Revue mensuelle suisse d'odonto-stomatologie: Rivista mensile svizzera di odontologia e stomatologia.
*__Revue odonto-implantologique.__ Q. France.
Revue d'odontologie, de stomatologie et maxillo-faciale. France.
Revue odontologique. *Now in* Revue d'odonto-stomatologie. France.
*__Revue d'odonto-stomatologie.__ Bi-M. France.
*__Revue d'odonto-stomatologie du Midi de la France.__ Q. France.

Revue d'orthopédie dento-faciale. Q. France.
Revue de stomatologie. Bi-M. France.
*****Revue de stomatologie et de chirurgie maxillo-faciale.**
8 a year. France.
*****Revue stomato-odontologique du Nord de la France.** Q.
France.
Revue trimestrielle d'implantologie. Q. Switzerland.
Rheinisches Zahnärzteblatt. 24 a year. W. Germany.
Riogrande odontológico. Bi-M. Brazil.
*****Rivista italiana di stomatologia.** M. Italy.
Rivista mensile svizzera di odontologia e stomatologia.
See Schweizerische Monatsschrift für Zahnheilkunde: Revue
mensuelle suisse d'odonto-stomatologie: Rivista mensile
svizzera di odontologia e stomatologia.

*****SAAD digest: Society for the Advancement of Anaesthesia
in Dentistry.** Great Britain.
*****SOLAIAT: Sociedad odontologico Latino-Americano de
implantes aloplasticos y transplantes.** Venezuela.
*****Scandinavian journal of dental research/Odontologisk
tidskrift.** Bi-M. Denmark.
*****Scandinavian Society of Forensic Odontology newsletter.**
Denmark.
*****Schweizerische Monatsschrift für Zahnheilkunde: Revue
mensuelle suisse d'odonto-stomatologie: Rivista men-
sile svizzera di odontologia e stomatologia.** M.
Switzerland.
*****Science et recherche odonto-stomatologiques.** France.
Selecciones odontológicas. Argentina.
*****Selecões odontologicas.** Brazil.
Selecta dentalia. Sweden.
Semaine dentaire. *Now called* Information dentaire. France.
Sintese odontológica. Q. Brazil.
*****Sociedad española de ortodoncia: actas.** Spain.
*****Société odonto-stomatologique du Nord-Est:** revue
annuelle. A. France.
*****South Carolina dental journal.** M. U.S.A.
**Sovetskoe medicinskoe referativnoe obozrenie. Stomato-
logija.** A. U.S.S.R.
Stom. Rivista di stomatologia infantile. Italy.
*****Stoma.** Greece.
**Stoma. Zeitschrift für die wissenschaftliche Zahn-
Mund- und Kieferheilkunde.** *Now in* Z.W.R. W. Germany.
*****Stomatologia.** Bi-M. Greece.
Stomatologia. Q. Italy.
*****Stomatologia.** Bi-M. Rumania.

Stomatologic titles: West Virginia University School of Dentistry. Dead. U.S.A.
*****Stomatologica.** Q. Italy.
*****Stomatologicke zpravy.** Czechoslovakia.
Stomatologický věstník. 10 a year. Czechoslovakia.
*****Stomatologija.** Bi-M. Bulgaria.
*****Stomatologija.** Bi-M. U.S.S.R.
Stomatologika chronika. See A cta stomatologica hellenica
Stomatology references, current medical literature. Dead U.S.A.
*****Stomatoloski glasnik srbije.** Q. Yugoslavia.
*****Suomen Hammaslääkäriseuran Toimituksia. Finska Tandläkarsällskapets Forhandlingar.** Q. Finland.
*****Svensk tandläkare-Tidskrift.** M. Sweden.
Sveriges Tandläkarförbunds Tidning. *Now called* Tandläkatidningen. Sweden.
*****Syrian dental journal.** Syria.

*****Tandlægebladet.** M. Denmark.
*****Tandläkartidningen.** 24 a year. Sweden.
Tandplejen. Dead. Denmark.
Tandtechnisch takblad. Netherlands.
*****Tandteknikern.** M. Sweden.
*****Technicien belge en prothèse dentaire.** Q. Belgium.
Technique dentaire. *See* Zahntechnik: La technique dentaire: L'odontotecnica
*****Temas odontológicos.** Q. Colombia.
*****Temple dental review and Garretsonian.** U.S.A.
*****Texas Dental Assistants' Association bulletin.** U.S.A.
*****Texas dental journal.** M. U.S.A.
*****Tidens tann.** Norway.
*****Tidsskrift for praktiserende Tandlaeger.** Denmark.
Tijdschrift voor tandheelkunde. M. Netherlands.
Transactions of the American Dental Association. A. U.S.A.
Transactions of the American Association of Industrial Dentists. A. U.S.A.
*****Transactions of the British Society for the Study of Orthodontics.** A. Great Britain.
Transactions of the Canadian Dental Association. A. Canada.
Transactions of the European Orthodontic Society. *See* European Orthodontic Society reports.
Transactions of the National Dental Association. *Now called* Transactions of the American Dental Association. U.S.A.

Transactions of the Odontological Society of Great Britain. Dead. *Now in* Proceedings of the Royal Society of Medicine. Great Britain.

Transactions of the Royal Schools of Dentistry, Stockholm and Umea. Sweden.

*****Tribuna odontológica.** Q. Argentina.

*****Tribuna odontologica do sindicato dos odontologistas do Estado da Guanabara.** Brazil.

Türk odontoloji bülteni. Turkey.

Venezuela odontológica. Bi-M. Venezuela.

*****Virginia dental journal.** U.S.A.

Voix buccale. Bi-M. France.

*****Voix dentaire.** M. France.

Washington State Dental Association newsletter. U.S.A.

*****Washington State dental journal.** U.S.A.

*****West Virginia dental journal.** Q U.S.A.

*****Western Dental Society bulletin.** U.S.A.

*****World news on maxillofacial radiology.** Chile.

Yearbook of dentistry. A. U.S.A.

*****Z.W.R. Zahnärztliche Welt. Zahnärztliche Rundschau. Zahnärztliche Reform. Das Deutsche Zahnärzteblatt. Stoma.** 2 a month. W. Germany.

Zahnärztliche Fortbildung. Germany.

*****Zahnärztliche Mitteilungen.** 24 a year. Germany.

*****Zahnärztliche Nachrichten Sudwurttemberg-Hohenzollern.** W. Germany.

*****Zahnärztliche Praxis.** 24 a month. Germany.

Zahnärztliche Rundschau. *Now in* Z.W.R. W. Germany.

Zahnärztliche Welt. *Now in* Z.W.R. W. Germany.

Zahnärztliche Zeitschrift. *Afterwards called* Zahnärztliche Rundschau. Germany.

*****Zahnärztlicher Informations-Dienst.** W. Germany.

*****Zahnarzt.** Bi-M. W. Germany.

*****Zahnmedizin in Bild.** E. Germany.

*****Zahntechnik.** W. Germany.

*****Zahntechnik: La technique dentaire: L'odontotecnica.** Bi-M. Switzerland.

Zahntechniker: Le mécanicien dentiste. Bi-M. Switzerland.

Zeitschrift für Dentistik und Zahntechnik. M. Austria.

Zeitschrift für Stomatologie. *Now called* Österreichische Zeitschrift für Stomatologie. Austria.

*****Zobozdravstveni vestnik.** Bi-M. Yugoslavia.